Basic Pharmacology
Understanding Drug Actions *and* Reactions

CRC PRESS
PHARMACY
EDUCATION
SERIES

Basic Pharmacology: Understanding Drug Actions and Reactions
Maria A. Hernandez and Appu Rathinavelu

Essentials of Human Physiology for Pharmacy
Laurie Kelly

Managing Pharmacy Practice: Principles, Strategies, and Systems
Andrew M. Peterson

Pharmacoethics: A Problem-Based Approach
David A. Gettman and Dean Arneson

Pharmaceutical Care: Insights from Community Pharmacists
William N. Tindall and Marsha K. Millonig

Essentials of Law and Ethics for Pharmacy Technicians
Kenneth M. Strandberg

Essentials of Pharmacy Law
Douglas J. Pisano

Essentials of Pathophysiology for Pharmacy
Martin M. Zdanowicz

Pharmacy: What It Is and How It Works
William N. Kelly

Pharmacokinetic Principles of Dosing Adjustments: Understanding the Basics
Ronald Schoenwald

Strauss's Federal Drug Laws and Examination Review, Fifth Edition
Steven Strauss

Pharmaceutical and Clinical Calculations, Second Edition
Mansoor Khan and Indra Reddy

Inside Pharmacy: Anatomy of a Profession
Ray Gosselin, Jack Robbins, and Joseph Cupolo

Understanding Medical Terms: A Guide for Pharmacy Practice, Second Edition
Mary Stanaszek, Walter Stanaszek, and Robert Holt

Pharmacokinetic Analysis: A Practical Approach
Peter Lee and Gordon Amidon

Guidebook for Patient Counseling
Harvey Rappaport, Tracey Hunter, Joseph Roy, and Kelly Straker

Basic Pharmacology
Understanding Drug Actions *and* Reactions

MARIA A. HERNANDEZ Ph.D.
Pharmaceutical and Administrative College of Pharmacy
Nova Southeastern University
Ft. Lauderdale, Florida, U.S.A.

APPU RATHINAVELU Ph.D.
Pharmaceutical and Administrative College of Pharmacy
Nova Southeastern University
Ft. Lauderdale, Florida, U.S.A.

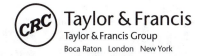

Taylor & Francis
Taylor & Francis Group
Boca Raton London New York

A CRC title, part of the Taylor & Francis imprint, a member of the
Taylor & Francis Group, the academic division of T&F Informa plc.

Published in 2006 by
CRC Press
Taylor & Francis Group
6000 Broken Sound Parkway NW, Suite 300
Boca Raton, FL 33487-2742

No claim to original U.S. Government works
Printed in the United States of America on acid-free paper
10 9 8 7 6 5 4 3 2 1

International Standard Book Number-10: 1-58716-160-5 (Hardcover)
International Standard Book Number-13: 978-1-58716-160-5 (Hardcover)

Library of Congress Cataloging-in-Publication Data

Catalog record is available from the Library of Congress

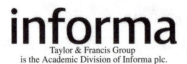

Taylor & Francis Group
is the Academic Division of Informa plc.

Visit the Taylor & Francis Web site at
http://www.taylorandfrancis.com

and the CRC Press Web site at
http://www.crcpress.com

DEDICATION

To All That Taught Me the Importance of Living,
Loving, Learning, and Leaving a Legacy:

Jesus Christ, my Savior and Friend

My parents, Ana Hernàndez and Dr. Rodolfo Hernàndez Miliani

My daughters, Michelle and Laura Rodriguez

My teachers

My Christian family

My coworkers

My students

(Dedication by: MAH)

Dedicated to my Family

(Dedication by: AR)

PREFACE

This book is designed for first-year pharmacy students as part of the basic science curriculum. The purpose of this book is to introduce students to the principles of chemistry and biology necessary to understand drug interactions at the cellular level. Special emphasis is devoted to the following topics:

1. Chemical and physical properties of drugs
2. Drug absorption and distribution
3. Drug interactions with cellular receptors
4. Drug metabolism and elimination

Professional pharmacy schools accept students from varied academic backgrounds, including students returning to academic life after several years of full-time employment. New pharmacy schools are also on the rise, and the basic science training of the entering classes is very diverse, creating the need for a foundational course that applies concepts learned in other settings to drugs in physiological systems. This book was designed with this student diversity in mind; we start out reviewing chemical principles as they apply to drug molecules (Chapters 1 through 7), especially those most commonly prescribed. Extensive use of drug structures helps to illustrate chemical concepts learned in general and organic chemistry courses. The second section of the book (Chapters 8 to 11) covers the dynamics of receptors in mediating the pharmacologic effects of drugs. The theories proposed in the scientific literature to explain drug–receptor interactions are described, and the qualitative relationship between drug binding and the cellular effects produced is explained.

Altogether, the concepts described in this book provide the framework for more advanced pharmacology and therapeutics courses. It is our desire that pharmacists will come back to this book to review the principles that make their contribution to the health care team unique.

ACKNOWLEDGMENTS

This book would not have been possible without the assistance and cooperation of some very talented people: my colleague, Dr. Jolanta Czerwinska, who made many drawings and is designing the online version of this book; my students, who learned to draw more chemical structures than they thought they would in a lifetime, Natalie Campbell and Sabrina Mussari; and my friend and very skilled graphic artist, Isa Kollgaard.

We are also indebted to the leaders of the College of Pharmacy at Nova Southeastern University for allowing us to enjoy the time and resources to bring this project to completion.

MH

Dr. Rathinavelu is most grateful to his family for their immense love, care and support which transformed into essential sources of energy, enthusiasm and persistence required for completing this project. He thanks the president of Nova Southeastern University, Mr. Ray Ferraro, Jr., for his leadership, Dr. Fred Lippman, R.Ph., Ed.D., Chancellor of Health Professions Division at NSU for his vision and Dr. Andres Malave, Ph.D., Dean of the College of Pharmacy at NSU for his mentorship, which altogether provided the stimulus and the quest for achieving excellence. He would also like to thank Dr. George L. Hanbury II, Ph.D., Dr. Ron Chenail, Ph.D., Mr. Joel Berman, Esq., and Dr. Irv Rosenbaum, Ed.D., for their constant encouragement. Finally, Dr. Rathinavelu would like to thank Dr. William D. Hardigan, Ph.D. for showing great faith in his abilities, all his friends for creating an undiminished enthusiasm towards greater success, and the Faculty of the Department of Pharmaceutical and Administrative Sciences at NSU College of Pharmacy for their continued support.

AR

CONTENTS

SECTION I   PHYSICOCHEMICAL PROPERTIES OF DRUGS

1   Fundamental Chemical Properties of Drugs 3
Introduction 3
The Periodic Table and Properties of Drugs 3
The Periodic Table and Chemical Reactivity............................ 10
Chemical Bonds... 16
Magnitude of Ionic Charge 18
Polyatomic Ions.. 19
Covalent Bonds.. 20
Coordinate Covalent Bonds 25
Resonance Structures... 27
Shapes of Drug Molecules 28
Electronegativity 33
Polarity of Chemical Bonds 33
Molecular Polarity 34
Further Reading.. 35

2   Acid–Base Properties of Drugs...37
Hydrolysis of Salts 38
Conjugate Acids and Conjugate Bases.................................... 41
Strength of Acids and Bases.. 43
Resonance and Inductive Effects... 47
Inductive Effects... 47
Resonance Effects 49
The Henderson–Hasselbach Equation...................................... 53
Further Reading.. 60

3   Structural Determinants of Drug Action................................61
Structurally Nonspecific Drugs.. 61
Volatile Anesthetics 61
Structurally Specific Drugs 63
Isosterism and Isosteres... 68
Structural Changes in Drug Molecules.................................... 71
Further Reading.. 76

4 Chemical Approaches to the Treatment of Cancer 77
Normal vs. Malignant Cells 77
Cell Cycle and Chemotherapy 78
From Chemical Warfare to Chemotherapy 79
Anticancer Drugs 80
Alkylating Agents 81
Antimetabolites 84
DNA Intercalators 87
DNA Crosslinking Agents 89
Further Reading 90

SECTION II   PRINCIPLES OF BIOPHARMACEUTICS

5 Administration and Absorption of Drugs 93
Drug Administration 93
Properties of the Drug 94
Drug Solubility 94
Polymorphism 97
Particle Size 98
pK_a 98
Therapeutic Objective 100
Onset of Action 100
Long-Term Administration 100
Restriction to a Local Site 101
Drug Absorption 101
Physiological and Physicochemical Factors in Drug Absorption 103
Drug Transport across Membranes 103
Passive Diffusion 103
Active Transport 104
Facilitated Transport 104
Ion Pair Transport 105
Endocytosis, Pinocytosis, Phagocytosis, and Exocytosis 105
pH of Body Compartments 105
Other Factors That Affect Absorption 107
Blood Flow to the Absorption Site 107
Surface Area Available for Absorption 108
Contact Time at the Absorption Surface 108
Drug Absorption, Bioavailability, and First-Pass Metabolism 108
Further Reading 110

6 Distribution and Excretion of Drugs 111
Factors in Drug Distribution 111
Capillary Permeability 112
Blood Perfusion 114
Perfusion and Permeability 114
Drug Structure and Compartment pH 116
Plasma Protein Binding 116
Intracellular Binding 117

Patterns of Distribution 117
Determination of the Volume of Distribution 120
Clearance and Elimination Rate... 122
Clearance and the Maintenance Dose Rate............................... 122
Half-Life and the Steady State 125
Bioavailability 127
Drug Elimination.. 130
    The Enterohepatic Cycle 130
    Renal Excretion 131
    Renal Processes... 132
Further Reading... 133

7   **Metabolic Changes of Drugs..135**
Cytochromes P450 136
    Inhibition of Drug Metabolism 138
    Induction of Drug Metabolism... 138
    Environmental and Genetic Factors in Metabolism by CYP450 139
    Clozapine and CYP1A2 Activity.. 142
    Genetic Polymorphism and *CYP2D6* 142
    CYP2D6 and Codeine.. 143
    Genetic Polymorphism and *CYP2C19*................................. 143
    Drug Interactions via the *CYP2C19* Isoform:
    Omeprazole–Diazepam Interaction 143
    CYP3A Family.. 143
    CYP3A4 and Grapefruit Juice.. 144
Redox Reactions and the CYP450 Enzyme Complex 144
NAD$^+$/NADH System... 145
FAD/FADH System... 147
The Cytochrome P450 Cycle... 147
Phase I and Phase II Reactions of Drug Metabolism.................... 149
    Phase I Reactions... 149
        Oxidations Using CYP450 Enzymes 149
        Oxidation using Other Enzymes...................................... 163
        Reduction 166
        Hydrolysis Reactions 167
    Phase II Reactions (Conjugation) 171
Dose-Dependent Toxicity of Acetaminophen 178
Further Reading... 186

SECTION III   PRINCIPLES OF DRUG–RECEPTOR AND DRUG–ENZYME INTERACTIONS

8   **Drug Receptors and Pharmacodynamics..............................189**
Mechanisms of Drug Action 189
Chemical Signaling and Receptor Function................................. 189
    Chemical Signaling.. 189
    Autocrine, Paracrine, and Endocrine Function..................... 192
    Nature of the Signaling Molecules (Ligands)........................ 192

Different Kinds of Receptors.. 194
    Extracellular Receptors.. 196
    Intracellular Receptors 196
    Plasma Membrane–Bound Receptors 196
    Three Types of Plasma Membrane–Bound Receptors.................... 196
Models of Drug–Receptor Interaction 198
    Drug–Receptor Interactions... 198
    Key Features of Binding Sites.. 198
    Lock-and-Key Fit 198
    Induced Fit 199
Affinity and Intrinsic Activity 200
    Affinity... 200
    Intrinsic Activity.. 200
Agonists, Antagonists, and Partial Agonists 201
    Agonists.. 201
    Antagonists... 201
    Partial Agonist 201
    Ligand Structure and Activity Relationship 201
    Why is the Receptor Concept Important?.. 202
Differential Effects of Agonists 202
    Differential Effects of Epinephrine 202
    Selective Actions of Adrenergic Agonists and Antagonists 205
    Atypical Receptors... 208
Cholinergic Neurotransmission 209
    Synthesis and Release of Acetylcholine 210
    Differential Effects of Acetylcholine through Cholinergic Receptors... 211
    Muscarinic and Nicotinic Actions of Acetylcholine.......................... 212
    The Location and Function of Acetylcholine Receptors.................... 213
    Cholinomimetics.. 214
    Cholinergic Agonists and Antagonists 215
    Clinical Use of Direct-Acting Cholinomimetics................................ 215
    Antimuscarinic 221

9   **Drug-Induced Enzyme Inhibition 223**
Drug Effects Mediated through Enzyme Inhibition 223
Competitive, Uncompetitive, and Noncompetitive Inhibition.................... 225
    Competitive Inhibition 225
    Uncompetitive Inhibition.. 226
    Noncompetitive Inhibition.. 228
    Allosteric Regulation 228
    Cooperativity... 229
    Feedback Inhibition 229
Examples of Drug–Enzyme Interactions 230
    Acetylcholinesterase 230
        Butyrylcholinesterase (BuChE)... 231
        The Active Center of Cholinesterase 232
        Anticholinesterase Drugs 234

Types of Cholinesterase Inhibitors 234
Reversible Anticholinesterases... 234
Irreversible Anticholinesterases 235
Effects of Anticholinesterase Drugs 236
Uses of Anticholinesterase Drugs 238
Antiocholinesterases for the Treatment of Glaucoma 238
Anticholinesterase for the Treatment of Myasthenia Gravis........... 239
Poisonous Effects of Irreversible Anticholinesterases 241
Cholinesterase-Regenerating Compounds 241
Transpeptidase-Penicillinase Inhibition Producing
Pharmacological Effects... 243
Transpeptidase.. 243
Bacterial Cell Wall Synthesis 243
Peptidoglycans.. 245
Transpeptidase.. 246
Transpeptidase Inhibitors.. 248
Penicillins... 250
Penicillinases.. 251
Beta-Lactamase Inhibitors 251
Suicide Inhibition of Enzymes 254
Suicide Inhibition of Thymidylate Synthetase (TS)............................ 254
Suicide Inhibition of Xanthine Oxidase (XO) 255
References.. 258

10   Drug–Receptor Dynamics and Theories 259
Occupation Theory (Clark) 259
Modified Occupancy Theory (Ariëns).. 264
Rate Theory (Paton) 264
Relationship between Concentration and Response.............................. 269
Concentration–Effect Curves 269
Drug Antagonism 270
Competitive Antagonism... 271
Schild's Equation 275
What Is the Importance of This Mathematical Relationship?.................... 278
Irreversible Antagonism... 280
Noncompetitive Antagonism 281
Partial Agonists... 282
Various Factors That Can Regulate a Drug's Effect 285
Potency and Efficacy 286
Potency... 286
Efficacy... 287
Dose–Response Curves.. 288
Graded Dose–Response Curves 288
Quantal Dose–Response Curves 290
Statistics That Can Be Derived from the Quantal
Dose–Response Curve 291
Therapeutic Index.. 293

Time–Action Curves 296
    Phase I: Time to Onset of Action 297
    Phase II: Time to Peak Effect 297
    Phase III: Duration of Action 297
    Phase IV: Residual Effects 297
Sample Problems 297
Practice Problems 303
Answers for the Problems 305
References 306

11 Receptor Regulation and Signaling Mechanisms 307
Spare Receptors 307
Overshoot 308
Down Regulation 309
Other Factors That Can Affect Drug Response 312
    Tolerance 312
    Tachyphylaxis 312
    Idiosyncratic Drug Response 313
Receptor Signaling and Second Messenger Systems 313
    Four Basic Mechanisms of Receptor Signaling 313
    The Four Major Types of Second Messengers 315
Hormones Acting through Intracellular Receptors 318
    Mechanism of Action 318
    Ligands Acting through Cell Surface Receptors 320
        Protein Kinases 320
        Phosphorylation and the Effects of Phosphorylation 320
        Two Types of Protein Kinases 320
        Examples of Receptor Signaling by Activation
        of Tyrosine Kinases 322
        Phosphorylation-Induced Receptor Down Regulation and
        Receptor Desensitization 323
Receptor-Coupled (Membrane-Bound) Guanylate Cyclase (GC) 325
Soluble Guanylate Cyclase 326
Receptors Linked to G-Proteins and Second Messenger Production 327
Activation of Adenylate Cyclase and G-Protein Function 329
Downstream cAMP Second Messenger Pathway 331
Ca^{2+}/Phosphoinositide/PKC Signaling Pathway 331
What Is the Purpose of G-Proteins or Any Other Second
Messenger System? 334
Ligand-Gated Ion Channels 334
Signaling through Voltage-Dependent Ion Channels 336
    Voltage-Dependent Sodium (Na^+) Channel 336
    Voltage-Gated Potassium (K^+) Channel 337
Ligand-Gated Sodium Channel 337
Calcium Channels 338
Location(s) of the Voltage-Sensitive Ca^{2+} Channels (VSCC) 339

How Does Calcium Contract the Skeletal Muscles and the
Vascular Smooth Muscles? 342
Chloride Channel 344
  GABA Receptors... 344
    Structure of GABA$_A$ Receptors 344
    GABA Binding Site.. 346
    Benzodiazepine Binding Site 348
    Barbiturates Binding Site 348
    Picrotoxin Binding Site 349
    GABA Antagonists... 349
  References 350

Index...**353**

I

PHYSICOCHEMICAL
PROPERTIES OF DRUGS

1

FUNDAMENTAL CHEMICAL PROPERTIES OF DRUGS

INTRODUCTION

Pharmaceutical manufacturers currently perform most of the drug formulations any given patient may need, work that in the past used to be the main professional practice of the pharmacist. The degree of sophistication of their knowledge of the action of drugs in living organisms has given pharmacists the opportunity to become the chemical experts in the healthcare team. And rightfully so; they contribute to providing the best therapy for a patient because their unique training allows them to look at the chemical structure of a drug and identify potential drug interactions and additional sensitivities based on a patient's profile. One example of this is the cross-sensitivity to saccharin experienced by those allergic to sulfonamides. Looking at the chemical structures allows one to discern that the reason for the cross-sensitivity is the similarities in certain functional groups in the two substances.

It is this explosion of knowledge in the molecular actions of drugs that warrants the need to introduce the core concepts in a single foundational course. These concepts will be essential to the in-depth coverage of drug classes in subsequent pharmacology and therapeutics courses.

We begin our discussion of these core concepts by reviewing the chemistry involved in the actions of drug molecules.

THE PERIODIC TABLE AND PROPERTIES OF DRUGS

Most drugs are organic compounds that behave as weak acids or bases in the aqueous medium of the living organism. But prior to understanding drug molecules in solution, we must first review how drug molecules are composed in terms of atomic structure. Indeed, a great way to review the atomic structure and composition of drug molecules is by learning the usefulness of the periodic table of the elements. Elements are listed in the periodic table on the basis of their atomic structure. However, the atom may not be the preferred structural unit for an element. Some elements, such as helium (He), can exist in monoatomic form, but free isolated atoms are rarely found in nature. Under normal conditions atoms aggregate to form diatomic molecules (e.g., oxygen, O_2), or triatomic molecules (e.g., ozone, O_3). Sulfur atoms readily collect in groups of eight; elemental sulfur is therefore described as S_8. Elements may also exist as aggregates of a larger number of atoms.

Four elements from the periodic table constitute at least 99% of the makeup of living organisms: hydrogen (H), oxygen (O), nitrogen (N), and carbon (C). It is not surprising, then, that these are the same elements most commonly found in drugs. Other elements that are also essential for life include calcium (Ca), phosphorus (P), potassium (K), sulfur (S), chlorine (Cl), magnesium (Mg), iron (Fe), iodine (I), fluorine (F), manganese (Mn), selenium (Se), zinc (Zn), molybdenum (Mo), copper (Cu), cobalt (Co), chromium (Cr), arsenic (As), nickel (Ni), silicon (Si), and boron (B).

Atoms of different elements may combine to form various molecules. We describe the molecule of Aricept® (donepezil), for example, as containing 24 carbon atoms, 30 hydrogen atoms, one chlorine atom, one nitrogen atom, and three oxygen atoms. This composition is then abbreviated in a notation called the *molecular formula* and is denoted as $C_{24}H_{30}ClNO_3$.

The *structural formula* of a drug describes the way the atoms are connected to one another, and this more "graphic" representation of the drug allows visualization of the structural segments known as *functional groups*. The functional groups found within a molecule are largely responsible for the activity and specificity we find in drugs. The structural formula of Aricept® is shown in Figure 1.1.

Drug molecules are, nevertheless, very simple molecules compared to many of those found in our bodies. Consider, for example, the molecule of insulin, with a molecular formula of $C_{254}H_{377}N_{65}O_{76}S_6$. A drug with as many atoms as insulin would be so difficult to prepare by synthetic methods that it would be impractical for any pharmaceutical company to manufacture.

Let us consider another drug, this time Celebrex® (celecoxib). We see that it has a molecular structure of $C_{17}H_{14}F_3N_3O_2S$, and looking at its structural formula, we see that while the nitrogen atom was attached only to carbon in Aricept®, nitrogen is bound to sulfur (S) and another nitrogen atom in Celebrex®, as shown in Figure 1.2.

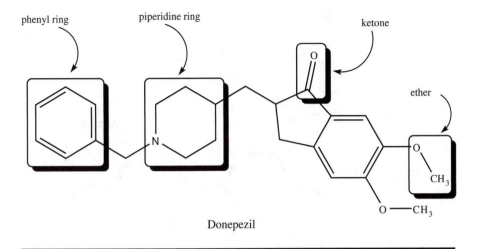

Donepezil

Figure 1.1   Structural formula of donepezil showing its functional groups.

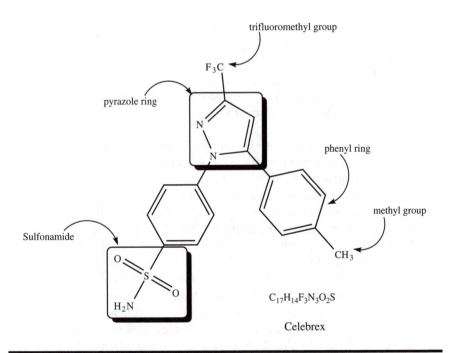

$C_{17}H_{14}F_3N_3O_2S$

Celebrex

Figure 1.2   Structural and molecular formula of Celebrex®.

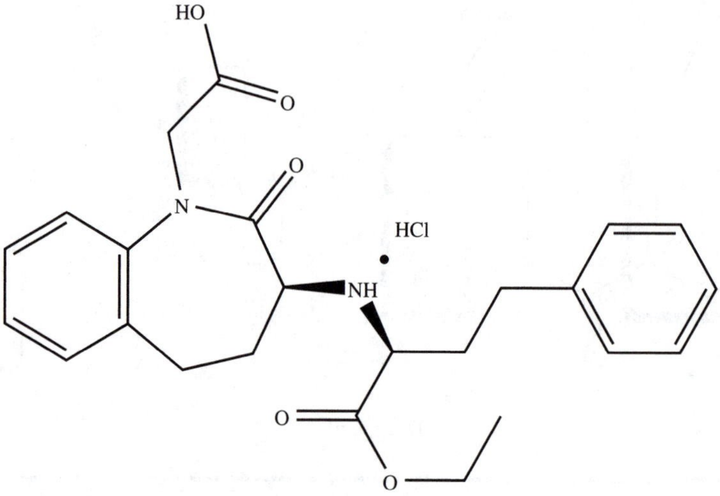

$C_{24}H_{28}N_2O_5 \cdot HCl$

Benazepril

Figure 1.3

Example 1.1

Name the functional groups present in the drug molecules shown in Figure 1.3 and Figure 1.4.

Answer: You may want to use your organic chemistry textbook to double-check your answers. Benazepril has the following functional groups: 1) two phenyl rings; 2) a carboxylic acid ester; 3) a carboxylic acid; 4) an amide, and 5) a secondary amine. These functional groups are indicated in Figure 1.5. The structure shown indicates that benazepril is formulated as its hydrochloride salt (HCl). Acid–base reactions will be studied later, but recall from general chemistry that an acid reacts with a base to form a salt. In this case the "basic" atom is the nitrogen atom in the amine functional group. Amines are basic functional groups while carboxylic acids are acidic functional groups.

Cipro® (ciprofloxacin) has the following functional groups: 1) one carboxylic acid; 2) one ketone; 3) one phenyl ring; 4) two tertiary amines; 5) one secondary amine; 6) one cyclopropane

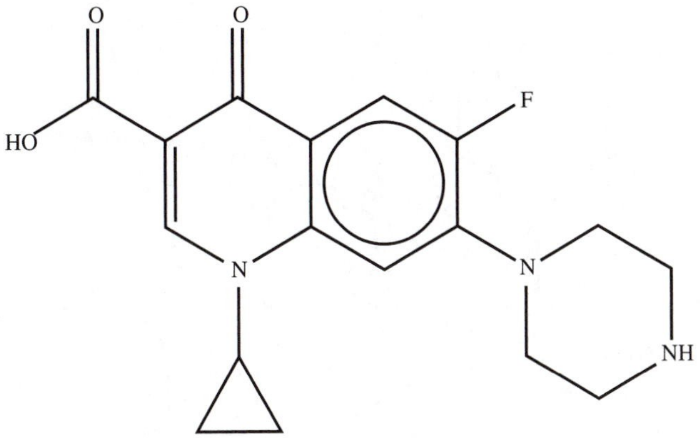

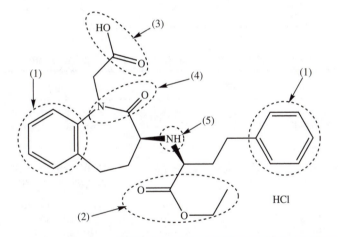

$$C_{17}H_{18}FN_3O_3$$
Cipro

Figure 1.4

HCl

Figure 1.5

ring; 7) one halogen (F). These functional groups are indicated in Figure 1.6.

A list of the functional groups most commonly found in drug molecules is given in Table 1.1.

The reasons why the atoms in drug molecules bind to one another in the particular ways they do is explained by their chemical reactivity or their electronic configuration determined by the element's position in the periodic table.

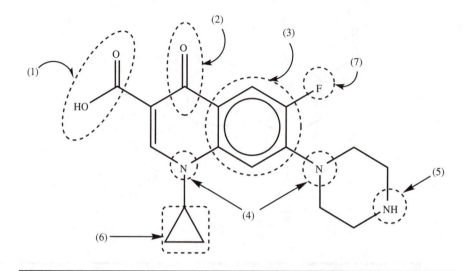

Figure 1.6

Table 1.1   Some Common Functional Groups in Drug Molecules

Functional Group	Structure	Drug Examples
Amine (R^2, R^3 = H, alkyl, aryl)	R_1—$N(R_2R_3)$	Zestril®; Zithromax®; Vasotec®; Paxil®
Quaternary amine (Salts)	(R_2R_1)—N^+—(R_3R_4)	Ipratropium bromide®; Cepacol®; Phemeride®
Azo	R—$N{=}N$—R'	Colazal™; Prontosil™
Carboxylic acid	R—CO_2H	Tequin®; Vasotec®; ibuprofen®; Zestril®
Ester	R—CO_2R'	Ritalin®; Tricor®; Vioxx®; Xalatan®; Adalat®
Amide	R—$CONH_2$	Sonata®; acetaminophen®; Glucotrol®; indomethacin®
Imide	$\underset{R}{\overset{O}{\|}}{-}NH{-}\underset{R'}{\overset{O}{\|}}$	Macrobid®; Avandia®; phenytoin®; Viagra®
Alcohol	R—OH	Metrogel®; Allegra®; pseudoephedrine®; Lescol®

Table 1.1 Some Common Functional Groups in Drug Molecules (continued)

Functional Group	Structure	Drug Examples
Ether	R——O——R'	Prilosec®; Serzone®; Flomax® Toprol®; Zebeta®; Skelaxin®
Phenol (Ar = Aromatic Rings)	Ar——OH	Detrol®; Amoxil®; acetaminophen; Asacol®
Aldehyde	$\begin{array}{c} \text{R—C—H} \\ \parallel \\ \text{O} \end{array}$	Xenical®
Ketone	$\begin{array}{c} \text{R—C—R'} \\ \parallel \\ \text{O} \end{array}$	Rhinocort®; nabumetone; Percodan®; Tricor®; warfarin
Cyano	R–C≡N	Sonata®; cimetidine®; Milrinone®
Sulfonic acid	R——SO_3H	Cardura®; Norvasc®
Sulfonamide (R2, R3 = H, alkyl, aryl)	$\begin{array}{c} \text{O} \\ \parallel \\ R_1 - \text{S} - NR_2R_3 \\ \parallel \\ \text{O} \end{array}$	Celebrex®; Viagra®; Zestoretic®; Amaryl®; Zaroxolyn®; Flomax®
Sulfoxide	$\begin{array}{c} \text{O} \\ \parallel \\ \text{R–S—R'} \end{array}$	Aciphex®; Prilosec®
Sulfone	$\begin{array}{c} \text{O}_{\diagdown} \;\; {}_{\diagup}\text{O} \\ \text{S} \\ R_1 \diagup \;\; \diagdown R_2 \end{array}$	Vioxx®
Thioether	R——S——R'	Zyprexa®; Axid®; Ceftin®
Nitro	R——NO_2	Adalat®; Macrobid®; Axid®; Metrogel®; clonazepam
Carbamate	$\begin{array}{c} \text{H} \quad \text{O} \\ \mid \quad\;\; \parallel \\ \text{R—N—C—O——R'} \end{array}$	Claritin®; Skelaxin®; Ceftin®
Urea	$\begin{array}{c} \text{O} \\ \parallel \\ R_1R - \text{N—C—N—}R_3R_2 \end{array}$	Amaryl®; Serzone®; Glucotrol®
Phosphonic acid	$\begin{array}{c} \text{O} \\ \parallel \\ \text{—R—P—OH} \\ \mid \\ \text{OH} \end{array}$	Fosamax®

$$^{19}_{9}F$$

Figure 1.7

We shall now turn our attention to the usefulness of the periodic table in describing the electronic configuration of the atoms that comprise drug molecules.

THE PERIODIC TABLE AND CHEMICAL REACTIVITY

The periodic table is an arrangement of all known elements in increasing order of atomic number. Common representations of the periodic table include the symbol of the element along with its atomic number and mass number. The atomic representation of the element fluorine is shown in Figure 1.7.

This representation of the fluorine atom tells us the number of sub-atomic particles present: nine protons, nine electrons, and 10 neutrons. The atomic number is equal to the number of protons in the nucleus (subscript), which equals the number of electrons outside the nucleus. The number of neutrons is found by subtracting the atomic number (9) from the mass number (19).

Number of neutrons = mass number – atomic number

Exercise 1.1

Find the elements C, O, H, N in the periodic table and write the symbol for each atom, indicating the name and number of all subatomic particles.

Protons and neutrons are located in the nucleus, while electrons move about the nucleus and are attracted to the positively charged protons. A more adequate representation of the movement of electrons about the nucleus is given by the use of orbitals. These graphical representations of probability functions are called *s* orbitals, *p* orbitals, *d* orbitals, and *f* orbitals. The shapes of *s*, *p*, and *d* orbitals are shown in Figure 1.8; they indicate the volume in space around the nucleus where the electron is most likely to be found. There are three *p* orbitals, five *d* orbitals, and seven *f* orbitals.

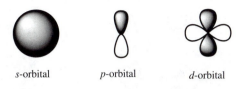

s-orbital   p-orbital   d-orbital

Figure 1.8   Shapes of three types of atomic orbitals.

An increment of one in atomic number in consecutive positions along a row (period) in the periodic table means that each consecutive element has one more proton in its nucleus and one more electron in its orbitals than its predecessor. Just as there are four types of orbitals, there are four sections in the periodic table that correspond to the type of electron subshell (orbital) that is being filled with each increment in atomic number. A detailed description of these energy levels (electron shells, n = 1, 2, 3, 4) and sublevels (electron subshells: 1s; 2s, 2p; 3s, 3p, 3d; etc.) is beyond the scope of our discussion, so let us focus on the utility of the periodic table in describing the chemical reactivity of elements found in drugs. For this, we must understand how the electron configuration depends on position in the periodic table, and how it is that the electron distribution determines how atoms combine to form drug molecules.

The maximum numbers of electrons that a subshell can hold are as follows: two (s orbitals), six (p orbitals), 10 (d orbitals), and 14 (f orbitals). This is reflected in the periodic table by showing four areas corresponding to the four types of orbitals (see Figure 1.9): 1) s orbital area: two electrons, two columns; 2) p orbital area: six electrons, six columns; 3) d orbital area: 10 electrons, 10 columns; and 4) f orbital area: 14 electrons, 14 columns.

Elements in the same group (column) in the periodic table have similar chemical reactivity due to the fact that their electron configurations are very similar: a single electron in the 2s subshell for lithium (Li), a single electron in the 3s subshell for sodium (Na), a single electron in the 4s subshell for potassium (K). Similar analyses can be made for every other group (column) in the periodic table. Li, Na, and K all tend to lose this last electron when combining in chemical reactions with nonmetals. The metal magnesium (Mg) belongs to the IIA family in the periodic table and loses two electrons to the nonmetal oxygen (O) to form the common antacid magnesium oxide, molecular formula MgO. Similar oxides with elements from the IA family would have molecular formulas of different atomic compositions, to reflect the fact that they can only lose one electron to oxygen. Oxides of sodium and potassium have the molecular formulas Na_2O and K_2O. (Note that the subscript of "1" is always understood but not written in chemical nomenclature.)

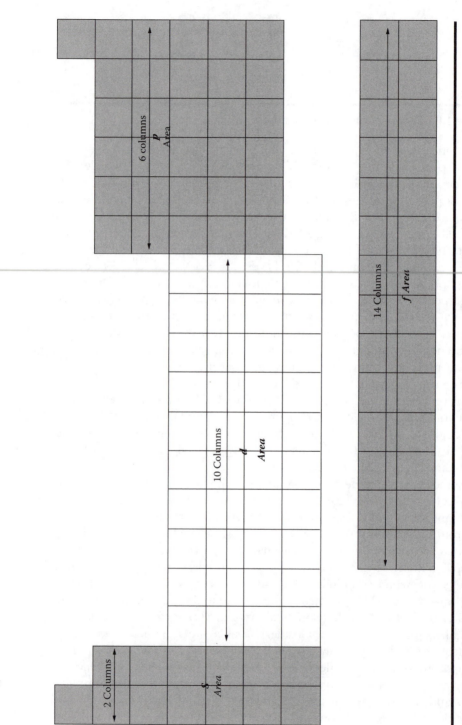

Figure 1.9 Relationship between position in the periodic table and electron configuration.

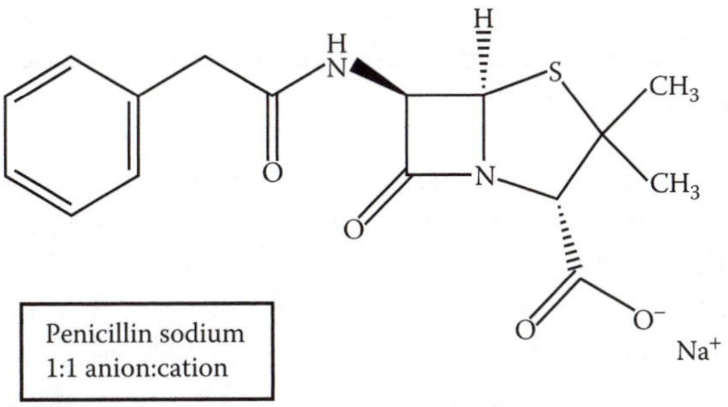

Penicillin sodium
1:1 anion:cation

Figure 1.10

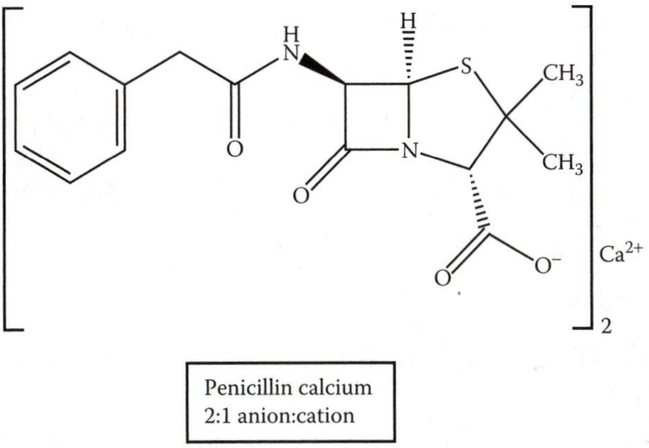

Penicillin calcium
2:1 anion:cation

Figure 1.11

In a more complex example that we will examine closely later, the electron configuration as depicted in the periodic table tells us that penicillin potassium has a 1:1 relationship in ion composition, while penicillin calcium has a 2:1 relationship in ion composition (see Figure 1.10 and Figure 1.11).

Sodium has one electron in the outermost electron shell, the $3s$ subshell, therefore it loses this electron to the nonmetal oxygen when combining to form salts such as penicillin sodium. Calcium, on the other hand, belongs to the IIA family of the periodic table and thus has two electrons in its outermost electron shell, the $4s$ subshell. Upon reaction with the nonmetal oxygen, calcium loses its two electrons to form the divalent cation. This requires two carboxylate ions to form, each taking up one electron to form a singly negatively charged anion.

Elements can be classified according to their electron configurations as noble gases, representative elements, transition elements, and inner transition elements, as shown in Figure 1.12:

The *noble gases* are in the far right column of the periodic table; they have filled p subshells (except for helium, He). Their filled subshells explain their lack of reactivity.

The *representative elements* are all the elements in the s and p areas of the periodic table (excluding the noble gases). Most drugs are composed of representative elements. The representative elements most commonly found in our bodies and in drugs are carbon (C), hydrogen (H), oxygen (O), and nitrogen (N).

The *transition elements* are in the d area of the periodic table. Many vital *trace* elements are found in this class.

The *inner transition* elements are in the f area of the periodic table. Drugs do not include elements in this class, and we will only mention them here.

A second classification of the elements describes them as metals or nonmetals based on selected physical properties such as luster, electrical and thermal conductivity, and malleability. Metals are good conductors of heat and electricity, have luster, and are malleable. Nonmetals, on the other hand, lack all of these properties. Chemical periodicity is observed for metallic and nonmetallic character in the following manner:

■ Metallic character increases from top to bottom within a group in the periodic table.

■ Metallic character increases from right to left within a period of the periodic table.

The opposite trend is valid for nonmetals.

The elements sodium (Na), potassium (K), magnesium (Mg), and calcium (Ca) are *metals* that are commonly found in drugs and form positively charged ions when combined with *nonmetal* elements such as oxygen (O) and sulfur (S).

Two other properties that exhibit chemical periodicity with the position of the element on the periodic table are atomic radius and electronegativity. Atomic radius is a measure of the "size" of the element's atom, and electronegativity is a measure of the relative attraction of an atom for electrons that are shared in a bond. Atomic radius varies according to the following scheme:

■ Atomic radius decreases from left to right within a period of the periodic table.

■ Atomic radius increases from top to bottom within a group in the periodic table.

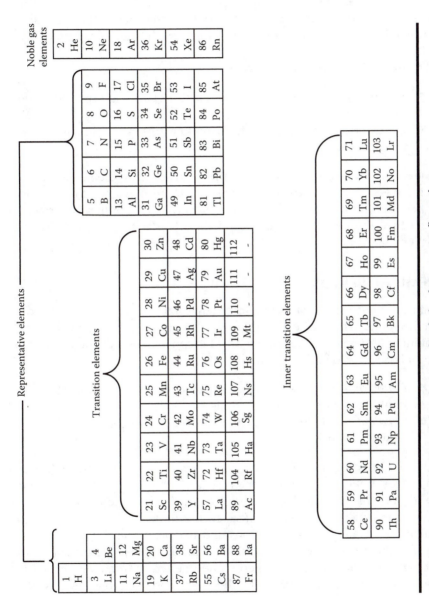

Figure 1.12 Classification of the elements by their electron configuration.

The reason for the increase in atomic radius going down within a group is easy to understand just based on the much larger atomic numbers of consecutive elements. The atomic number increases only by one with each consecutive element along a period, but as the nuclear charge increases, electrons enter the same (outermost) shell. The increased nuclear charge draws these electrons closer to the nucleus, resulting in smaller atomic size.

Electronegativity varies as follows:

- Electronegativity increases from left to right along a period of the periodic table.
- Electronegativity increases from bottom to top within a group of the periodic table.

The trend is more consistent within the representative elements than in other classes. The most electronegative of all the elements, fluorine (F), has been arbitrarily assigned an electronegativity of 4.0; this generates a scale where the rest of the elements fit in accordance to their measured bond energies.

CHEMICAL BONDS

Chemical bonds are the attractive forces that hold atoms together in more complex units. They arise from the interactions of the electrons in the combining atoms. Chemical bonds can be conveniently divided into two broad classes, ionic and covalent:

- *Ionic bonds* result when there is *transfer* of one or more electrons from an atom or group of atoms to another.
- *Covalent bonds* result from the *sharing* of one or more electrons between atoms.

These two bonding models are useful in describing ionic and molecular compounds, but in reality most bonds are not 100% ionic or 100% covalent; instead, they have some degree of both ionic and covalent character.

Two fundamental concepts crucial to the understanding of ionic and covalent bonds are valence electrons and the octet rule.

Valence electrons are the electrons in an atom that are available for bonding. For representative elements (the ones most frequently found in drugs) and noble gases, these are the outermost electrons, that is, the electrons with the highest shell number (n).

The valence electrons in an atom are the most important of all its electrons in determining its bonding characteristics. They can be determined from the atom's electron configuration.

Mg: Ca:

___

Figure 1.13

Example 1.2

Explain how to determine the number of valence electrons in the atoms Mg, Ca, Al, and O, commonly found in antacid drugs.

Solution: Looking at the periodic table, we find the element magnesium in group IIA, period 3.

The following are three generalizations related to valence electrons:

1. Representative elements in the same group of the periodic table have the same number of valence electrons.
2. The periodic table group number is the same as the number of valence electrons for representative elements.
3. The maximum number of valence electrons is eight for representative elements. Only the noble gases, starting with Ne, achieve this full shell configuration.

The shorthand representation of valence electrons around an atom is called an electron-dot structure. The generalizations mentioned above explain why Ca and Mg both have two valence electrons, since they belong to group II, and their electrons dot structures are as shown in Figure 1.13. Aluminum is in group III and oxygen in group VI. Their valence electrons are 3 and 6, respectively.

The closed-shell configurations of the noble gases are considered to be the most stable; that is, they do not undergo spontaneous change readily. For this reason, the noble gases are the most unreactive of all the elements. Other atoms tend to attain the closed-shell configuration of the noble gases through compound formation; this observation has been named the *octet rule*. A formal description of the octet rule is as follows:

Octet rule: Upon compound formation, atoms lose, gain, or share electrons in such a way that allows all atoms involved to attain a noble gas electron configuration.

The octet rule is very useful in predicting the combining ratios of atoms involved in compound formation. It explains, for example, why two (and not some other number) hydrogen atoms are bound to oxygen in the molecule of water and why the ratio is 1:1 in MgO and 2:1 in penicillin calcium.

We will now further examine the two most common types of bonds, ionic and covalent.

Ionic bonds result from the transfer of electrons from one atom to another. The resulting species are called "ions" and are electrically charged as a result of the transfer of electrons:

- The atom that loses its electron(s) ends up positively charged and is called a *cation*.
- The atom that accepts the electron(s) ends up negatively charged and is called an *anion*.

Cations frequently found in drugs include Na^+, Li^+, K^+, Mg^{+2}, and Ca^{+2}. These are all metal elements.

Anions frequently found in drugs include Cl^-, O^{-2}, S^{-2}, and CO_3^{-2}. These are all nonmetal elements.

Ionic bonds form between a metal and a nonmetal. The use of electron dot structures helps to visualize the formation of the ionic bonds through the electron transfer. The ionic bond in NaCl is formed by the transfer of one electron from sodium to chlorine.

Looking back at the periodic table and locating both Na and Cl we see that sodium has one more electron than the noble gas neon (Ne), while chlorine has one less electron than noble gas argon (Ar). When these two atoms combine to form an ionic bond, the path which requires less energy, that is to say the favored path, is for sodium to transfer one electron to chlorine. This process affords a complete octet for both Na and Cl. Sodium achieves the electron configuration of noble gas Ne by transferring one electron to chlorine, which then achieves the electron configuration of noble gas Ar. This same reasoning can be applied to ionic bond formation between other metals and nonmetals within the representative elements. Metals are located in the periodic table in such a way that they can achieve noble gas configurations by losing electrons to a nonmetal. Nonmetals are located in the periodic table in a way that allows achieving noble gas configuration by gaining electrons.

MAGNITUDE OF IONIC CHARGE

Metals can lose electrons to acquire an octet of electrons. The magnitude of the positive charge on the metal ions in groups IA to IIIA, for example, is the same as the group number:

- Group IA metals form cations of single positive charge: Na^+, K^+, Rb^+, Cs^+.
- Group IIA metals form cations with two positive charges: Mg^{+2}, Ca^{+2}, Sr^{+2}, Ba^{+2}.
- Group IIIA metals form cations with three positive changes: Al^{+3}, ga^{+3}, In^{+3}.

Nonmetals can gain electrons to acquire an octet. The magnitude of the negative charge on the nonmetal ions in Groups VIA to VIIA is the same as [group number − 8]:

- Group VIIA metals form anions of single negative charge (VII − 8): F^-, Cl^-, Br^-, I^-.
- Group VIA metals form anions with two negative charges (VI − 8): O^{-2}, S^{-2}, Se^{-2}.

POLYATOMIC IONS

A different category of ions commonly found in nature and in drug molecules is that of polyatomic ions. Polyatomic ions are a group of atoms held together by covalent bonds; these ions have a net charge. The net charge can be positive as in the ammonium ion, NH_4^+, or negative as in the sulfate ion, SO_4^{-2}. Polyatomic ions never exist alone but rather are always associated with a counterion(s) of opposite charge in proportions such that the net charge is zero. For this reason, one SO_4^{-2} will associate with 2 NH_4^+ in order to maintain neutrality in the ionic compound.

Exercise 1.2

Identify the polyatomic ions in timolol maleate, shown in Figure 1.14.

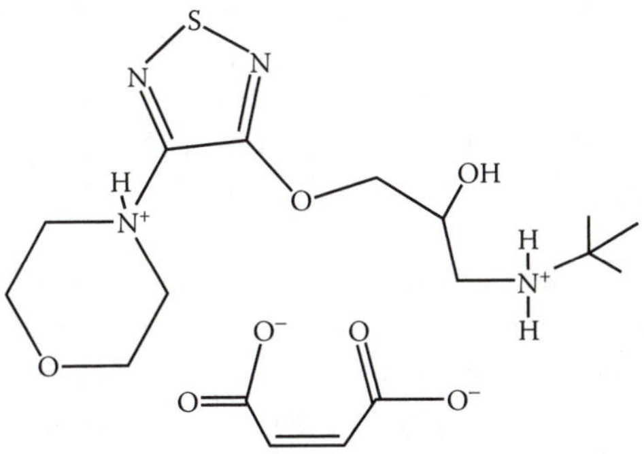

Timolol maleate

Figure 1.14

COVALENT BONDS

Covalent bonding occurs when two atoms share electrons in order to attain the octet of their closest noble gas in the periodic table. The atoms in covalent compounds usually have *bonding* and *nonbonding* electrons. The bonding electrons are those valence electrons that are shared between the atoms. A line between the atoms sharing them in a structural formula commonly represents them. The nonbonding electrons are valence electrons not involved in electron sharing. Nonbonding electrons are not usually written in structural formulas of drug molecules found in the pharmaceutical literature.

A comparison with ionic bonds is useful at this point:

Covalent Bond	Ionic Bond
Forms between atoms of two nonmetals	Forms between atoms of a metal and a nonmetal
Electron sharing occurs upon bonding (between identical or different nonmetals)	Electron transfer occurs upon bonding (metal to nonmetal)
Molecular compounds result. Structural unit is the molecule.	Ionic compounds do not exist as discrete molecules. Extended array of + and – ions.

Exercise 1.3

Label bonds 1, 2, 3 as covalent or ionic in the drug structure shown in Figure 1.15.

A single line represents a single covalent bond. However, single covalent bonds are not adequate to explain covalent bonding in all molecules. Sometimes, atoms must share two or three pairs of electrons in order to acquire the octet configuration. This gives rise to multiple bonding, including:

- Double bonds, when two atoms share two pairs of valence electrons
- Triple bonds, when two atoms share three pairs of valence electrons

Double and triple bonds in drug structures are also represented by lines; a double bond between two atoms is depicted by a double line and a triple bond by a triple line. The number of covalent bonds an atom can form equals the number of electrons it needs to achieve a noble gas configuration.

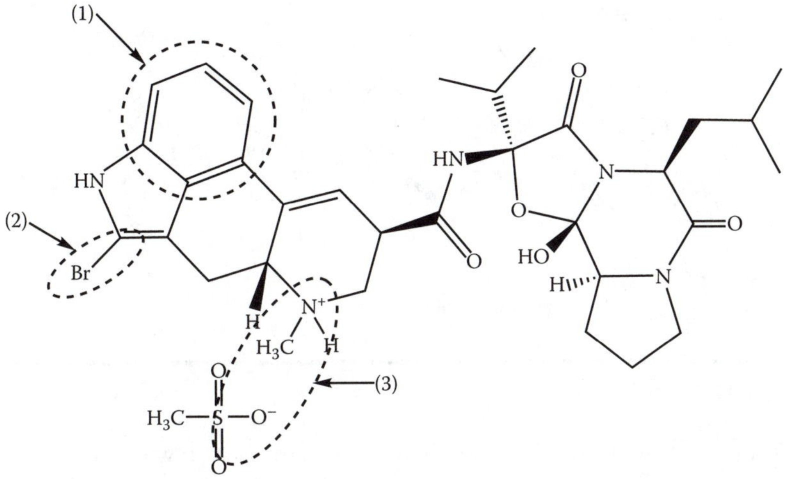

Bromocriptine mesylate

Figure 1.15

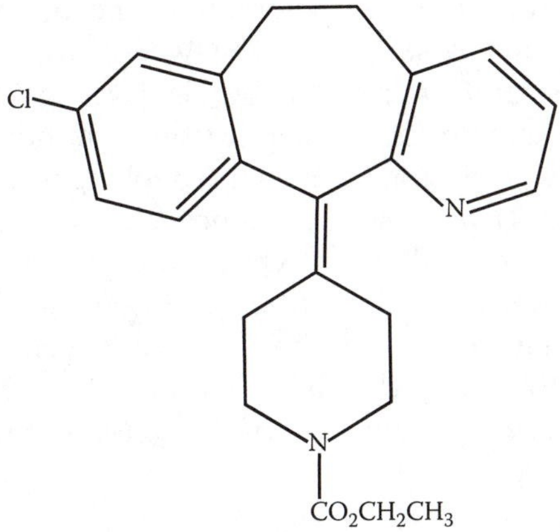

Claritin

Figure 1.16

Exercise 1.4

The drug structures in Figure 1.16 and Figure 1.17 include multiple bonds. Identify double and/or triple bonds in each structure.

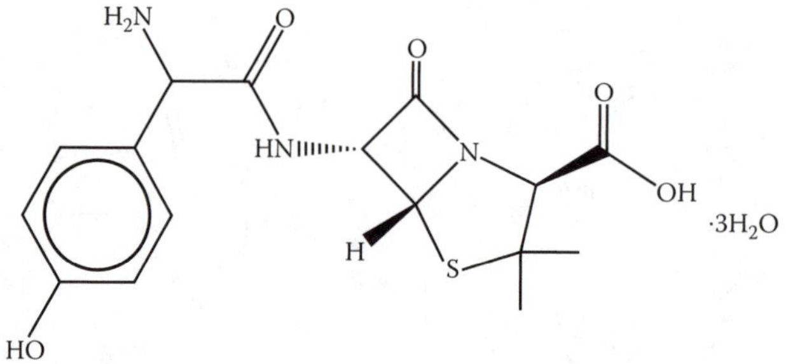

Amoxicillin

Figure 1.17

Drug structures are depicted in the literature in a way that assumes the specialist's understanding of the types of bond that are formed between the different atoms. A knowledge of electron configurations and valence electrons' participation in bond formation allows the recognition of the types of bonds formed, even when they are not entirely written out in the structural formula.

The functional group –COOH is an abbreviated form that a pharmacist should be able to recognize as representing one double bond between carbon and oxygen and a single bond between carbon and –OH.

Not all elements can form multiple bonds. Hydrogen and the halogens (group VIIA), for example, can only form single bonds because they are short only one electron from achieving noble gas configuration. The halogens (F, Cl, Br, I) have seven valence electrons and one vacancy, while hydrogen has one valence electron and one vacancy. Double and triple bonding becomes possible when an atom needs two and three electrons, respectively, to achieve the octet. However, whether or not an atom forms a multiple bond depends also on the other atom to which it will bond. These *bonding behaviors* can be illustrated for O, N, and C in the following manner:

◼ Oxygen can obtain an octet by sharing electrons in either two single bonds or one double bond, as shown in Figure 1.18. For example, oxygen atoms with both types of bonding behaviors can be found in Aricept®, as shown in Figure 1.19. One oxygen atom is found in a carbonyl group on the five-member ring and the other two are methoxy ethers (–OCH$_3$) in the phenyl ring.
◼ Nitrogen can obtain an octet by sharing electrons in one of three bonding modes: three single bonds, one single and one double bond, or one triple bond, as shown in Figure 1.20. Nitrogen is versatile. For example, in Claritin®, as shown in Figure 1.21, we

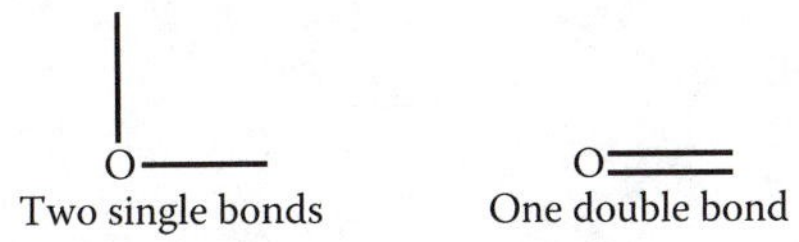

Figure 1.18

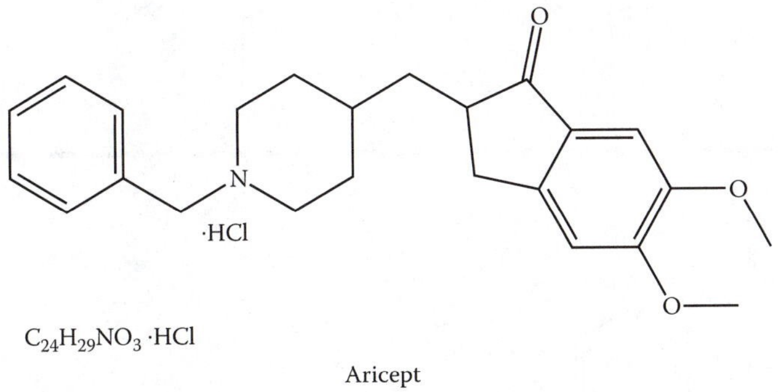

$C_{24}H_{29}NO_3 \cdot HCl$

Aricept

Figure 1.19

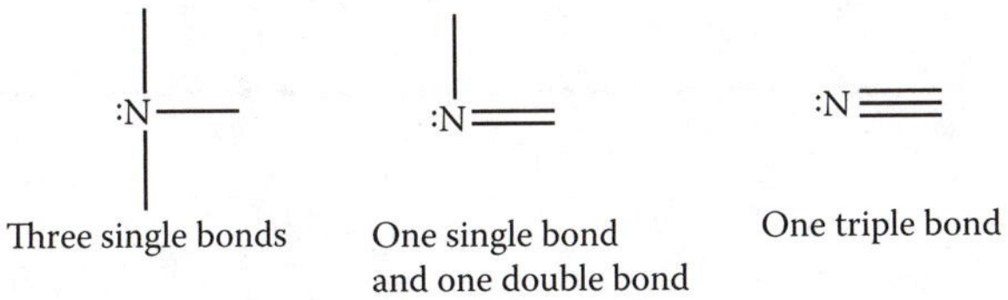

Figure 1.20

find the first two binding modes, while in Milrinone, as shown in Figure 1.22, all three binding modes of nitrogen are found. The triple bond is that in the –CN group. This functional group is called a nitrile or cyano group.

■ Carbon can obtain an octet by sharing electrons in one of four binding modes, as shown in Figure 1.23:
  – 4 single bonds
  – 1 double and 2 single bonds
  – 2 double bonds
  – 1 single and 1 triple bond

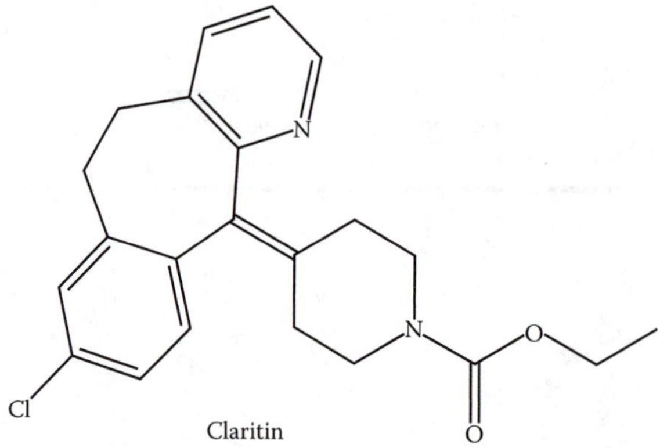

Claritin

Figure 1.21

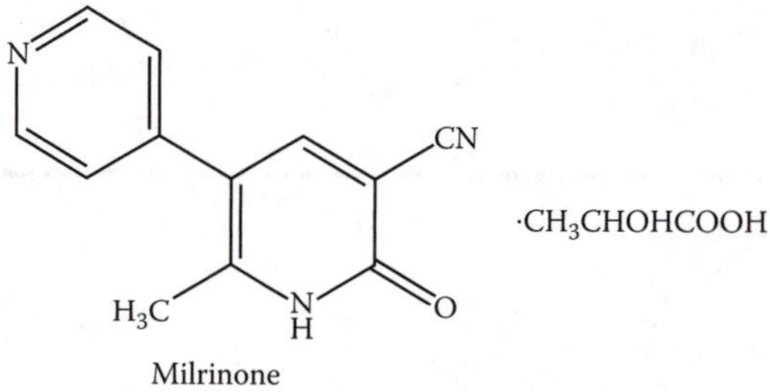

Milrinone

·CH₃CHOHCOOH

Figure 1.22

| 4 single bonds | 2 single bonds & 1 double bond | 2 double bonds | 1 single bond & 1 triple bond |

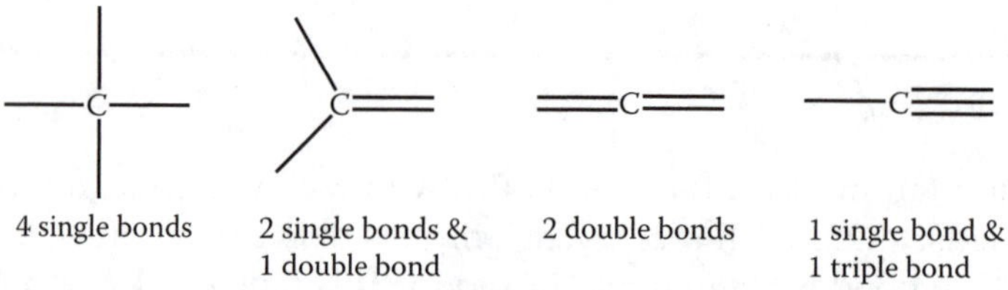

Figure 1.23

Carbon is indeed the most versatile element and for this reason, it is the main component of organic matter. Figure 1.24, Figure 1.25, and Figure 1.26 show examples of the many ways in which carbon may be bonded within drug molecules.

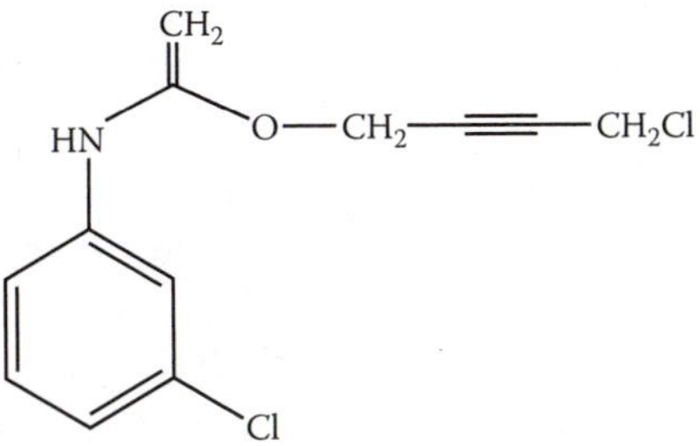

Barban

Figure 1.24

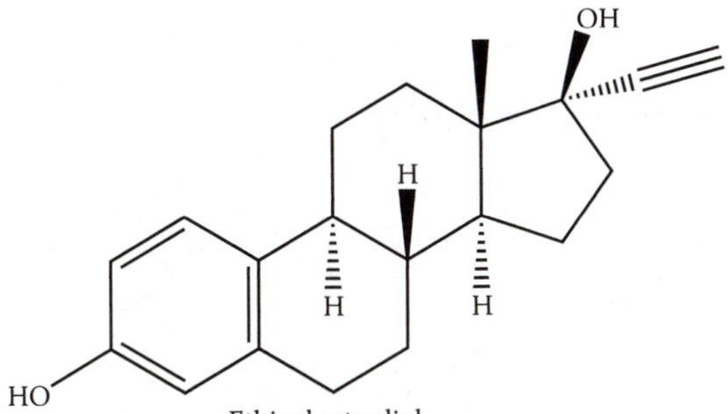

Ethinyl estradiol

Figure 1.25

COORDINATE COVALENT BONDS

The covalent bonds discussed so far are formed between atoms contributing an equal number of electrons to the bond. There is another type of covalent bond in which the electrons shared all come from a single element. Such a bond is called coordinate covalent bond. Nitrogen and sulfur are usually found participating in this type of bonding. The ammonium ion, NH_4^+, contains a coordinate covalent bond; its formation can be viewed as the reaction of hydrogen ion (H^+) and ammonia (NH_3). Examples of drugs containing coordinate covalent bonds include the antibacterial quaternary ammonium compounds shown in Figure 1.27 and Figure 1.28.

The nitrogen atom in quaternary ammonium compounds no longer has a nonbonding pair of electrons. Both electrons are involved in coordinate covalent bonding.

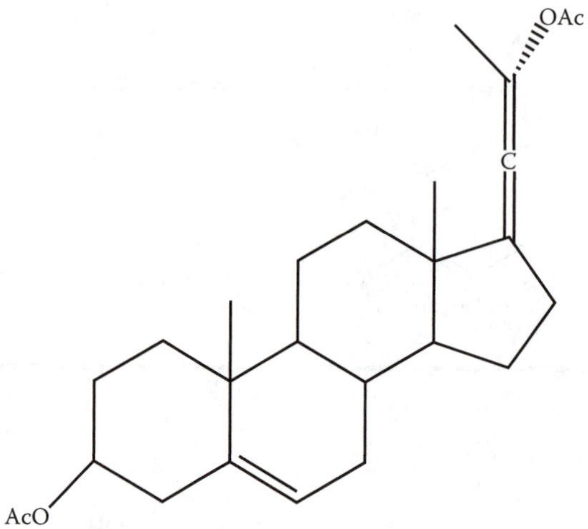

Steroidal allene acetate

Figure 1.26

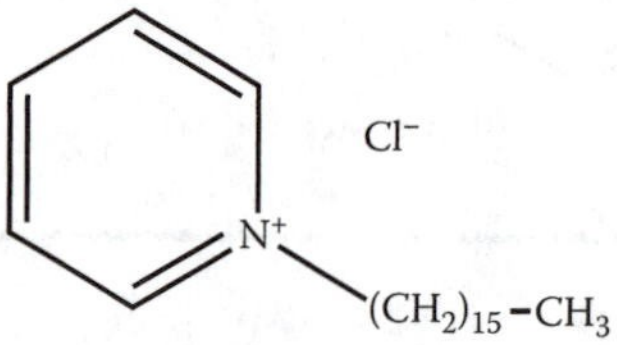

Cetylpyridinium chloride

Figure 1.27

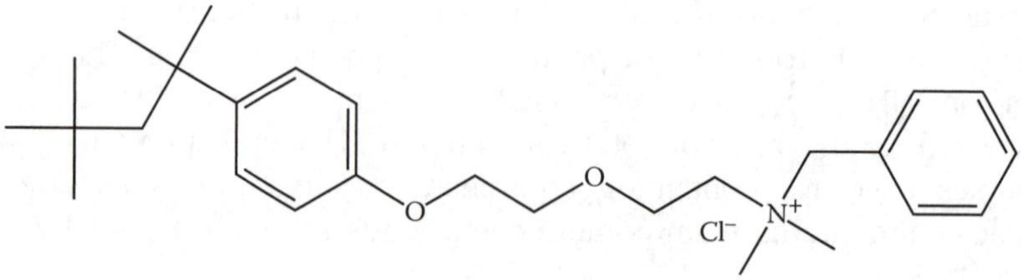

Benzethonium chloride

Figure 1.28

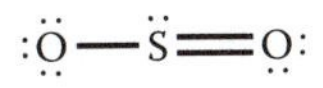

$$:\ddot{O} - \ddot{S} = \ddot{O}:$$

Figure 1.29

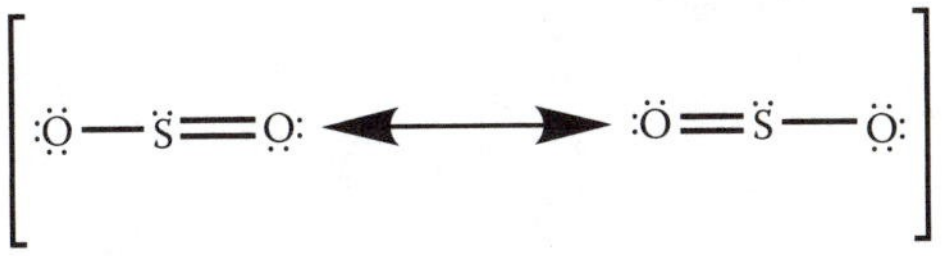

$$\left[:\ddot{O} - \ddot{S} = \ddot{O}: \longleftrightarrow :\ddot{O} = \ddot{S} - \ddot{O}: \right]$$

Figure 1.30   Resonance Structures for SO$_2$

RESONANCE STRUCTURES

Two bond properties that can be determined experimentally are bond strength and bond length. They are inversely related; the stronger the bond, the shorter the distance between the atoms. Triple bonds are stronger than double, and double bonds are stronger than single bonds. For this reason, triple bonds are shorter than double and the double bonds are shorter than single bonds.

Most electron dot structures of molecules give information that is consistent with the available experimental data on bond length and strength. However, for some molecules no single electron dot structure adequately accommodates the available experimental information. One example of this is the molecule of sulfur dioxide (SO$_2$). An electron dot structure for this molecule that satisfies the octet rule is shown in Figure 1.29. This structure suggests that the S–O single bond would be weaker and longer than the S=O double bond, which is experimentally not true. The two sulfur-oxygen bonds have equal strength and length and are intermediate between a single and a double bond. This bonding cannot be represented by a single electron dot structure, but by two electron dot structures, which are called *resonance structures*.

Resonance structures are two or more electron dot structures for a molecule or ion, which contain the same number of electrons within the same arrangement of atoms and differ only in the location of the electrons.

The bonding situation for SO$_2$ then is more adequately represented by two resonance structures, as shown in Figure 1.30. It is customary to connect resonance structures by a double-headed arrow.

The existence of resonance forms also explains the bonding in many drug molecules. For example, many drugs and several amino acids contain aromatic or heteroaromatic rings, and although alternating double bonds are drawn (see below), each bond in the ring is intermediate between single and double bond. Examples are shown in Figure 1.31 and Figure 1.32.

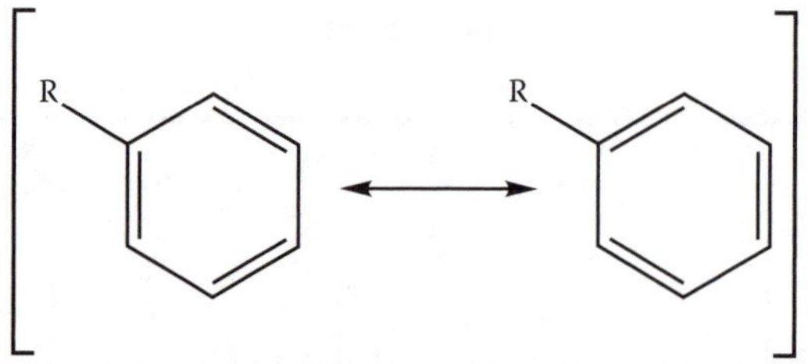

Drug X

Figure 1.31

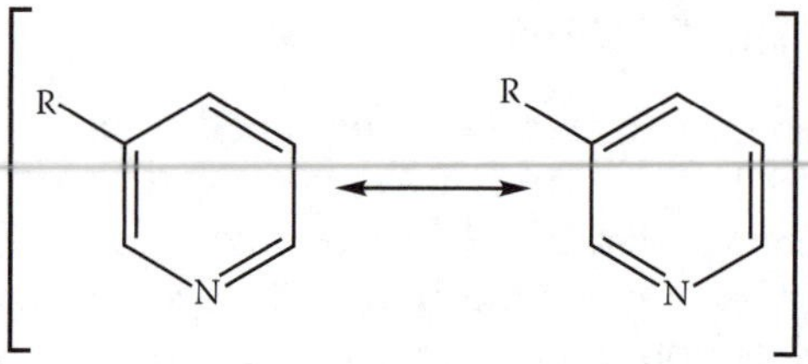

Drug Y

Figure 1.32

Another important concept is that of conjugation or *delocalization* of electron density into unsaturated systems. Functional groups such as amine (NR_2) and hydroxyl (OH) have nonbonding electrons on nitrogen and oxygen, respectively, that can be delocalized into an aromatic ring or a conjugated system of multiple bonds. This *delocalization* is represented by curved arrows, such as those in Figure 1.33, showing that electron density can flow from the electron-rich atom into the unsaturated system or aromatic ring from which it is separated by no more than a single bond.

Notice that only one nitrogen in eseroline is conjugated to the aromatic ring, and therefore it can delocalize its nonbonding electrons into this unsaturated system. This property of certain electron-rich atoms is important in evaluating the relative acidity or basicity of drug molecules and explains to a great extent how a drug distributes in the body.

SHAPES OF DRUG MOLECULES

Molecular geometry is determined by the three-dimensional arrangement of atoms in a molecule. Small changes in the shape of a drug molecule, caused by adding or removing atoms, can significantly affect the activity or toxicity of a drug. It is possible to predict the molecular geometry of

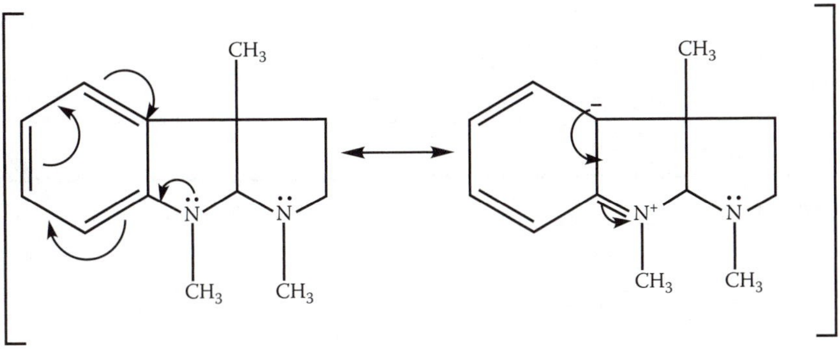

Eseroline resonance structures

Figure 1.33

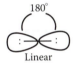

180°

Linear

Figure 1.34

a drug molecule from its electron dot structure by a procedure called valence-shell-electron-pair-repulsions (VSEPR). The central concept in VSEPR theory is that electron pairs in the valence shell of atoms arrange themselves so as to minimize repulsion. Two, three, and four electron pairs can arrange themselves in the following manner in order to minimize repulsion:

- Two electron pairs will minimize repulsion by positioning themselves opposite to each other across the nucleus at a 180° angle. This electron arrangement is called *linear*. It is illustrated in Figure 1.34.
- Three electron pairs will minimize repulsion by positioning themselves in the corners of an equilateral triangle. This electron arrangement is called *trigonal planar*, and the corresponding angles are 120°. See Figure 1.35.
- Four electron pairs will minimize repulsion by positioning themselves in the corners of a tetrahedron. This electron arrangement is called *tetrahedral*, and the corresponding angle between any two electron pairs is 109°. See Figure 1.36.

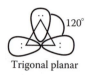

Trigonal planar

Figure 1.35

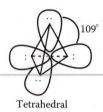

Tetrahedral

Figure 1.36

The geometry around a central atom in a drug molecule can be found by first determining the number of electron pairs around it, taking into account these two simple rules:

1. Double and triple bonds about a central atom count as "one" VSEPR electron pair because they take up the same region in space.
2. Nonbonding and bonding electron pairs are regarded as equal in VSEPR analysis.

Using these conventions, the VSEPR electron pair count around central atoms is as follows for the drug molecule shown in Figure 1.37.

The sulfonamide functional group in Celebrex has four VSEPR electron pairs: two double bonds and two single bonds, therefore the geometry is tetrahedral around the sulfur atom. The geometry around the ring nitrogen atoms is trigonal pyramidal for N1 (three single bonds + one nonbonding pair) and nonlinear or angular for N2 (one single, one double, and one nonbonding electron pair).

This example highlights the relationship between the number of VSEPR electron pairs and molecular geometry. This relationship can be summarized as shown in Figure 1.38, Figure 1.39, and Figure 1.40.

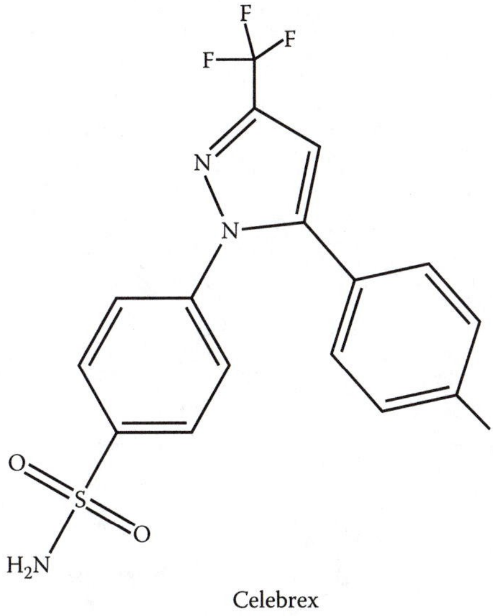

Celebrex

Figure 1.37

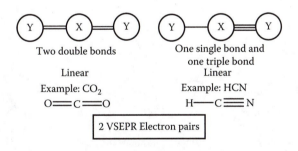

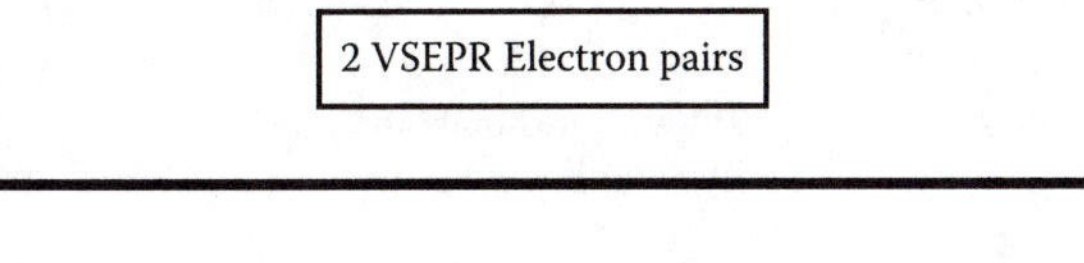

Two double bonds

Linear

Example: CO_2

$$O{=}C{=}O$$

One single bond and
one triple bond
Linear

Example: HCN

$$H{-}C{\equiv}N$$

2 VSEPR Electron pairs

Figure 1.38

The molecular geometry of the NH_2 group (N central atom) in Celebrex® (see above) is trigonal pyramidal (three single bonds, one nonbonding pair). Functional groups CF_3 and CH_3 are tetrahedral around the central carbon atom.

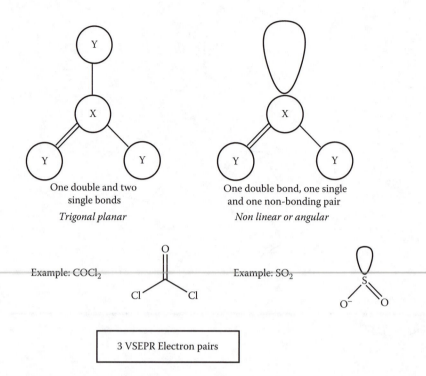

Figure 1.39

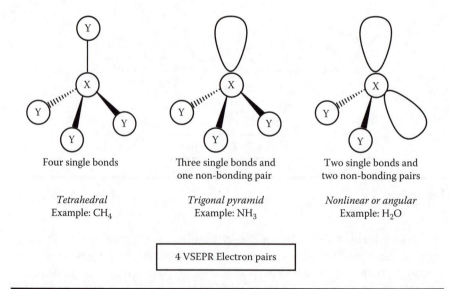

Figure 1.40 Relationship between number of VSEPR electron pairs and molecular geometry.

ELECTRONEGATIVITY

The covalent and ionic models described so far represent extremes in a continuum of bonding arrangements that is possible between atoms. The concepts of *electronegativity* and *bond polarity* go hand in hand to explain many of the properties of drugs that are crucial for their absorption and distribution in the human body.

Electronegativity is a measure of the attraction that an atom has for shared electrons in a bond relative to its bonding partner. The electronegativity scale, developed by Dr. L. Pauling, is commonly used and takes fluorine as the reference element with the highest electronegativity of 4.0. Trends in the electronegativity values in the periodic table are as follows:

- Electronegativity increases from left to right within a period of representative elements.
- There is a regular increase in 0.5 units from left to right in the second period.
- Electronegativity generally increases from bottom to top within a group.

POLARITY OF CHEMICAL BONDS

The different electronegativities of atoms participating in chemical bonds affect the way the bonding electrons are shared between them. When two atoms involved in a chemical bond have very different electronegativities, the bond between them is "polarized"; that is, the more electronegative atom attracts the electrons more strongly. This results in electrons spending more time around the atom with greater electronegativity, which in turn causes a partial negative charge to be formed in this atom, and a partial positive charge to be formed in the least electronegative atom.

Bond polarity is a measure of the inequality in electron sharing between atoms participating in a chemical bond:

- A *nonpolar covalent* bond is one in which there is equal sharing of electrons.
- A *polar covalent* bond is one in which electron sharing is unequal.

The unequal sharing of electrons in a polar covalent bond is usually represented by a vector pointing from the δ+ towards the δ– atom. This is shown for the HCl molecule in Figure 1.41. Both hydrogen atoms in a H_2 molecule share electrons equally; this is also shown in Figure 1.41.

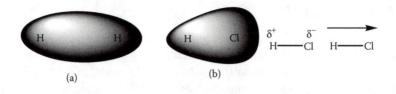

(a)   (b)

Figure 1.41 Equal sharing of electrons in H_2 (a), vs. unequal electron sharing in HCl (b).

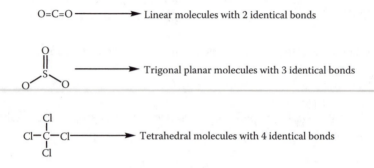

Figure 1.42 Unpolar molecules with polar bonds.

Calculating the difference in the electronegativities of the atoms involved and using the following convention allows us to determine the degree of polarity of a bond:

1. Nonpolar covalent bonds are formed between two atoms that have a difference in electronegativity less than or equal to 0.5.
2. Polar covalent bonds are formed between two atoms that have a difference in electronegativity greater than 0.5 but less than 2.0.
3. Ionic bonds are formed between two atoms that have a difference in elctronegativity greater than or equal to 2.0.

In ionic bonds, the degree of bond polarity is such that there is actually electron transfer from the least electronegative atom to the most electronegative atom.

MOLECULAR POLARITY

Molecular polarity arises from unequal distribution of electronic charge in a molecule and depends on two factors: bond polarities and molecular geometry.

A molecule may have polar bonds and yet be nonpolar as a whole. The effects of polar bonds cancel each other in symmetrical molecules, resulting in a nonpolar molecule. Some examples are given in Figure 1.42.

The nonlinear (angular) triatomic H_2O molecule has two polar bonds that do not cancel each other; the water molecule has a net polarity due to its angular geometry. It is the combined characteristics of its electronic configuration, bonding patterns, and molecular shape that make water the key component of physiological media, where the actions and reactions of drug molecules take place.

FURTHER READING

1. *Chemical Principles* by Steven S. Zumdahl. Houghton Mifflin College Div; 5th Edition (2004).
2. *Review of Organic Functional Groups: Introduction to Medicinal Organic Chemistry* by Thomas L. Lemke. Lippincott Williams & Wilkins; 4th Edition (2003).

2

ACID–BASE PROPERTIES
OF DRUGS

Most drugs currently in the market are small organic molecules that behave in aqueous solutions as weak acids or bases. We must therefore review acid–base theory in order to understand their behavior in the dilute aqueous solutions that represent physiological conditions. Upon dissolution in water, drug molecules *ionize* to different degrees, depending on their chemical structures. Unlike strong acids like HNO_3 or strong bases like NaOH, which ionize completely upon dissolution in water, weak acids or bases will be a mixture of an ionized species (cation or anion) and a molecular (nonionized) species in *equilibrium*. Therefore, the ionization of many drugs in the aqueous solutions of body fluids is an equilibrium process.

The acid–base theory that will work best for our purposes is that of Brønsted–Lowry:

An *acid* is a substance that can donate a proton (H^+).
A *base* is a substance that can accept a proton (H^+).

When an acid or base is dissolved in water, the following acid–base reaction takes place and equilibrium is established:
For acid HA:

$$HA + H_2O \rightleftharpoons H_3O^+ + A^- \tag{2.1}$$

For base B:

$$B: + H_2O \rightleftharpoons BH^+ + OH^- \tag{2.2}$$

The equations above indicate that water can act as either proton acceptor or donor, depending on the other reaction component. Equilibrium is established when the rate of the forward reaction equals the rate of the reverse reaction. The corresponding equilibrium constants are:
For acids:

$$K_{eq} = \frac{\left[H_3O^+\right]\left[A^-\right]}{\left[HA\right]\left[H_2O\right]} \tag{2.3}$$

For bases:

$$K_{eq} = \frac{\left[BH^+\right]\left[OH^-\right]}{\left[B\right]\left[H_2O\right]} \tag{2.4}$$

The concentration of water in any given physiological fluid is not affected by the solutes present, since they are all very dilute conditions. Water concentration remains constant at 55 M, based on a density of 1 g/mL and a molecular weight of 18 g/mole of water. Substituting this water concentration in Equation (2.1) and Equation (2.2) above yields expressions that will be more useful for our analysis of drugs in physiological fluids. The acid dissociation constant, K_a, is defined as follows:

$$K_a = 55\ K_{eq} = \frac{\left[H_3O^+\right]\left[A^-\right]}{\left[HA\right]} \tag{2.5}$$

Likewise, the base association constant, K_b, is defined as follows:

$$K_b = 55K_{eq} = \frac{\left[BH^+\right]\left[OH^-\right]}{\left[B\right]} \tag{2.6}$$

Clearly, the more that the above equilibria, as shown in Equation (2.1) and Equation (2.2), lie to the right-hand side, the larger K_a and K_b will be, the stronger the acid or base, and the more ionized they will be.

HYDROLYSIS OF SALTS

Many drugs are formulated as salts, a process that involves taking the weak acid or base and reacting it with base or acid, respectively, in order to generate an ionic compound or salt. When salts are dissolved in water, the ions dissociate completely and associate with water molecules to form *solvated* anions and cations. One common error is to confuse low solubility with low percent dissociation, but these two processes are totally different. Barium sulfate, for example, has very low water solubility, but whatever amount does dissolve is 100% ionized into Ba^{+2} and SO_4^{-2}. The same applies to many drugs formulated as salts. They may have varying degrees of water solubility, but whatever amount is dissolved in water is 100% ionized into the component ions. Indeed, the decision to formulate a drug as a salt, usually adding one more step in the manufacturing process, comes from the need to obtain greater solubility in body fluids. The salt is usually more soluble than the parent compound, although some exceptions will be discussed in a later chapter.

Another caveat to add at this point is that whether the drug is administered as a free acid or base or as its salt, dissolution in water will bring about the corresponding acid–base equilibrium. The equilibrium constant will be satisfied, regardless of whether we begin with the parent compound or one of its salts. The reaction of potassium acetylsalicylate (aspirin, potassium salt) and water is shown in Equation (2.7), abbreviating the acid as HA, the salt as KA.

$$KA + H_2O \rightleftharpoons K^+_{(hydrated)} + A^-_{(hydrated)} \qquad (2.7)$$

Once in solution, A^- will pick up H^+ (from water dissociation) to form HA. We can write this reaction as:

$$A^- + H^+ \rightleftharpoons HA \qquad (2.8)$$

But as soon as H^+ is withdrawn from the solution this way, the H_2O dissociates some more to replace that H^+. This reaction we have seen before:

$$H_2O \rightleftharpoons H^+ + OH^- \qquad K_w = \frac{\left[H^+\right]\left[OH^-\right]}{\left[H_2O\right]} \qquad (2.9)$$

Adding both these reactions gives us the net reaction for the hydrolysis of A^-:

$$A^- + H_2O \rightleftharpoons HA + OH^- \qquad (2.10)$$

This is the so-called *hydrolysis* reaction, and its equilibrium constant, commonly designated by K_h (hydrolysis constant), can be written as follows:

$$K_h = \frac{[HA][OH^-]}{[A^-]} = 55 \, K_{eq} \tag{2.11}$$

We leave out the water from the denominator because as usual its activity stays constant. Multiplying the numerator and denominator by $[H^+]$ yields a value for K_h equal to K_w/K_a.

The hydrolysis reaction above will be similar for all salts of drugs that are weak acids and have been reacted with a strong base (e.g., KOH) to form a salt. It also explains why an aqueous solution of the salt of a weak acid is slightly basic, i.e., OH^- is generated upon hydrolysis. This last point is not significant in physiological fluids since the latter are commonly buffered, so they can resist pH changes.

A similar situation arises when the salt we are considering is formed from a parent drug that is a weak base (e.g., epinephrine), and a strong acid (HCl). Let us abbreviate epinephrine as RNH_2 and its chloride salt as $RNH_3^+Cl^-$ or $RNH_2 \cdot HCl$. Upon dissolution of this salt in water there is complete ionization of the salt, as follows:

$$RNH_3^+Cl^- + H_2O \rightarrow RNH_3^+ + Cl^- \tag{2.12}$$

The Cl^- does not affect the water dissociation equilibrium (Equation 2.9), but the RNH_3^+ can because some of it can combine with OH^- to produce RNH_2 and H_2O by the reaction:

$$R - NH_3^+ + OH^- \rightleftharpoons RNH_2 + H_2O \tag{2.13}$$

Adding this reaction and the water dissociation we get the following net reaction:

$$RNH_3^+ \rightleftharpoons RNH_2 + H^+ \tag{2.14}$$

This last equation looks like a simple dissociation of a protonic acid, and this is the way we will consider the ionization equilibrium of basic drugs in physiological fluids. In this manner, we can view acids and bases on a similar framework of ionization equilibrium, a perspective that will be convenient for our purposes.

The equilibrium expression for Equation (2.14) has the form:

$$K = \frac{\left[RNH_2\right]\left[H^+\right]}{\left[RNH_3^+\right]} \tag{2.15}$$

Multiplying numerator and denominator by [OH⁻] we get:

$$K = \frac{\left[RNH_2\right]\left[H^+\right]\left[OH^-\right]}{\left[RNH_3^+\right]\left[OH^-\right]} = \frac{\left[H^+\right]\left[OH^-\right]}{\left[RNH_3^+\right]\left[OH^-\right]/\left[RNH_2\right]} = \frac{K_w}{K_b} = K_a \tag{2.16}$$

Although it would be most proper to call K the hydrolysis constant for the amine RNH_2, for the purposes of our discussion we will call it the dissociation constant (K_a) of the cationic form of the amine, or RNH_3^+.

Equation (2.16) expresses the inverse relationship between the base strength (K_b) of the parent compound and the acid strength of its protonated, cationic form:

A strong base (large K_b) has a protonated, cationic form that is a weak acid (low K_a).

A weak base (small K_b) has a protonated, cationic form that is a strong acid (high K_a).

CONJUGATE ACIDS AND CONJUGATE BASES

The two acids and two bases involved in a Brønsted–Lowry equilibrium situation can be grouped into two conjugate acid–base pairs. A *conjugate acid–base pair* is two species that differ from each other only by one proton. The two conjugate acid–base pairs in Equation (2.1) and Equation (2.2) above are shown in Figure 2.1.

The *conjugate base* of an acid is the species that remains when an acid loses a proton. It is abbreviated CB. The *conjugate acid* of a base is the species formed when the base accepts a proton. It is abbreviated CA.

Exercise 2.1

Write the equation for the ionization of acetic acid (CH_3COOH) in water and identify the corresponding conjugate acid–base pairs.

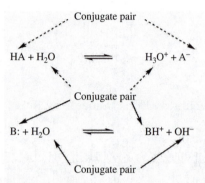

Figure 2.1

Answer: The reaction of acetic acid in water is described in Equation (2.17). Note that only the hydrogen on the carboxyl group can be donated, i.e., the hydrogens on the methyl (CH_3) group are not "acidic."

$$CH_3COOH + H_2O \rightleftharpoons CH_3COO^- + H_3O^+ \qquad (2.17)$$

The two conjugate acid–base pairs in this reaction are as follows:

1. CH_3COOH **(CA)** / CH_3COO^- **(CB)**
2. H_3O^+ **(CA)** / H_2O **(CB)**

One must draw upon knowledge of general and organic chemistry to determine which functional groups in drug molecules can take part in an acid–base reaction. The easiest functional groups to recall as acidic are the carboxyl groups and as basic functional groups are the amines. Sometimes, however, NH groups can be acidic, as in phenytoin. This special nitrogen functional group is called "imide" (Table 1.1 in Chapter 1).

Exercise 2.2

Write the equation for the ionization of phenytoin in water and identify the corresponding conjugate acid–base pairs.

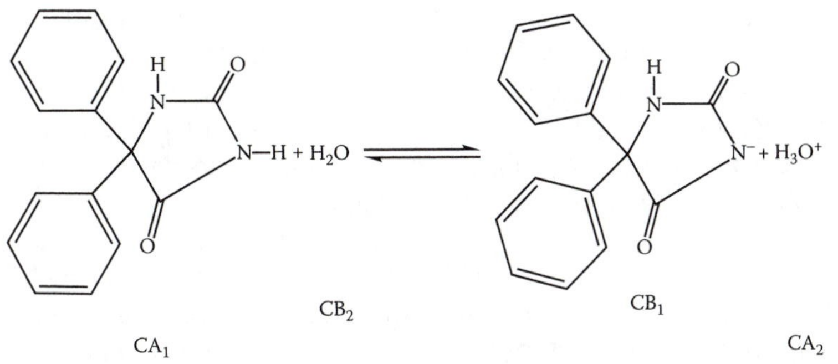

Figure 2.2

Answer: The NH groups in phenytoin are acidic because they are adjacent to two strongly electron-withdrawing carbonyl groups. One of the NH groups is subject to electron-withdrawing effects of two carbonyls, while the other is under the influence of only one carbonyl group. The reaction of phenytoin in water is described in Figure 2.2.

The two conjugate pairs are CA_1/CB_1 and CA_2/CB_2, as shown in the figure.

Exercise 2.3

Write the equation for the ionization of ephedrine hydrochloride in water and identify the corresponding conjugate acid–base pairs. (See Figure 2.3.)

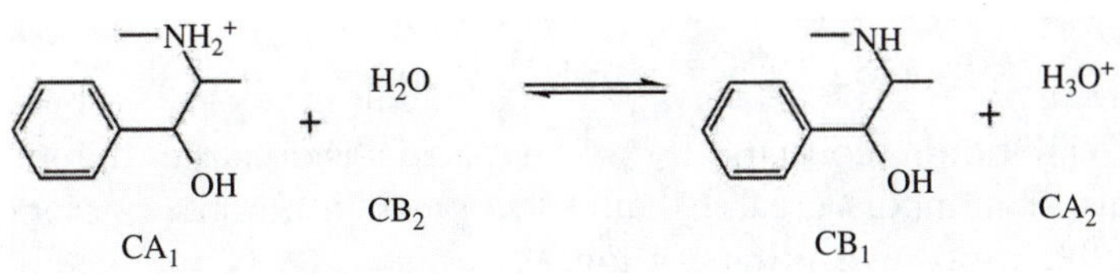

Figure 2.3

STRENGTH OF ACIDS AND BASES

Brønsted–Lowry acids vary in their ability to transfer a proton to water upon dissolution, i.e., they vary in their ability to "ionize" in aqueous solutions.

A *strong acid* is one that can transfer 100% or close to 100% of its acidic hydrogen atoms to water upon dissolution. This process generates many hydronium (H_3O^+) ions in solution, and the equilibrium in Equation (2.1) lies far to the right. The actual concentration of unionized species HA present in solution may be so small that it cannot be measured, and the resulting K_a (Equation 2.5) is very large.

A *weak acid* is one that transfers only a small portion of its acidic hydrogen atoms to water upon dissolution. The amount of hydronium ions thus generated is much less than in the case of strong acids. The actual percentage of proton transfer for weak acids depends on the molecular structure, the molecular polarity, and the strength and polarity of individual bonds in the molecule. A weak acid generates a small amount of hydronium ions, and the equilibrium in Equation (2.1) is far to the left, toward the nonionized species HA. The resulting K_a is small number.

$$HA + H_2O \rightleftharpoons H_3O^+ + A^- \tag{2.1}$$

$$K_a = 55\ K_{eq} = \frac{\left[H_3O^+\right]\left[A^-\right]}{\left[HA\right]} \tag{2.5}$$

When comparing two acids for their relative strength it is usually the magnitude of the difference (as a power of 10) in their K_a that is most informative. For example, if acid A_1 has a K_a of 5.1×10^5 and acid A_2 has a K_a of 3.4×10^2, we can say that acid A_1 is approximately 1000 times stronger than acid A_2. This approximation is all we need in many cases. It is also more convenient for our purposes to use the logarithm of K_a rather than K_a itself when comparing acid strengths.

The logarithm of a number is the exponent to which 10 is raised to generate the number:

$$\log 10^x = x \quad \text{and} \quad \log 10^{-x} = -x$$

The equilibrium constant for strong acids is a large number, and logarithms of numbers greater than 1 are positive numbers. Strong acids therefore have positive values of log K_a.

Weak acids, on the other hands, such as many drug molecules, have K_a values in the range between 0 and 1. Logarithms of K_a values in this range are negative numbers.

For example, if acid HA_1 donates 1 in 1000 of its acidic hydrogen atoms to water, its K_a will be 1×10^{-3}, and the log K_a will equal -3. An even weaker acid may donate only one in a million of its acidic hydrogen atoms to water; its K_a will be 1×10^{-6} and its log K_a will equal -6. Scientists have found it more convenient to compare different acids' strengths in terms of positive numbers, and therefore the $-\log K_a$ that is used. In analogy with pH, which is the $-\log[H^+]$, the $-\log K_a$ is called the pK_a of the acid. A small pK_a means a large K_a (strong acid), just as a small pH means a large $[H^+]$. In the example of the two acids above, the pK_a values will be 3 and 6 respectively, and the acid with the smaller pK_a of 3 is stronger than the acid with the larger pK_a of 6.

Many published tables in the literature list the pK_a values of acids as a means of comparing their relative strength. Table 2.1 gives some examples of strong acids (large K_a, small pK_a) and weak acids (small K_a, large pK_a).

Just as there are strong acids and weak acids, there are also strong bases and weak bases. Strong bases are limited to the hydroxides of group IA and IIA in the Periodic Table. Weak bases include many of the drug molecules that possess an amine functional group: RNH_2. When comparing two bases, the one with a smaller pK_b is the stronger of the two. We will not, however, find many tables published with pK_b values to compare base strengths. Instead, scientists have found it more convenient to compare relative acid strengths for all proton-donating species, HA for acids and BH^+ for bases. We will use four common drugs to illustrate — the weak acids aspirin and acetaminophen and the weak bases amphetamine and diazepam (Figure 2.4).

Table 2.1 Relative Strength of Selected Acids

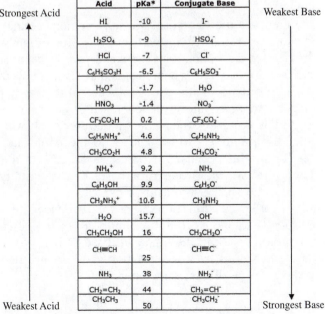

	Acid	pKa*	Conjugate Base	
Strongest Acid	HI	-10	I-	Weakest Base
	H_2SO_4	-9	HSO_4^-	
	HCl	-7	Cl-	
	$C_6H_5SO_3H$	-6.5	$C_6H_5SO_3^-$	
	H_3O^+	-1.7	H_2O	
	HNO_3	-1.4	NO_3^-	
	CF_3CO_2H	0.2	$CF_3CO_2^-$	
	$C_6H_5NH_3^+$	4.6	$C_6H_5NH_2$	
	CH_3CO_2H	4.8	$CH_3CO_2^-$	
	NH_4^+	9.2	NH_3	
	C_6H_5OH	9.9	$C_6H_5O^-$	
	$CH_3NH_3^+$	10.6	CH_3NH_2	
	H_2O	15.7	OH-	
	CH_3CH_2OH	16	$CH_3CH_2O^-$	
	CH≡CH	25	CH≡C-	
	NH_3	38	NH_2^-	
	$CH_2=CH_2$	44	$CH_2=CH^-$	
Weakest Acid	CH_3CH_3	50	$CH_3CH_2^-$	Strongest Base

* Approximate Values

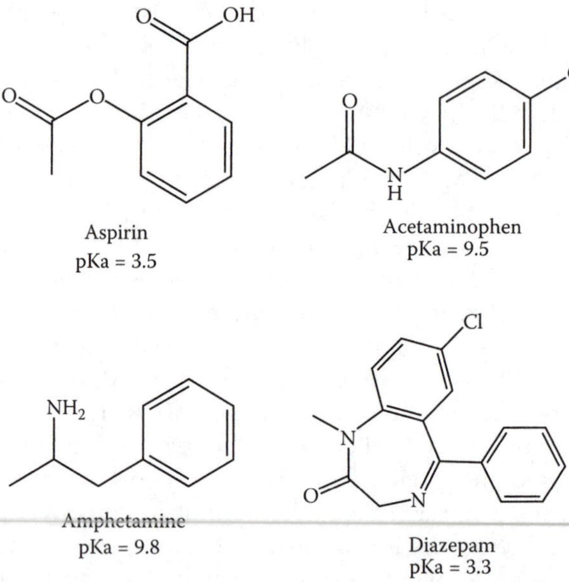

Figure 2.4

The comparison of aspirin and acetaminophen is straightforward, as explained before; aspirin, with the smaller pK_a, is a stronger acid than acetaminophen.

In order to compare the two bases we must remember that it is their conjugate acids that we are dealing with when we use their pK_a values. The conjugate acid of diazepam, with the small pK_a, is stronger than the conjugate acid of amphetamine, which means that diazepam is the weaker base of the two. In order to make a judicious use of the many pK_a tables in the literature, one must know the chemical structure of the acidic species listed, and by inspecting the nature of the functional groups present decide whether the pK_a refers to an acid or to the conjugate acid of a base. We must know this because for bases, as we saw in the example above, the larger the pK_a, the stronger the base. This is contrary to acids; the larger the pK_a, the weaker the acid.

In summary, for calculation purposes, we can view all acid–base reactions in aqueous solutions from the standpoint of the conjugate acid form losing a proton to form the conjugate base. When we do this we can always use pK_a values in our calculations and do not need to deal with K_b or pK_b values at all. Just remember:

- For acids: the stronger the acid, the smaller the pK_a.
- For bases: the stronger the base, the larger the pK_a.

RESONANCE AND INDUCTIVE EFFECTS

Functional groups in drug molecules can affect the ionization equilibrium, i.e., can make an acid a stronger or a weaker acid. These electronic effects of functional groups are classified as resonance and inductive effects and represent the contribution that resonance stabilization and electronegativity have on ionization.

INDUCTIVE EFFECTS

The C-C bond in ethane (CH_3–CH_3) has no polarity because it involves two equivalent carbon atoms. However, the C–C bond in chloroethane (Cl–CH_2–CH_3) is polarized by the presence of the electronegative chlorine atom. This polarization is the sum of two effects: first, the Cl atom (electronegativity of 3.0) takes some of the electron density of the carbon atom (electronegativity of 2.5) it is attached to, i.e., it polarizes that covalent bond so that the electrons spend more time close to the Cl atom than to the C atom. The carbon attached to chlorine then compensates this withdrawal of electron density by drawing the electrons from the C–C bond closer to itself. This results in the polarization of the C–C bond.

> *Inductive effect* is the polarization of one bond caused by the polarization of an adjacent bond.

The effect is greatest for adjacent bonds, but can also be felt farther away.

The inductive effect of a substituent in a drug molecule makes it a stronger or weaker acid (relative to the unsubstituted acid), depending on whether the substituent is electron-donating or electron-attracting relative to hydrogen. Polarization of bonds is an effect through space; therefore, it decreases in strength the larger the distance from the acidic group.

Functional groups can be classified as electron-withdrawing (–I) or electron-donating (+I) relative to hydrogen. A nitro group (NO_2, –I), for example, will draw electrons to itself more than a hydrogen atom would if occupying the same position in the drug molecule. Table 2.2 shows functional groups commonly found in drug molecules that can have –I or +I effects.

Exercise 2.4

Nitroacetic acid is stronger than acetic acid. The pK_a values are 4.76 and 1.68. Assign the pK_a to each acid and explain your choice.

Table 2.2 Inductive Effect of Functional Groups

+I Groups		-I Groups		
$-CH_3$		$-NO_2$	$-NH_3^+$	$-NR_3^+$
$-CH_2R$		$-C{\equiv}N$	$\overset{\displaystyle O}{\underset{\displaystyle \parallel}{-C}}-H$	$\overset{\displaystyle O}{\underset{\displaystyle \parallel}{-C}}-R$
$-CHR_2$		$\overset{\displaystyle O}{\underset{\displaystyle \parallel}{-C}}-OH$	$-SR$	$-SH$
$-CR_3$		$\overset{\displaystyle O}{\underset{\displaystyle \parallel}{-C}}-OR$	$-OR$	$-OH$
		$\overset{\displaystyle O}{\underset{\displaystyle \parallel}{-C}}-NH_2$	$-F\ ,\ Cl-$	$-Br\ ,\ I-$
$-C\underset{O^-}{\overset{O}{\diagup}}$		$-\overset{O\ \ O}{\underset{R}{S}}$	$-HC{=}CH_2$	$-C{\equiv}CH$

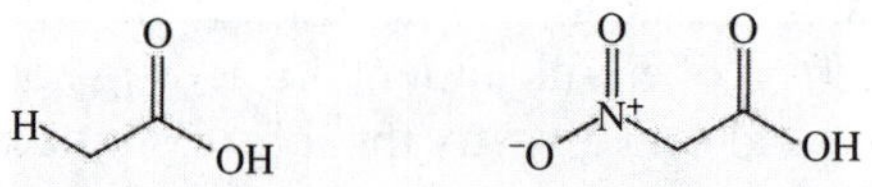

Acetic acid	Nitroacetic acid
pKa = 4.76	pKa = 1.68

Figure 2.5

The smaller pK_a belongs to the stronger acid, i.e., nitroacetic acid (see Figure 2.5.) The only difference in the structure of these two molecules is the substitution of NO_2 for H. The NO_2 group is a strong electron-withdrawing, –I group. It withdraws electron density from the carboxyl group, but the withdrawal is more effective in the carboxylate (CB) form of the acid than in its protonated CA form. Spreading the negative charge has a stabilizing effect, and the equilibrium favors the greater thermodynamic stability of the CB form. The nitro substitution then increases the acidity of the parent compound by displacing the ionization equilibrium toward formation of the stabilized anionic form (CB).

–I groups increase the acidity of uncharged acids such as acetic acid because these groups spread the negative charge of the anion. However, –I groups increase the acidity of any acid, no matter what the charge. For example, if the acid has a charge of +1, as in $RNH_3^+Cl^-$, a –I group destabilizes the positive center by increasing and concentrating the positive charge of the acid. This destabilization is relieved when the proton is lost; therefore, the neutral, deprotonated CB form of the acid is favored, and the ionization equilibrium shifts toward it. A –I group substitution in $RNH_3^+Cl^-$ makes the parent amine a weaker base. In general we may say that:

■ Functional groups that withdraw electrons by the inductive effect (–I) increase acidity and decrease basicity.
■ Functional groups that donate electrons by the inductive effect (+I) decrease acidity and increase basicity.

RESONANCE EFFECTS

Resonance or conjugative effects result from the high mobility of π-electrons and their delocalization in a system of conjugated double bonds. Functional groups that increase the electron density of conjugated systems are called +R (electron-donating), and those that decrease electron density are called –R (electron-withdrawing). An example of resonance effects is found in the higher acidity of carboxylic acids compared to primary alcohols.

Carboxylic Acid   2 Resonance Structures

$$(2.18)$$

$$RCH_2OH \rightleftharpoons RCH_2O^- + H^+ \qquad (2.19)$$

The carboxylate anion ($RCOO^-$) is stabilized by resonance not available to the RCH_2O^- ion or to RCOOH. The $RCOO^-$ ion is stabilized not only by the existence of two resonance structures but also by the fact that the negative charge is spread over two oxygen atoms, rather than concentrated on a single oxygen atom as in RCH_2O^-. Table 2.3 shows functional groups commonly found in drug molecules that can have –R or +R effects.

Exercise 2.5

Assign pK_a values to each nitrogen atom (1 and 2) in the drug shown in Figure 2.6: pK_a = 8.1 and pK_a = 2.0.

Table 2.3 Resonance Effect of Functional Groups

+R, +I Groups	-R, -I Groups	+R, -I Groups
—O⁻	—NO$_2$	—F
—S⁻	—C≡N	—Cl
	$-\overset{\overset{\displaystyle O}{\|\|}}{C}-OH$	—Br
	$-\overset{\overset{\displaystyle O}{\|\|}}{C}-OR$	—I
	$-\overset{\overset{\displaystyle O}{\|\|}}{C}-NH_2$	—NH$_2$
	$-\overset{\overset{\displaystyle O}{\|\|}}{C}-H$	—NR$_2$
	$-\overset{\overset{\displaystyle O}{\|\|}}{C}-R$	—SH
	—CF$_3$	—SR
	$-\overset{\overset{\displaystyle O\diagdown\|\diagup O}{}}{S}-R$	$-HN-\overset{\overset{\displaystyle O}{\|\|}}{C}\diagdown R$
		—OH
		—OR
		$-O-\overset{\overset{\displaystyle O}{\|\|}}{C}\diagdown R$

The non-bonding electron pair on nitrogen 1 can be less readily donated to a proton than the non-bonding electron pair on nitrogen 2, due to resonance into aromatic ring. This makes nitrogen (N1) less basic (does not want to get protonated), and displaces the equilibrium toward the deprotonated form. What makes the base weaker makes its conjugate acid stronger: the stronger acid wants to dissociate more fully; this happens with the CA of nitrogen 1. Therefore, the stronger the acid, the smaller the pK_a; CA of nitrogen 1 has pK_a of 2.0. If you see it as a base, then remember that the stronger the base, the larger the pK_a, and for this reason, nitrogen 2 has the pK_a of 8.1.

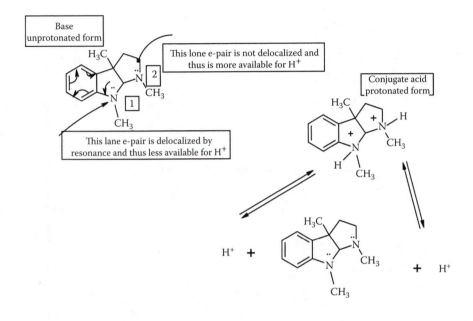

Figure 2.6

Exercise 2.6

Rank the acids in Figure 2.7 from strongest to weakest.

To compare relative acidities, consider the number and types of inductive and resonance effects present.

- **C** is the strongest acid because it has two electron pullers (–I, –R) that stabilize the anion.
- **A** follows because it has one electron puller (–I).
- **B** follows because it has one electron puller (–I), whose effect is slightly counteracted by the +I group (e- pusher).
- **D** is last because it has only an electron pusher (+I), which destabilizes the anion.

The order of acidity, from strongest to weakest, is C > A > B > D.

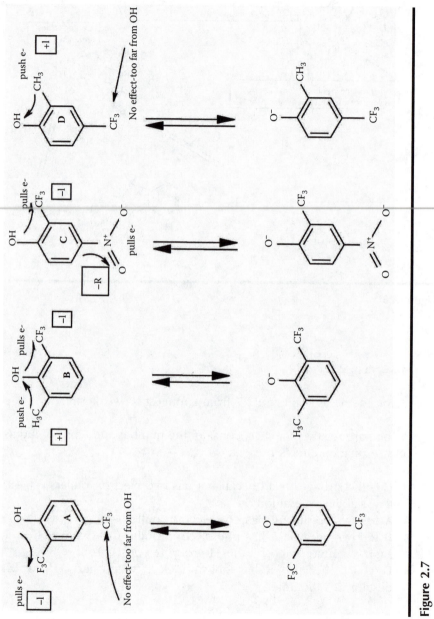

Figure 2.7

THE HENDERSON–HASSELBACH EQUATION

The use of conjugate acid/conjugate base terminology is expedient for the purpose of deriving a most useful equation in pharmacology: the Henderson–Hasselbach equation.

A brief review of math principles regarding logarithms is in order. The logarithm of the product of two numbers equals the sum of the logarithm of each number:

$$Log\ (a)*(b) = \log a + \log b$$

The logarithm of the quotient of two numbers equals the logarithm of the numerator minus the logarithm of the denominator:

$$Log\ (a)/(b) = \log a - \log b$$

Therefore:

$$Log\ (a)(b)/(c) = \log a + \log b - \log c$$

Consider the general acid–base reaction in aqueous solution:

$$CA \rightleftharpoons H^+ + CB \tag{2.20}$$

where CA is the *acidic form* or *protonated form* of any given drug, and CB is the *basic form* or *deprotonated form*.

The pertinent equilibrium expression for the above reaction is:

$$K_a = \frac{\left[H^+\right]\left[CB\right]}{\left[CA\right]} \tag{2.21}$$

Taking the logarithm on both sides of the equation we obtain:

$$Log\ K_a = \log [H^+][CB]\ /\ [CA]$$

or

$$Log\ K_a = \log [H^+] + \log [CB] - \log [CA]$$

Multiplying both sides of the equation by −1 we obtain:

$$-\log Ka = -\log [H^+] - \log [CB] + \log [CA]$$

Substituting "−log" by its equivalent, "p":

$$pK_a = pH + \log [CA] - \log [CB]$$

And finally, combining logarithm parts of this equation we obtain the Henderson–Hasselbach equation:

$$pK_a = pH + \log \frac{[CA]}{[CB]} \qquad (2.22)$$

This equation can be used substituting equivalent terms for CA and/or CB, protonated/deprotonated form, and ionized/deionized forms. For example, another useful way of expressing the Henderson–Hasselbach equation is as follows:

For acids and bases:

$$pK_a = pH + \log \frac{[\text{Protonated Form}]}{[\text{Deprotonated Form}]} \qquad (2.23)$$

For acids:

$$pK_a = pH + \log \frac{[\text{Unionized Form}]}{[\text{Ionized Form}]} \qquad (2.24)$$

For bases:

$$pK_a = pH + \log \frac{[\text{Ionized Form}]}{[\text{Unionized Form}]} \qquad (2.25)$$

Please note the terms used here and understand which of them are equivalent for acid–base reactions in aqueous solutions:

CA = acidic form = protonated form = ionized form (if drug is a base that acquired a proton, BH^+)
CA = acidic form = protonated form = unionized form (if drug is an acid that has not yet donated its proton, HA)
CB = basic form = deprotonated form = ionized form (if drug is an acid that donated its proton, A^-)
CB = basic form = deprotonated form = unionized form (if drug is a base that has not yet accepted a proton, B)

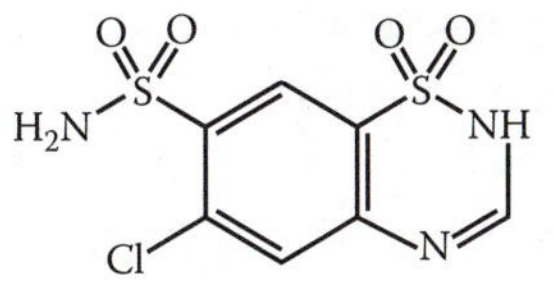

Chlorthiazide 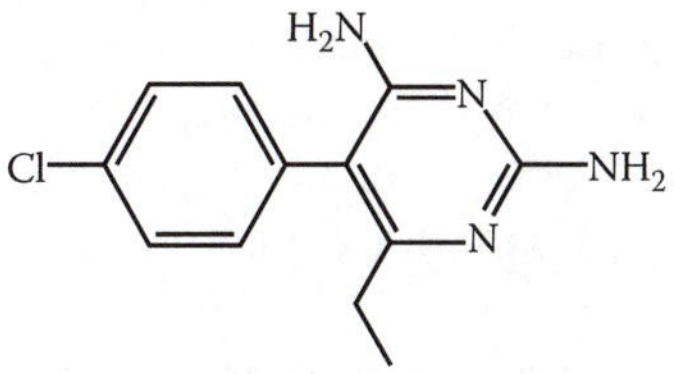   Pyrimethamine

Figure 2.8

In summary, while CA is always the protonated form and CB is always the deprotonated form, whether CA or CB will be an ionized or unionized species will depend on whether the original drug molecule was an acid or a base. You need to know which functional groups in drug molecules confer acidity or basicity, i.e., which functional groups in a molecule are *ionizable*.

Exercise 2.7

Write the reaction and equilibrium expression for the ionization of chlorthiazide and pyrimethamine in water.

Answer: The structures for these drugs (shown in Figure 2.8) can be found in a number of places, two of which are the Physician's Desk Reference (PDR) and chemfinder.com (http://chemfinder.cambridgesoft.com/).

Chlorthiazide has two "ionizable" functional groups; both the NH and the NH_2 next to the SO_2 groups are ionizable. Hydrogens on these nitrogen atoms are acidic, in contrast with the hydrogens on both NH_2 groups in pyrimethamine. Chlorthiazide is an acid and pyrimethamine is a base, even though both reactive centers are NH or NH_2 groups. The difference in reactivity lies in the effect of neighboring groups on the availability of nitrogen's nonbonding electron pair to accept a proton. Sulfonamides are most frequently acidic because the SO_2 has a strong –R and –I effect on the NH neighbor. Aromatic amines like pyrimethamine are weakly basic because the phenyl group has a moderate –R effect on any neighboring NH_2 group, but this effect is not yet so strong as to prevent involvement of nitrogen's nonbonding electron pair to accept a proton. Another aspect worth discussing at this point is relative ionizability within different possible reactive centers. Only one NH_2 group in pyrimethamine is basic enough to react with water; that is the one not in between the two ring nitrogens. The NH_2 next to the two ring nitrogens has its nonbonding electrons tied up in resonance delocalization with these two electronegative atoms. The other NH_2 group interacts with only one ring nitrogen and therefore can still donate its nonbonding electrons to a proton.

The pK_a values reported in the literature for chlorthiazide are 6.8 and 9.4; we will use the first one, 6.8, which corresponds to the most acidic hydrogen in the molecule, as shown below:

CA Form H_2O CB Form $+$ H^+ (2.26)

Protonated Form   Deprotonated Form

Chlorthiazide is an Acid

Unionized Form   Ionized Form

This reaction describes the ionization of chlorthiazide in water. The corresponding equilibrium expression, using Chlor-NH as an abbreviation for the CA form and Chlor-N⁻ for the CB form, is

$$K_a = \frac{\left[H^+\right]\left[\text{Chlor-N}^-\right]}{\left[\text{Chlor-NH}\right]} \tag{2.27}$$

In the case of pyrimethamine, which is a base, we will use the dissociation of its acidic form to describe the behavior of this drug in water, as shown in Figure 2.9. The corresponding equilibrium expression for this reaction is:

$$K_a = \frac{\left[H^+\right]\left[\text{PyrimNH}_2\right]}{\left[\text{PyrimNH}_3^+\right]} \tag{2.28}$$

The antimalarial drug pyrimethamine can be used to illustrate the effect of the ionization processes we have been discussing on the distribution of drugs among different compartments in the body. The urine typically has a pH of 6.0 while the blood has a pH of 7.4. The distribution of pyrimethamine between urine and blood is illustrated in Figure 2.10.

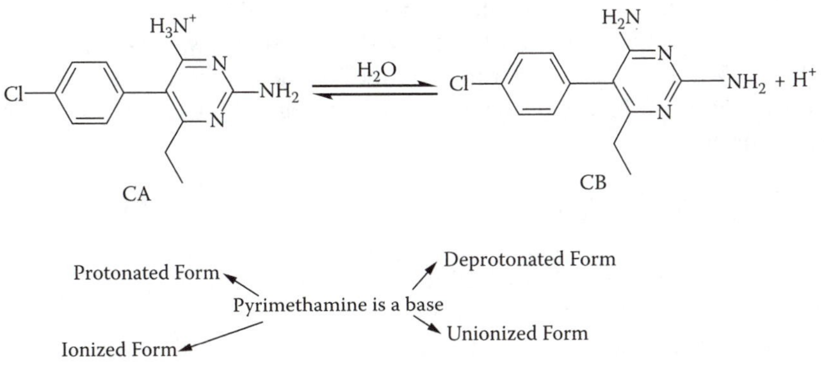

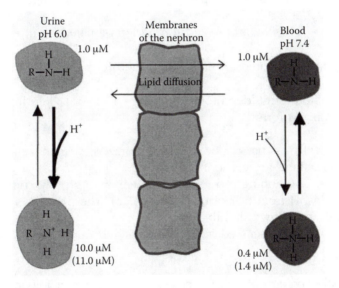

Figure 2.9

Figure 2.10 Effect of pyrimetamine's pK_a and compartment pH on drug distribution and excretion.

Figure 2.10 shows a hypothetical equilibration of pyrimethamine across the renal tubule (nephron), with a concentration of 1 μM. The acid–base equilibrium for this drug (Figure 2.9; Equation 2.28) will be established on both sides of the membrane. A weak base like pyrimethamine (pK_a = 7.0) is trapped in the urine because at a pH of 6 (lower than its pK_a), the protonated, ionized form predominates, and the total concentration of both species is higher in the urine (11.0 μM) than in the blood (1.4 μM). Therefore, if the goal is to enhance the excretion of pyrimethamine, one would administer a urine acidifier, since lowering the pH in the urine will shift even further the equilibrium toward the ionized, water-soluble form of the drug. In the case of pyrimethamine, using the concentration values given in Figure 2.10 for the Henderson–Hasselbach equation, we obtain (in the urine):

$$pK_a = 6 + \log[\text{protonated form}]/[\text{deprotonated form}] = 7.0$$

$$\log[\text{protonated form}]/[\text{deprotonated form}] = 1.0$$

$$[\text{protonated form}]/[\text{deprotonated form}] = 10 = [\text{ionized form}]/[\text{unionized form}]$$

This result tells us that for every one unionized pyrimethamine species in the urine, there are 10 ionized species. A similar process for the equilibrium in the blood compartment yields the following:

$$pK_a = 7.4 + \log[\text{protonated form}]/[\text{deprotonated form}] = 7.0$$

$$\log[\text{protonated form}]/[\text{deprotonated form}] = 7.0 - 7.4$$

$$[\text{protonated form}]/[\text{deprotonated form}] = 10^{-0.4} = 0.398 = [\text{ionized form}]/[\text{unionized form}]$$

This result tells us that for every one unionized pyrimethamine species in the urine, there are 0.4 ionized species.

A similar partitioning process takes place among body compartments that differ in pH from that of the blood (~7.4). The pH values of various body fluids are shown in Table 2.4.

The principles discussed above for pyrimethamine apply to all weak bases:

Renal excretion of a weak base is enhanced by acidifying the urine.

On the other hand, the opposite is true of weak acids:

Renal excretion of a weak acid is enhanced by basifying the urine.

These statements are easily understood by a mathematical examination of the Henderson–Hasselbach equation, coupled with an understanding of the acid–base properties of any given drug under consideration.

Table 2.4 pH Values of Several Body Fluids

Body Fluid	pH
Blood	7.4
Duodenum	5.5
Ileum	8.0
Saliva	6.4
Semen	7.2
Stomach	1.5
Urine	5.8
Premenopause Vagina	4.5
Postmenopause Vagina	7.0

One of the most important applications of the Henderson-Hasselbach equation is the manipulation of drug excretion by the kidney. Virtually all drugs are filtered at the glomerulus, and if the drug is present mainly in the lipid-soluble nonionized form when it passes by the renal tubule, a significant fraction will be reabsorbed by passive diffusion. If the goal is to enhance excretion of the drug, one must prevent its reabsorption from the renal tubules.

A list of common drugs that are weak acids or weak bases is given in Table 2.5.

In a later chapter we will discuss at greater length the effect of pK_a and compartment pH on the distribution and excretion of drugs.

Table 2.5   pKa Values for Selected Drugs

Weak Acids	pKa	Weak Bases	pKa
Amoxicillin	2.4	Alprenolol	9.6
Acetazolamide	7.2	Allopurinol	9.4, 12.3
Ampicillin	2.5	Amphetamine	9.8
Aspirin	3.5	Atropine	9.7
Chlorothiazide	6.8, 9.4*	Chlorpheniramine	9.2
Ciprofloxacin	6.1, 8.7*	Cocaine	8.5
Cephalexin	3.6	Codeine	8.2
Ethacrynic acid	2.5	Diazepam	3.0
Furosemide	3.9	Diphenhydramine	8.8
Ibuprofen	4.4, 5.2*	Amoxicillin	7.4
Levodopa	2.3	Ephedrine	9.6
Methotrexate	4.8	Epinephrine	8.7
Methyldopa	2.2, 9.2*	Imipramine	9.5
Penicillamine	1.8	Lidocaine	7.9
Pentobarbital	8.1	Methadone	8.4
Phenobarbital	7.4	Methamphetamine	10.0
Phenytoin	8.3	Methyldopa	10.6
Propylthiouracil	8.3	Metoprolol	9.8
Salicylic acid	3.0	Morphine	7.9
Sulfadiazine	6.5	Nicotine	7.9, 3.1*
Sulfapyridine	8.4	Norepinephrine	8.6
Theophylline	8.8	Phenylephrine	9.8
Tolbutamide	5.3	Pilocarpine	6.9, 1.4*
Warfarin	5.0	Pseudoephedrine	9.8
* denotes more than one ionizable group			

FURTHER READING

1. *Organic Chemistry* by T. W. Graham Solomons, Craig B. Fryhle. Chapter 3. Wiley; 8th Edition (2003).
2. *Review of Organic Functional Groups: Introduction to Medicinal Organic Chemistry* by Thomas L. Lemke. Appendix B. Lippincott Williams & Wilkins; 4th Edition (2003).
3. *Wilson and Gisvold's Textbook of Organic Medicinal and Pharmaceutical Chemistry* by John H. Block (Editor), John M. Beale, Jr. Chapter 2. Lippincott Williams & Wilkins; 11th Edition (2004).

3

STRUCTURAL DETERMINANTS OF DRUG ACTION

STRUCTURALLY NONSPECIFIC DRUGS

We label drugs as structurally nonspecific when there is no direct correlation between their chemical structure and their pharmacological action. Correlation does exist with their physicochemical properties, such as redox potential, solubility, and partition coefficient.

Three common features of structurally nonspecific drugs are:

1. They have vastly different chemical classes but share similar biological responses.
2. They are needed in relatively high concentrations to effect pharmacological action. This translates into high doses.
3. Within any given chemical class, small structural changes do not result in large changes in biological action.

Among the older antibacterial drugs shown in Figure 3.1, the diversity of chemical structures with bactericidal activity can be noted. Bactericidal concentrations for all these compounds are high, and for this reason they have been replaced with more effective antibacterial drugs.

Gastric antacids can also be considered structurally nonspecific drugs. Their activity on gastric acid is strictly a neutralization reaction, and various compounds of magnesium, calcium, sodium, and aluminum can be used for the same purpose. Their structural diversity is shown in Figure 3.2.

VOLATILE ANESTHETICS

The volatile (inhalation) anesthetics are an important class of drugs that can be considered structurally nonspecific. Although some effects of these

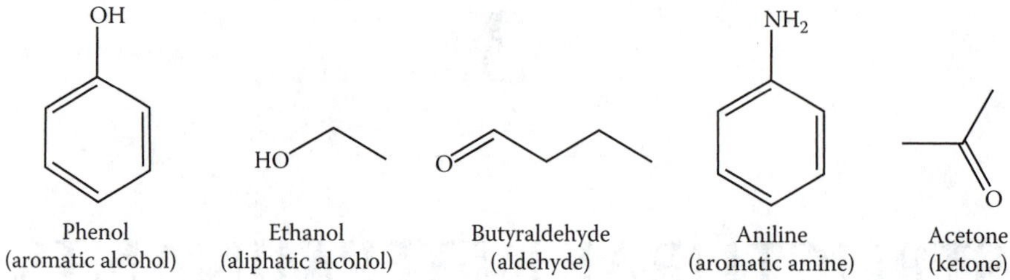

Figure 3.1 Different chemical classes with bactericidal activity.

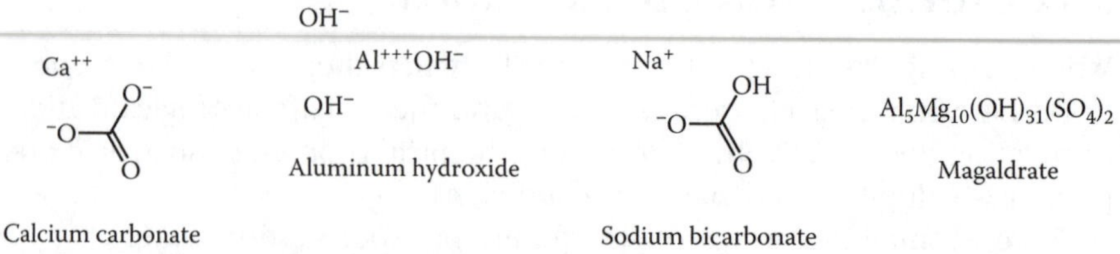

Phenol (aromatic alcohol)   Ethanol (aliphatic alcohol)   Butyraldehyde (aldehyde)   Aniline (aromatic amine)   Acetone (ketone)

Figure 3.2 Chemical structures of gastric antacids.

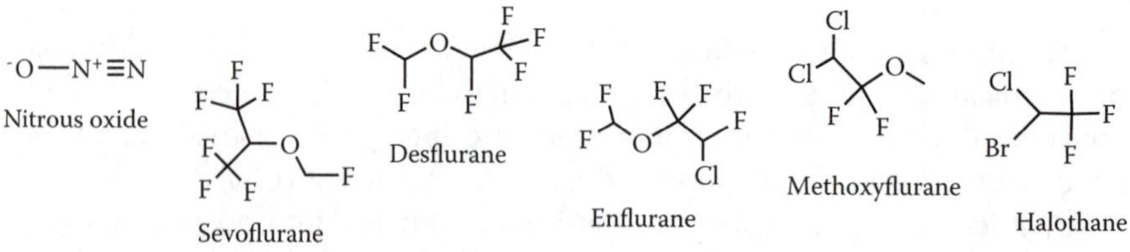

Calcium carbonate   Aluminum hydroxide   Sodium bicarbonate   Magaldrate $Al_5Mg_{10}(OH)_{31}(SO_4)_2$

Figure 3.3 Chemical structures of general anesthetics.

Nitrous oxide   Sevoflurane   Desflurane   Enflurane   Methoxyflurane   Halothane

drugs have recently been explained by interaction with GABA (γ-aminobutyric acid) receptors, at the high concentrations required for anesthesia they most likely disrupt nerve transmission through nonspecific interactions with synaptic membranes and their associated proteins. The structures of some of the volatile anesthetics are shown in Figure 3.3.

Again we note a variety of chemical structures, with similar biological actions.

The *lipid theory* developed by Meyer and Overton states that there is a direct correlation between the lipid solubility of an anesthetic agent and its anesthetic potency. A key parameter that measures the lipid solubility of an agent is its *n*-octanol/water partition coefficient (P). The n-octanol/water system resembles the constituents of the lipid bilayer in cell membranes.

$$P = \frac{(\text{Drug})_{n\text{-octanol}}}{(\text{Drug})_{water}} \tag{3.1}$$

A drug that is highly lipophilic will dissolve much more in *n*-octanol than in water, and the corresponding value of P will be high. The direct correlation between P and the minimal alveolar concentration (MAC) required for anesthesia can be seen in Table 3.1.

Table 3.1   Partition Coefficient and Anesthetic Potency

Volatile Anesthetic	MAC (%)	Partition Coefficient
Halothane	0.8	51
Enflurane	1.6	36
Sevoflurane	2.0	48
Desflurane	6.0	27
Nitrous Oxide	105.0	2.3

Although no complete agreement as to their mechanism of action exists, it is generally accepted that volatile anesthetics dissolve in the membrane lipids, forcing them into a disorganized fluid state (see Figure 3.4) that distorts ion channels. The net result is lack of synaptic transmission and loss of somatic sensation.

STRUCTURALLY SPECIFIC DRUGS

A major proportion of available drugs on the market fall into the category of structurally specific drugs. These are drugs for which specific structural features are required for biological action. The structural requirement is due to their interaction with specific "receptors." The drug molecule is said to be "complementary" in shape to its "receptor," which can be a

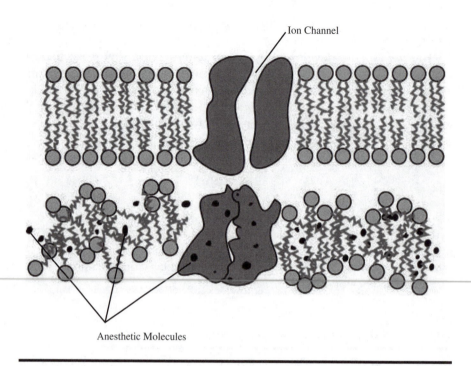

Ion Channel

Anesthetic Molecules

Figure 3.4 Effect of a general anesthetic on a lipoprotein membrane.

protein or nucleic acid. In many cases the structural requirement is so stringent that only one stereochemical isomer can bind to the receptor.

There are four different types of isomers:

1. Positional (e.g., pentobarbital, amobarbital)
2. Geometric [e.g., *cis* and *trans*-diethylstilbestrol (DES)]
3. Enantiomers (e.g., R(–) and S(+) epinephrine)
4. Diastereomers (two or more chiral centers, e.g., ephedrine)

Positional isomers are compounds of the same molecular formula that differ only in the position of a functional group in the drug molecule. Amobarbital and pentobarbital are positional isomers, differing only in the position of a $-CH_3$ group. Even this small change has an effect on biological action. See Figure 3.5.

Geometric isomers are compounds of the same molecular formula that differ only in the arrangement of functional groups around a double bond or a ring. They are also called configurational isomers since the difference is only in the arrangement (configuration) of certain groups in space. An example of the influence of this type of isomerism in biological activity can be seen with *cis*- and *trans*-diethylstilbestrol (DES). See Figure 3.6.

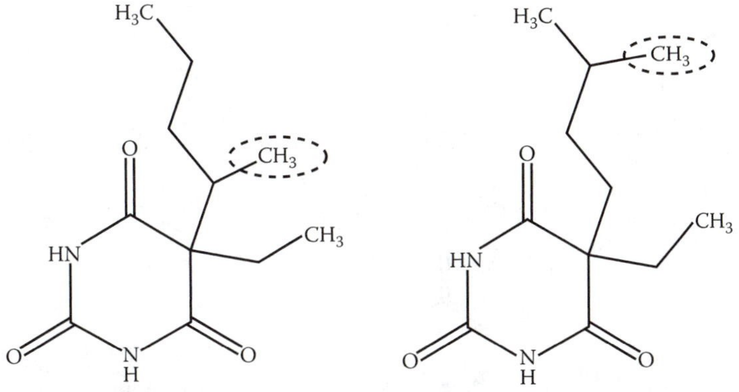

Figure 3.5 Positional isomers and biological activity.

Comparing the structures of *trans-* and *cis*-DES with that of estradiol makes it obvious that the *trans* isomer has a greater resemblance to the natural ligand of the estrogen receptor; therefore, it possesses greater estrogenic activity.

Another important type of isomerism arises when compounds of the same molecular formula differ in that they are mirror images of one another. Many things around us lack reflection symmetry (for example, our hands or a pair of shoes); they cannot be superimposed on one another. We call this phenomenon "chirality," and in the case of carbon compounds (and drugs) we recognize it by the presence of one or more (usually carbon) atoms, each of which forms noncoplanar bonds to *four different atoms or groups.* If a drug molecule has only one *chiral center,* then the only type of optical isomers possible is "enantiomers." An enantiomeric pair of isomers consists of two molecules that are nonidentical mirror images and differ only in the direction in which they rotate the angle of polarized light. When there are two or more chiral centers, other types of optical isomers are possible for drug molecules — "diastereomers." See Figure 3.7.

Thalidomide and Ritalin® (ethylphenidate) are examples of drugs that are manufactured as racemates (enantiomeric pairs), since resolution of the two enantiomers is not an easy task and adds considerable cost to the production process (and for the consumer). It is very likely that only one of the enantiomers has the desired pharmacological activity, therefore making the pharmaceutical product only 50% effective. (See Figure 3.8.) Some pharmaceutical firms are seeking patents on selected enantiomers of these two drugs.

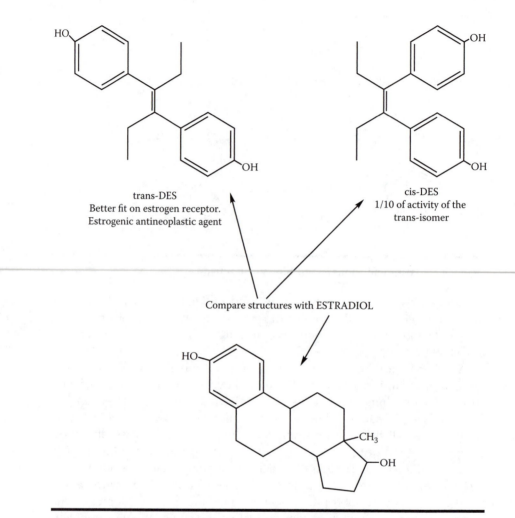

Figure 3.6 Geometric isomers and biological activity.

It is the widespread occurrence of different biological actions among optical isomers that has given ample support for the existence of receptors. Moreover, researchers have also been able to develop theories about the nature of drug–receptor interactions. Enantiomers have identical physicochemical properties, except for optical rotation, and are difficult to isolate pure from one another in the laboratory. Diastereomers, on the other hand, have different physical properties, such as melting point and solubility, for example, which makes them amenable to easy separation techniques in the laboratory.

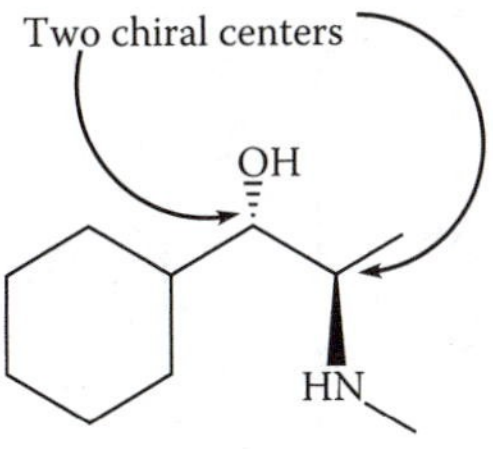

Ephedrine

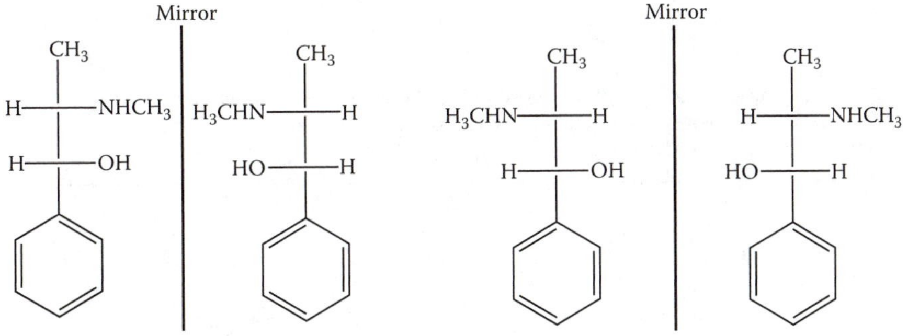

(1) (2) (3) (4)

Ephedrine Enantiomers

Pseudoephedrine Enantiomers

Diastereomers: (1) and (3); (1) and (4); (2) and (3); (2) and (4)

(1) 1R, 2S (-) Ephedrine - direct activity on both α, β adrenergic receptors.
(3) 1R, 2R (-) Ephedrine (diastereomer) α- adrenergic blocking activity.

Figure 3.7 Enantiomers and diastereomers of ephedrine.

Figure 3.9 shows a schematic representation of the interaction between the neurotransmitter epinephrine and its receptor in nerve cells. The postulated fit to the receptor shown in Figure 3.9 explains why L-epinephrine is 12 to 15 times more potent than D-epinephrine at constricting blood vessels: the area on the receptor labeled "Y" does not interact with the OH in D-epinephrine.

These schematic representations of drug–receptor interaction can achieve much greater degrees of sophistication through the use of supercomputers, which allow the analysis of ligand–receptor interactions occurring through familiar bonding patterns — covalent and noncovalent bonds (discussed in Chapter 1).

Table 3.2 shows the nature and strength of bonds formed between a drug or ligand and its receptor.

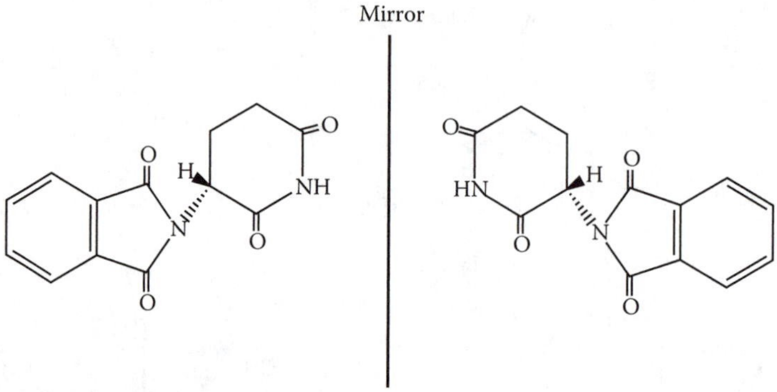

Mirror

Thalidomide enantiomers. Discontinued in 1962 because of birth defects; now used in cancer, Aids, leprosy. Most likely one enantiomer had desired biological action while the other had the observed toxicity.

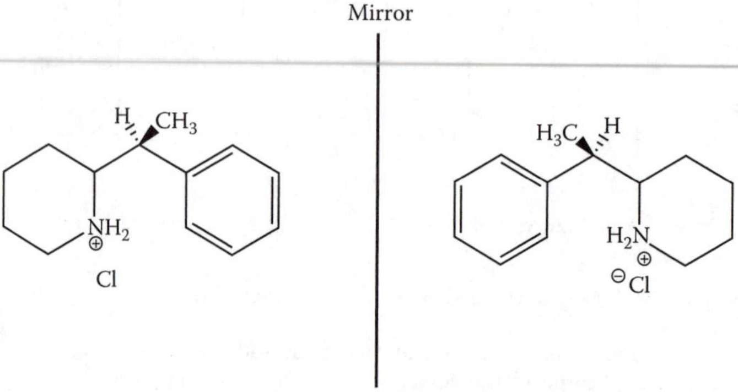

Mirror

Ritalin Renantiomers. Work is currently in progress to prove that only one enantiomer improves efficacy in treatment of attention-deficit-hyperactivity disorder.

Figure 3.8   Racemic pairs of thalidomide and Ritalin®.

ISOSTERISM AND ISOSTERES

The term "isosteres" refers to structural components in drug molecules that have similar steric and electronic characteristics and that can be interchanged within drugs that belong to the same pharmacological class. "Classical isosteres" refers to the concept as initially defined by Langmuir, who sought to explain similarities in physical properties of nonisomeric compounds. Classical isosteres are compounds or groups of atoms having the same number and arrangement of electrons. Examples of isosteres are the molecules of N_2 and CO, both of which have a total of 14 electrons and no charge, and which also have similar physical properties. Other examples cited by Langmuir were CO_2 and N_2O, and N_3^- and NCO^-.

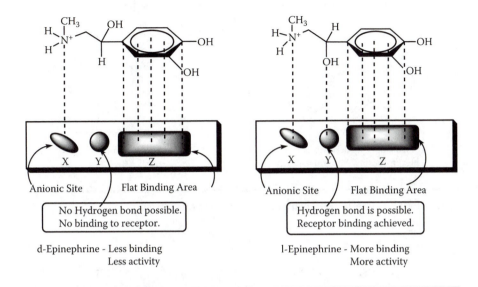

d-Epinephrine - Less binding
Less activity

l-Epinephrine - More binding
More activity

Figure 3.9 **Three-point model of the interaction of epinephrine with its receptor.**

Table 3.2   Drug-Receptor Interactions

Bond Type	Bond Energy (Kcal/mol)
1. Covalent bonds	40–110
2. Noncovalent bonds	0.5–7
2.1 Reinforced Ionic	10
2.2 Ionic bond	2–6
2.3 Hydrogen bond	1–7
2.4 Hydrophobic	1–2
2.5 Van der Waals	<1

Langmuir's concept of isosterism evolved to deemphasize the number of electrons in the structural components that could be considered isosteres. Hybridization during bond formation leads to significant differences in lengths, angles, and the polarity of bonds formed between atoms with the same number of peripheral electrons. The nitrogen atom has very different structural and electronic characteristics in the nitro group (NO_2, planar) than in ammonia and amines (NH_2R, trigonal pyramidal).

Nonclassical isosteres (bioisosteres) is the term used to refer to atoms or groups of atoms that have similar size, electronegativity, and stereochemistry

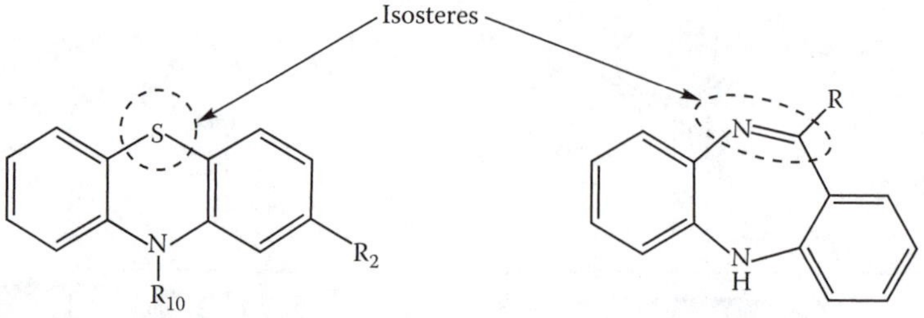

Isosteres

Phenothiazine derivatives
(Chlorpromazine, Mesoridazine)

Dibenzodiazepine derivatives
(Clozapine)

Figure 3.10 Isosteric replacements in antipsychotic drugs.

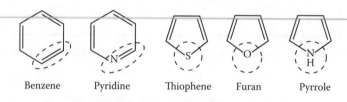

Benzene   Pyridine   Thiophene   Furan   Pyrrole

Figure 3.11 Vinylene isosteres in aromatic rings.

and that impart similar physical or chemical properties to drugs within a pharmacological class. Thiophene and benzene have similar properties, and the group –CH=CH– (vinylene) is a "ring equivalent" of divalent sulfur, –S–. An example of isosteric replacement of this type is seen in the phenothiazine ring system of tranquilizing agents. Exchanging the –S– for the vinylene group produced the dibenzodiazepine class of antipsychotic drugs. This change is shown in Figure 3.10.

The vinylene system in aromatic rings of drug molecules can be replaced by groups such as sulfur, oxygen, and NH, although the aromatic character of the rings may be decreased. Figure 3.11 shows some examples.

Isosteric replacement in a drug molecule may lead to a compound of similar activity (analog, agonist) or it may alter its effect to the extent that the structural analog is really an antagonist in its biological effect. An antagonist can bind to the receptor but does not elicit a response. Every pharmacological class must be considered individually, as prediction of agonist or antagonist behavior following isosteric replacement cannot be made. As an example, antibacterial activity is retained for all isosteres in the series shown in Figure 3.12.

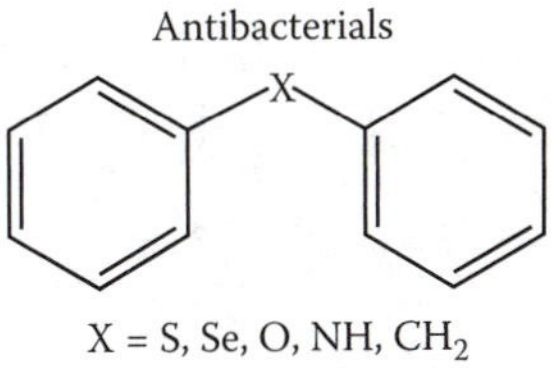

Antibacterials

X = S, Se, O, NH, CH$_2$

Figure 3.12   Antibacterials with various isosteric replacements.

Adenine   R = NH$_2$

Hypoxanthine   R = OH

6-Mercaptopurine R = SH

Metabolites

Antimetabolite

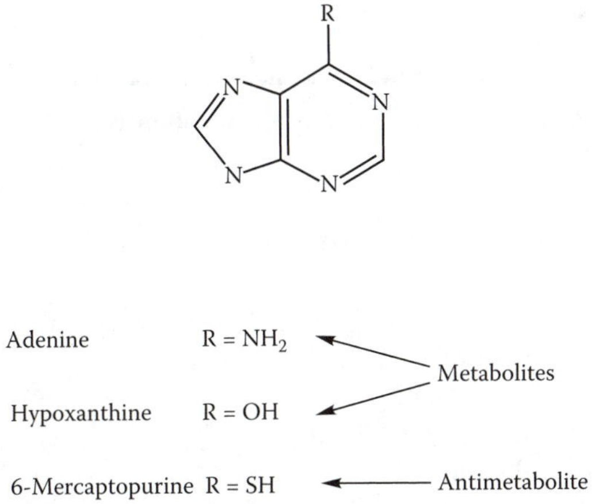

Figure 3.13   Isosteric replacements in adenine and hypoxanthine.

Similar isosteric replacements in adenine and hypoxanthine for an –SH group in 6-mercaptopurine yields an antimetabolite that is useful as an anticancer agent (see Figure 3.13). A weaker hydrogen bonding –SH group may cause decreased DNA base pair interactions during the replication phase, which decreases the rate of cellular synthesis.

Similar replacements in the structure of the metabolite folic acid yields the antimetabolites aminopterin and methotrexate. See Figure 3.14.

STRUCTURAL CHANGES IN DRUG MOLECULES

There are many structural changes in drug molecules that are performed later in their pharmaceutical development. Once a "lead" chemical entity has been identified for the desired pharmacological effect, minor changes in its structure and/or formulation provide optimal performance of the final product.

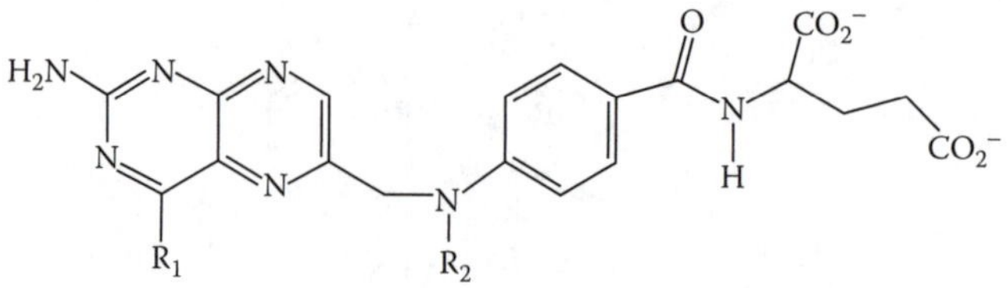

Figure 3.14 Folic acid and its isosteric antimetabolites.

Some of the reasons drug structures are changed in the final phase of their development include:

- To increase water solubility
- To increase lipophilicity
- To modify drug metabolism
- To improve the drug's taste

Examples of these changes are given below in Figure 3.15 through Figure 3.18.

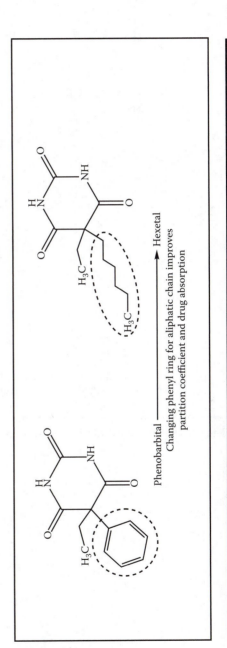

Figure 3.15 Chemical modification to improve lipophilicity.

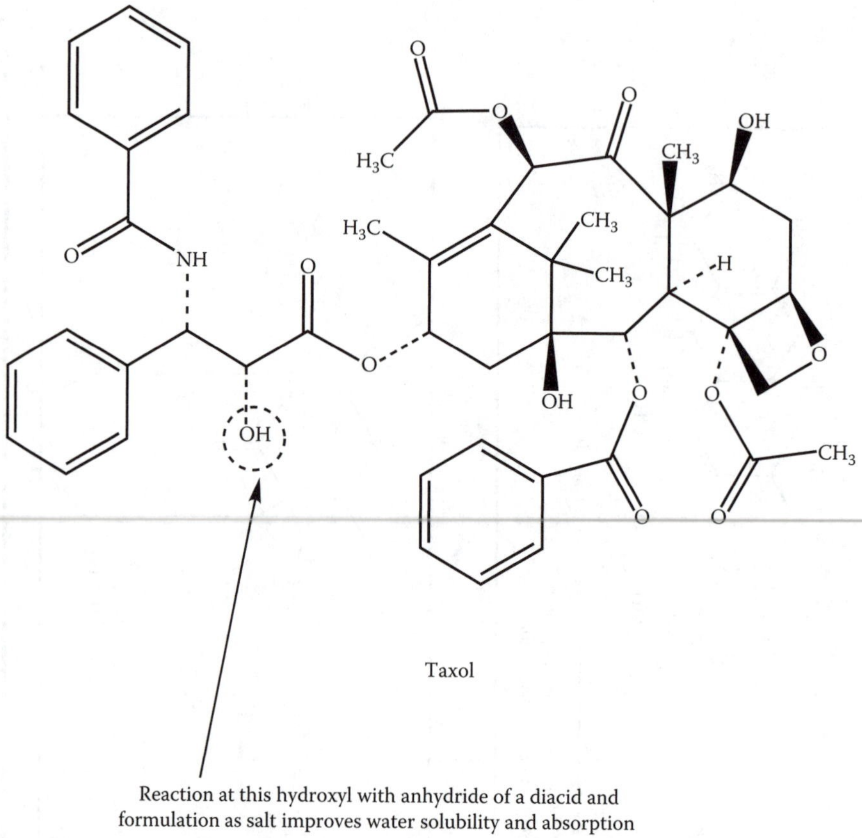

Taxol

Reaction at this hydroxyl with anhydride of a diacid and
formulation as salt improves water solubility and absorption

Figure 3.16 Chemical modification to improve water solubility.

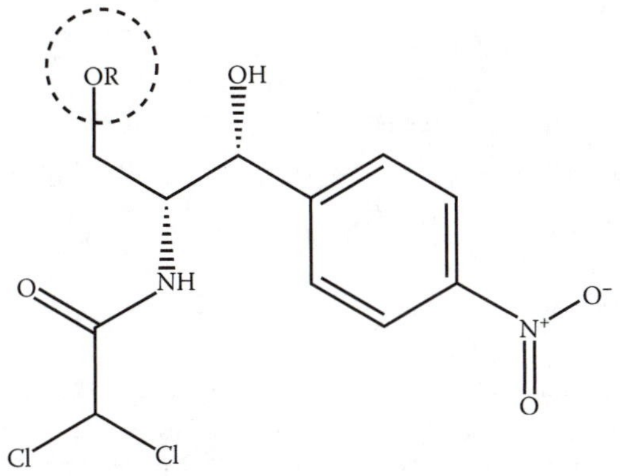

Chloramphenicol R = H

Chloramphenicol palmitate R = $-\overset{\displaystyle O}{\underset{\displaystyle \|}{C}}-(CH_2)_{14}-CH_3$

The palmitate ester is less water soluble, and the bitter taste of chloramphenicol is not detected in the mouth. The drug rather dissolves in the stomach, bypassing the taste receptors.

Figure 3.17   Chemical modification to improve drug taste.

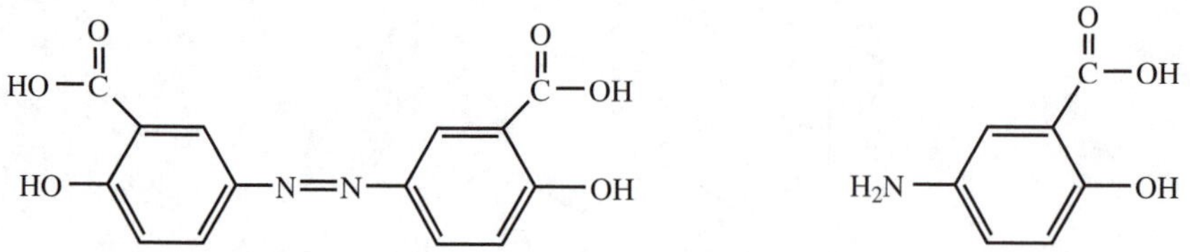

Olsalazine

Mesalamine

Mesalamine is used for ulcerative cholitis. It is degraded to inactive forms
before reaching the colon. Olsalazine (dimer) reaches the colon witho ut
degradation, and there it is metabolized by reduction of the -N=N- bond,
yielding the active drug, mesalamine.

Figure 3.18 Chemical modification to change drug metabolism.

FURTHER READING

1. *Essentials of Molecular Pharmacology* by Andrejus Korolkovas. John Wiley &
   Sons Inc. (1970).
2. *Remington: The Science and Practice of Pharmacy* by Alfonso R. Gennaro.
   Chapter 28. Lippincott Williams & Wilkins; 20th Edition (2000).

4

CHEMICAL APPROACHES TO
THE TREATMENT OF CANCER

The field of cancer chemotherapy has experienced tremendous growth in recent years; nonetheless, it still lacks the kind of breakthrough therapy that penicillin represented for antimicrobials. Steady progress in cancer research includes:

1. Understanding of the molecular biology of tumors
2. Better understanding of the mechanism of action of anticancer drugs

The techniques now available to carry out these tasks have allowed the rational design of new potential therapeutics. Molecular modeling techniques are providing a way to visualize drug–receptor interactions, while improved screening systems and large cooperative clinical trials allow fast evaluation of new drug candidates.

Only very rare cancers are considered "curable." These include Burkitt's lymphoma, choriocarcinoma, acute leukemia in children, Hodgkin's disease, Ewing's sarcoma, and testicular carcinoma. The most prevalent type of cancer in women, breast cancer, can at best be treated with a combination of drugs; moreover, the prognosis is not at all good for cancers of the liver, pancreas, lung, and colon.

NORMAL VS. MALIGNANT CELLS

Unfortunately for cancer patients, there are no significant differences between normal cells and cells in their tumors; therefore, selective toxicity is seldom achieved. This is not the case with bacterial infections; differences between human cells and bacteria (e.g., ribosomes, cell wall) are significant enough to allow the design of therapies that specifically kill the bacteria while leaving the normal cell unharmed. Also, the immune mechanisms that are so important in killing bacteria are virtually insignificant for cancer chemotherapy; cancer cells elude the immune surveillance system of the body.

A "complete" cure of cancer would require killing every malignant cell, which is very difficult to attain. Moreover, the few surviving cancer cells become resistant to the therapeutic agent used, creating the need for protocols that include three or more anticancer drugs with different mechanisms of action.

Unlike normal cells, cancer cells display an uncontrolled ability to proliferate and can invade surrounding tissues and establish new growth at distant sites in the body (metastasis). Cancer cells do not have the normal cell ability to differentiate, another aspect of a defective cell regulation pathway.

Not all types of cancer show high rates of proliferation. Acute leukemia cells, for example, have lower rates of proliferation than their normal counterparts in the bone marrow. The rates of cell proliferation can be very different depending on the type of tumor; solid tumors, for example, are very slow growing compared to lymphomas.

The uncontrolled proliferation of cancer cells can also be seen as a defect in cell homeostasis, which should maintain a balance between cell production and cell death. Much research is currently underway to understand the molecular pathways of programmed cell death (apoptosis) and the specific death signals bypassed by cancer cells that allow their survival.

CELL CYCLE AND CHEMOTHERAPY

The cell cycle is the period of time between cell birth and division. Before a cell can divide it must double all its parts, and DNA duplication is perhaps the most important event since the DNA must be copied exactly, and each daughter cell must receive a complete version of the genetic material.

The different stages in the cell cycle are shown in Figure 4.1. The stages vary greatly in duration among cell types, but typical time spans are as follows:

- *S phase*: 10 to 20 hours. This is the "synthesis" phase, where DNA replication occurs.
- *M phase*: 0.5 to 1 hour. This phase is where mitosis occurs; mitosis is the actual cell division where the two DNA copies separate.
- *G_1 and G_2 phases*: The duration of the G_2 phase is in the range of 2 to 10 hours. These are gaps that occur between mitosis and synthesis, which prepare the cell for the next phase.
- *G_0 phase*: A sub-phase of G_1 in which cells are resting, i.e., they are not preparing to divide.

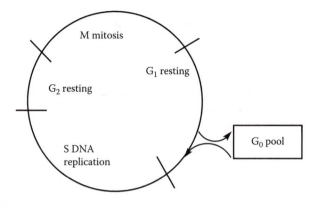

Figure 4.1   Cell cycle.

The most potent anticancer drugs act by damaging DNA; their effect is greatest during the S phase. Other anticancer drugs, such as Taxol, block the formation of the mitotic spindle in the M phase. For anticancer drugs to be most effective, a high percentage of tumor cells must be undergoing division (S and M phases). Normal tissues that proliferate rapidly such as hair follicles and bone marrow are especially susceptible to damage by anticancer drugs for the same reasons. On the other hand, slowly growing tumors with a low percentage of cells in the S and M phases (e.g., carcinomas of lung and colon) are not responsive to anticancer drugs. Rather, these cell types are mostly in the G_0 or resting phase.

Because G_0 varies greatly in length it causes also G_1 to vary substantially in different cell types as well as among different tumors.

FROM CHEMICAL WARFARE TO CHEMOTHERAPY

"Sulfur mustards" were chemicals used during World War I as powerful vesicants, producing blisters at tissues far from the site of contact. The name was given due to the odor of the chemical during the manufacturing process. Sulfur mustards were shown to be active against animal tumors, but they were indiscriminant in their actions and therefore had little therapeutic value. Figure 4.2 shows the structure of a sulfur mustard.

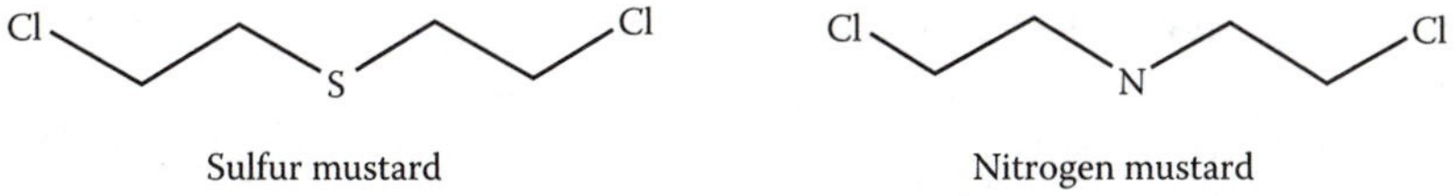

Sulfur mustard   Nitrogen mustard

Figure 4.2   Typical sulfur and nitrogen mustards.

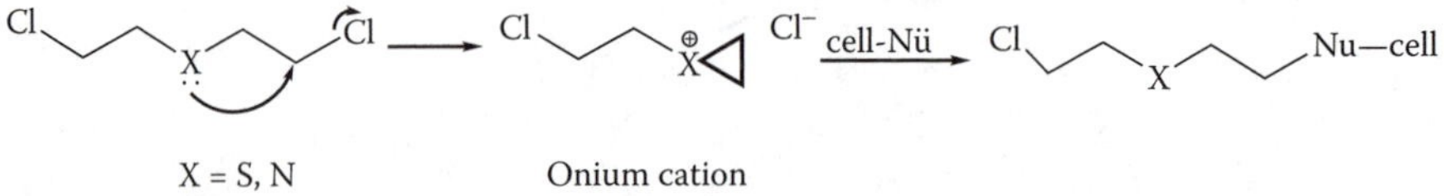

Figure 4.3 Onium cation formation.

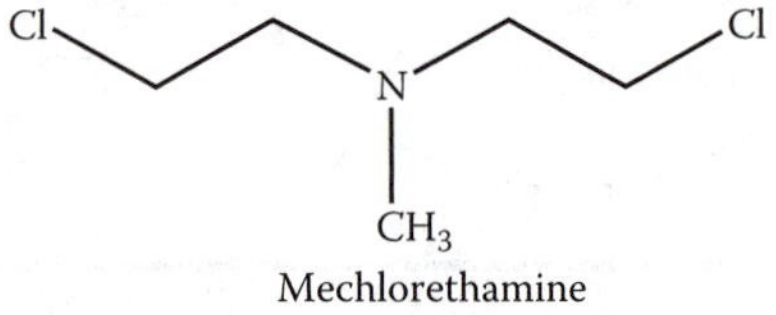

Mechlorethamine

Figure 4.4 Structure of mechlorethamine (Mustargen®).

Many "nitrogen mustards" were made between the two world wars in search for selective tumor toxicity. The structure of a nitrogen mustard is shown in Figure 4.2. Chemically speaking, these substances act by intramolecular nucleophilic displacement of one of the Cl atoms by the S or N atom in the molecule, leaving a very reactive cyclic "onium" cation. (See Figure 4.3.) The onium cation can then react with a nucleophile in the tumor cell (cell-Nu). One nitrogen mustard, meclorethamine, shown in Figure 4.4, showed selectivity toward lymphoid tissue, and after proper clinical trials, it was found useful against Hodgkin's disease and other lymphomas.

These substances are called "alkylating agents" because the net result is attachment of a substituted alkyl chain to a cellular nucleophile. The rate of the alkylation reaction depends on the nucleophilicity of atom X and is greatly enhanced if the nucleophile is ionized ($S^- > S$).

ANTICANCER DRUGS

Many other drugs have been developed for the treatment of cancer since the discovery of the sulfur and nitrogen mustards. We will discuss only a few in order to highlight the chemical aspects of their mechanisms of action. Several classifications of anticancer drugs are possible, but we will limit our discussion to the following types:

1. Alkylating agents
2. Antimetabolites
3. DNA intercalators
4. DNA crosslinking agents

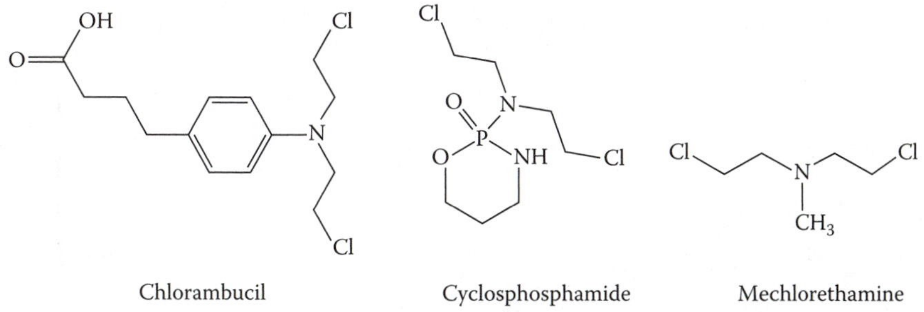

Chlorambucil   Cyclosphosphamide   Mechlorethamine

Figure 4.5   Structures of three alkylating agents.

Alkylating Agents

Alkylating agents were the first anticancer drugs developed and are still in use. They exert their effect at any point of the cell cycle and are called phase-nonspecific. Examples include mechlorethamine, cyclophosphamide, and chlorambucil. The structures of these three drugs are shown in Figure 4.5.

An electron-deficient group (Lewis acid) in the drug molecule reacts with an electron-rich group (Lewis base) in a crucial biomolecule, for example nitrogen 7 (N-7) of the DNA base guanine. This is shown in Figure 4.6. The Lewis acid in this case is called "aziridinium ion," which for aliphatic nitrogen mustards like Mustargen®, forms quickly by intramolecular displacement of Cl by N. See Figure 4.7.

On the other hand, aryl-substituted nitrogen mustards such as chlorambucil do not readily form the *aziridinium ion* due to decreased nucleophilicity of the nitrogen atom. This explains the fact that chlorambucil can be taken orally: it will survive the aqueous, acidic environment of the stomach and is generally stable in water. Such is not the case for mechlorethamine, which must be prepared just prior to use and administered by intravenous infusion.

Resonance structures such as (I) (Figure 4.8) explain the decreased nucleophilicity of the nitrogen in chlorambucil, compared to Mustargen® (mechlorethamine), and stabilize the molecule towards the formation of aziridinium ion, the true alkylating agent, and the reactive species that can also react with water to inactivate the drug.

Some alkylating agents are not active until they are changed by metabolism in the body. An example is cyclophosphamide, which is converted by the hepatic enzyme CYP 450 into the 4-hydroxy derivative, as shown in the first reaction in Figure 4.9.

The hydroxylated product is a carbinolamine, which can rearrange into the open-chain amino aldehyde form. This aldehyde can be further degraded into phosphoramide mustard and acrolein. It has been shown

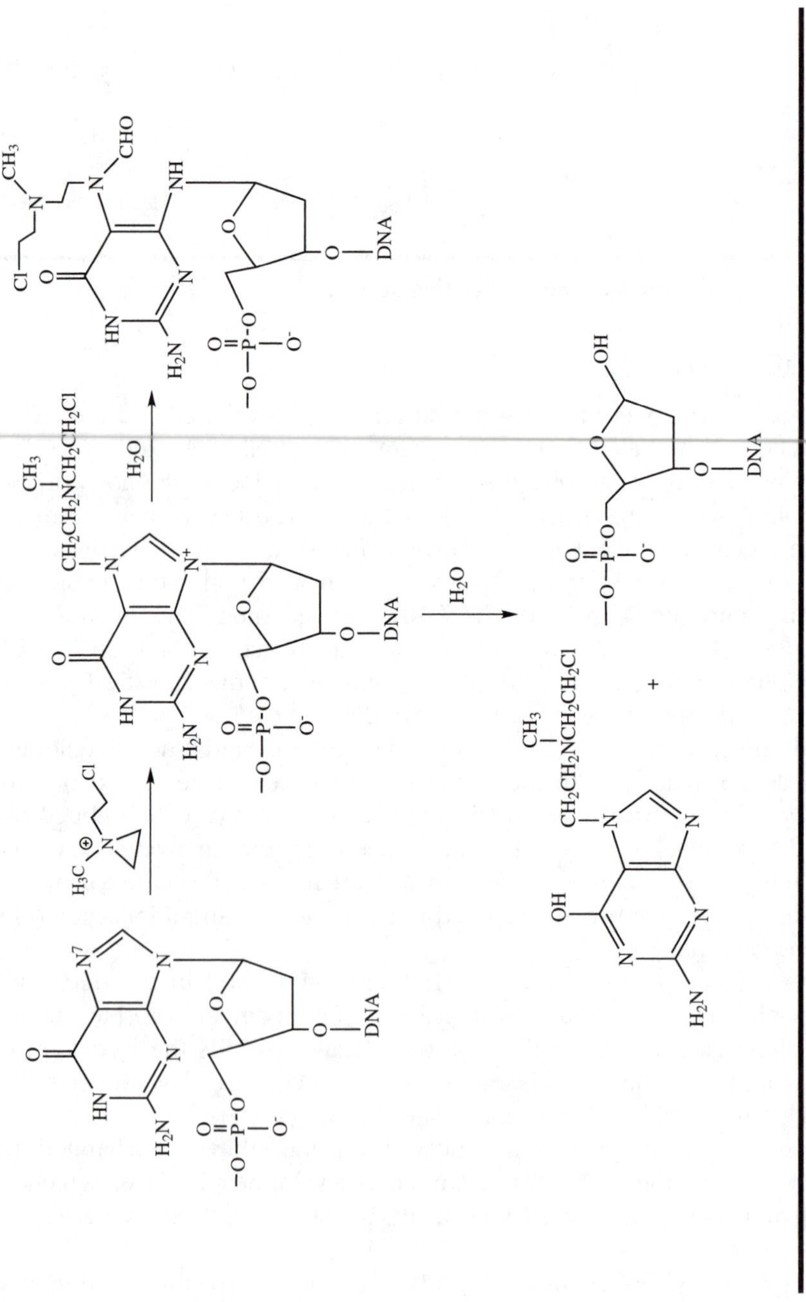

Figure 4.6 Alkylation of guanine in DNA by Mustargen®.

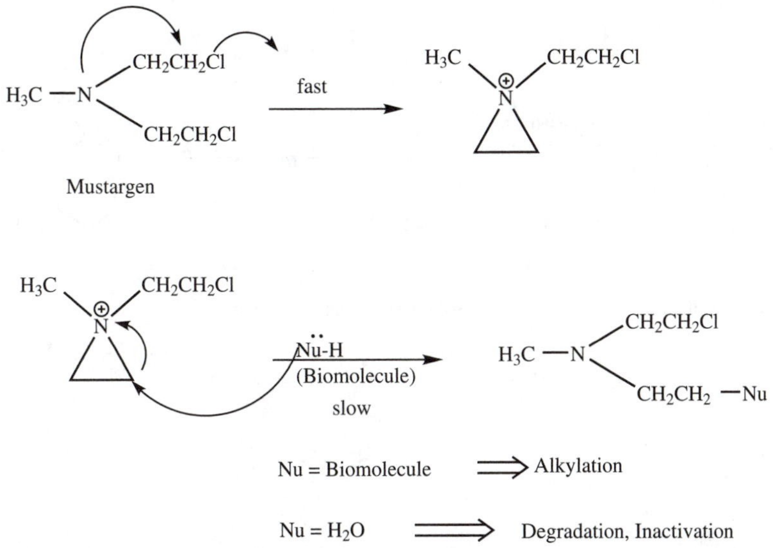

Figure 4.7 Aziridinium ion formation.

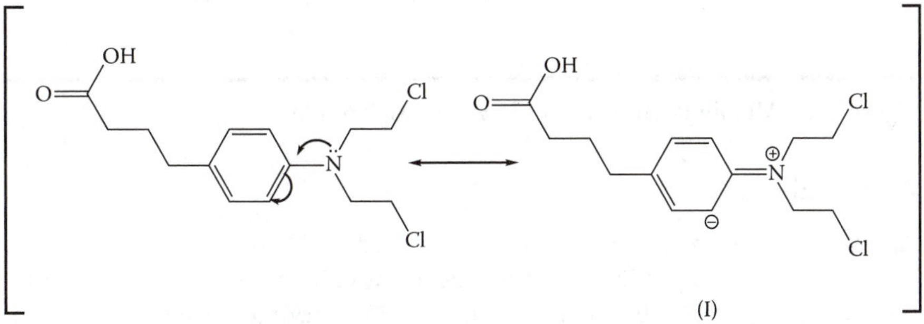

Figure 4.8 Chlorambucil is more stable than Mustargen.

that the formation of the aziridinium ion occurs via the conjugate base form of the phosphoramide mustard. Some neoplastic cells have very low pH, and selective toxicity can be attained by the resulting displacement of the equilibrium toward the conjugate acid (CA) form, with slower formation of the aziridinium ion. In other cells at higher pH, formation of the aziridinium ion is faster and degradation by other nucleophiles (including water) is more likely.

Bifunctional nitrogen mustards (two chloroethylene chains) such as those described above can crosslink DNA by repeating the same cycle of aziridinium ion formation and nucleophilic attack by a purine or pyrimidine base in the DNA.

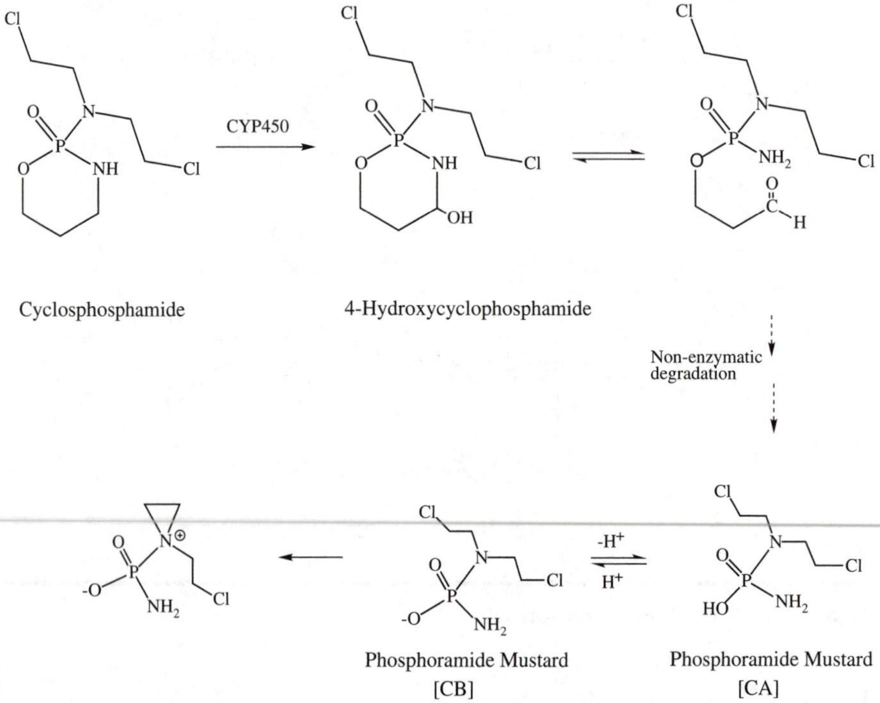

Figure 4.9 Metabolic activation of cyclophosphamide.

Antimetabolites

Antimetabolites are substances that antagonize a normal metabolite in the body, disrupting a pathway that is crucial for cell survival. Some examples we will discuss include 6-mercaptopurine, 5-fluorouracil (5-FU), and methotrexate. Antimetabolites are structurally similar to the metabolite antagonized, and many are enzyme inhibitors. Metabolic activation is also required for some of the drugs in this class. For example, 6-mercaptopurine is a *prodrug* that requires metabolic transformation into the ribonucleotide. In this form, the drug is a potent inhibitor of the enzyme involved in a rate-controlling step of the *de novo* synthesis of purines, which are bases in DNA. The metabolic transformation of this prodrug is shown in Figure 4.10.

Neoplasms that lack the enzyme HGPRTase (Hypoxanthine-Guanine PhosphoRibosyl Transferase) are consequently resistant to 6-mercaptopurine. The actions of 6-mercaptopurine are complex, as its metabolites can inhibit ≅20 enzymes.

The invention of 5-FU is a classical example of rational drug design. Heidelberger made the observation that in certain tumors uracil was used more than orotic acid as a precursor for pyrimidine biosynthesis; he

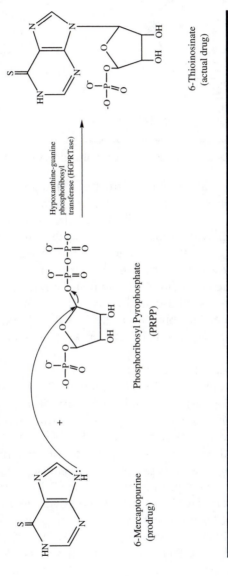

Figure 4.10 Metabolic activation of 6-mercaptopurine.

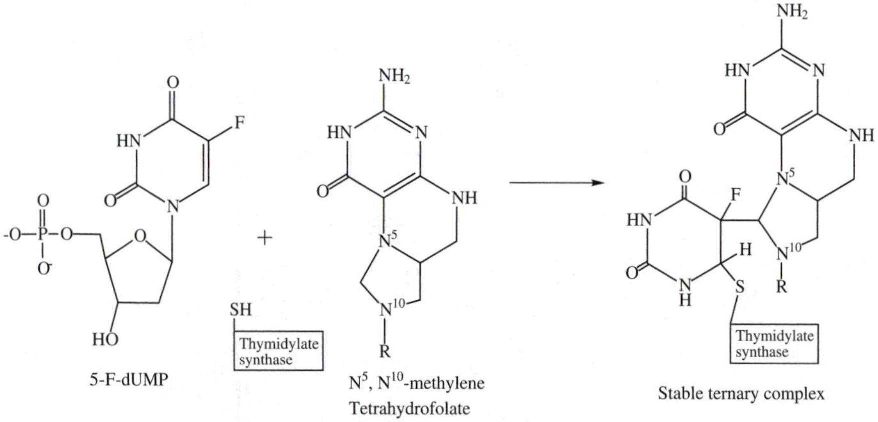

Figure 4.11   Ternary complex in the inhibition of thymidylate synthase by 5F-dUMP.

designed a molecule with only one structural change — the 5-position, where a $-CH_3$ group is transferred from N^5, N^{10} methylene tetrahydrofolate (THF) (Figure 4.11). Fluorine was chosen as the substituent because of its greater electronegativity compared to hydrogen and the effect of its greater inductive effect on the adjacent carbon, rendering the pyrimidine ring more susceptible to attack by the $-SH$ group in the enzyme.

The ternary complex of 5-Fluoro d-uridine monophosphate (5-F-dUMP) the enzyme thymidylate synthase, and N^5, N^{10}-THF resembles the transition state of the normal reaction, but due to the covalent bonds formed in the complex, the inhibition is considered irreversible: the $-C-F$ bond is stable (see Figure 4.11).

Metabolic activation of 5-fluorouracil to 5-fluoro-2′-deoxyuridylic acid can proceed by two routes described in Figure 4.12. One involves reaction of 5-FU with ribose-1-phosphate to give the riboside (**1**), which can then be phosphorylated by uridine kinase to give 5-fluorouridylic acid. The latter can be reduced by ribonucleotide reductase to yield the 2′-deoxy derivative (**3**). Another route is the direct conversion of 5-FU into 5-fluorouridylic acid by a phosphoribosyltransferase present in certain tumors. The pharmaceutical product floxuridine (5-flourouracil-2′-deoxyriboside) is phosphorylated to the active drug (**3**) by 2′-deoxyuridine kinase. The key metabolite (**3**) inhibits thymidylate synthase, a key enzyme in the conversion of uridine to thymidine; therefore, the cell is deprived of a key DNA base and the effect is called "thymine-less" death.

Methotrexate and related drugs are antimetabolites classified as "folate acid antagonists." They kill cells by inhibiting the enzyme dihydrofolate reductase. The structures of dihydrofolic acid, the natural substrate of this enzyme, and the antimetabolite methotrexate are shown in Figure 4.13. This class of antimetabolites binds so tightly to the enzyme that the

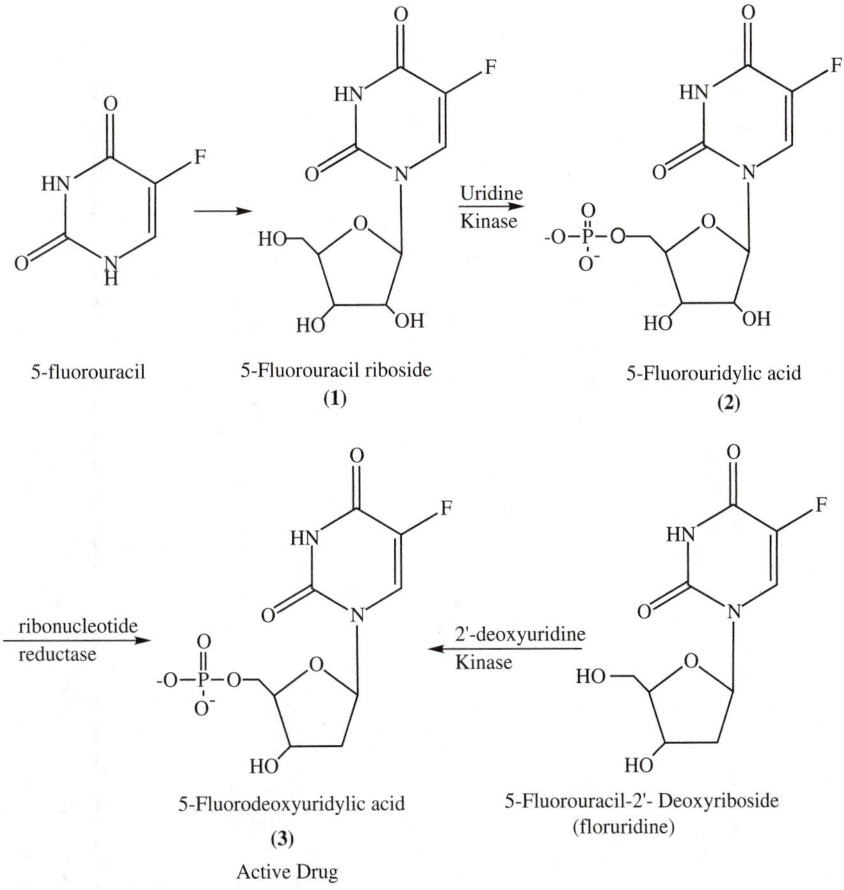

Figure 4.12   Metabolic activation of 5-fluorouracil.

inhibition is considered "irreversible," and DNA synthesis is inhibited by depriving the tumor cell of a key cofactor in the synthesis of thymine. Host toxicity is currently diminished by the implementation of "leucovorin rescue therapy." This consists of treating the patient with a high (almost lethal) dose of methotrexate, then "rescuing" the normal cells by administering leucovorin, an intermediate in tetrahydrofolate synthesis, which helps the normal cells bypass the blockade of tetrahydrofolate (THFolate) reductase, while cancer cells die.

DNA Intercalators

Another class of anticancer drugs acts by intercalating into the double helix of DNA molecules. This is the case for antibiotic doxorubicin

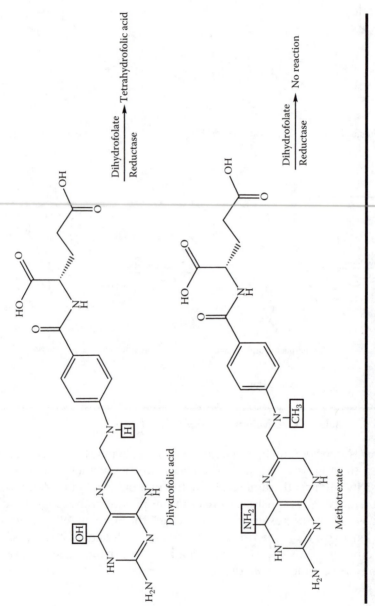

Figure 4.13 Methotrexate antagonizes dihydrofolic acid.

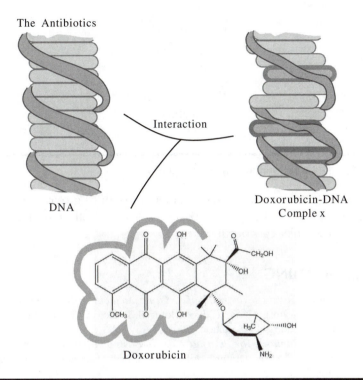

Figure 4.14   DNA intercalation by doxorubicin.

(Adriamycin®) and other members of this family with the anthracyclinone ring structure.

The intercalation process results in partial unwinding of the double helix in order to accommodate the flat anthracyclinone ring between successive DNA base pairs. (See Figure 4.14.) Forces that stabilize the intercalator into the DNA structure include hydrogen bonding to guanine –NH_2 groups, π-bonding between aromatic rings, and numerous van der Waals interactions. Many functions of DNA are affected by the intercalation of this type of drug. Single- and double-strand breaks occur, which can not be repaired by the enzyme topoisomerase II.

DNA Crosslinking Agents

The last class of anticancer drug that we will consider the DNA crosslinking agents. Platinum complexes such as cisplatin (Figure 4.15) have been found to be active against tumors and have a *cis* geometry about the pair of ligands with intermediate "leaving ability."

DNA adducts formed with cisplatin inhibit *DNA polymerase,* affecting replication and transcription and leading to breaks and miscoding. The

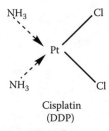

Cisplatin
(DDP)

Figure 4.15 DNA crosslinking agent "cisplatin."

interaction with DNA involves displacement of both Cl groups by nitrogen or oxygen atoms in the purine bases of DNA. Both intrastrand and interstrand crosslinks can occur.

FURTHER READING

1. *Wilson and Gisvold's Textbook of Organic Medicinal and Pharmaceutical Chemistry* by John H. Block (Editor), John M. Beale, Jr. Chapter 12. Lippincott Williams & Wilkins; 11th Edition (2004).
2. *Goodman & Gilman's The Pharmacological Basis of Therapeutics* by Joel Griffith Hardman, Lee E. Limbird, Alfred G. Gilman. Chapter 52. McGraw-Hill Professional; 10th Edition (2001).

II

PRINCIPLES OF BIOPHARMACEUTICS

5

ADMINISTRATION AND ABSORPTION OF DRUGS

The objective of drug therapy is to produce and maintain a therapeutic response while minimizing undesirable and/or toxic effects. When we consider *what the drug does to the body* we study its *pharmacodynamics* — the relationship between drug concentration at the site of action and the pharmacological response. In Chapter 4 we covered some aspects of the pharmacodynamics of anticancer drugs by studying their mechanisms of action.

If we consider *what the body does to the drug,* we study its *pharmacokinetics,* and we evaluate the time course of drug and metabolite concentrations in the body. Finally, the drug can have one of several formulations, or dosage forms. When we consider *what the dosage form does to affect drug activity*, we must evaluate it in the context of the science of *biopharmaceutics,* which allows us to understand how the physicochemical properties of the drug, the route of administration, and the dosage form affect the rate and extent of systemic absorption.

In this chapter we will present an overview of the biopharmaceutical principles involved in the administration and absorption of drugs, and in the following chapter we will present more detail on the pharmacokinetic variables of the absorption, distribution, and elimination of drugs.

DRUG ADMINISTRATION

Drugs can be administered in a number of ways, which are classified as follows:

- *Enteral* administration, which includes the oral, sublingual, and rectal routes (mouth to rectum — the gastrointestinal tract.)

- *Parenteral* administration, which includes the intravenous (IV), intramuscular (IM), and subcutaneous (SC) routes. These routes involve injections outside the gastrointestinal tract.

Other forms of drug administration include such routes as topical (skin surface), intranasal (in the nose), and intrathecal (in the spine).

Oral administration of a drug is the most common route, although it has some disadvantages, such as variability in amount absorbed and a complicated pathway to the target tissue. The advantages still outweigh the disadvantages, however, as it is possible to manufacture a wide variety of oral dosage forms in a cost-effective manner, giving the physician an ample range of therapeutic options.

Drugs are distributed throughout the body in the water phase of the blood plasma, regardless of their site of entry. A drug must first enter the blood (except those applied topically for a local effect), and then it can reach the target organ at a rate determined by the blood flow through that organ. The drug must then cross the vascular endothelium, traverse through interstitial fluid, and then get inside the cells of that particular organ.

Some of the drug molecules may be bound to proteins in the blood plasma and thus may not be freely diffusible out of the plasma. It is generally true that the amount of a drug in the tissues in which it acts is only a small part of the total amount of the drug present in the body. A large proportion of the drug remains in solution in various compartments or is localized in subcellular particles, in fat depots, or at macromolecular surfaces. Approximately 80% of the cell mass is water, and only a very small fraction of the cell's dry weight is represented by specific receptors; therefore, only a small fraction of drug is associated with receptors. Moreover, the receptors are macromolecules of high molecular weight, each bearing one and sometimes several drug binding sites. Therefore, even with high drug–receptor affinity at complete receptor occupancy (providing that the drug interacts reversibly), most of the drug molecules will be in the aqueous phase in equilibrium with those bound to the receptor.

The following factors need to be considered when choosing a route of administration for a drug:

1. Properties of the drug
2. Therapeutic objectives

Properties of the Drug

Drug Solubility

Drug solubility is the mass of drug that can be dissolved per unit volume of solvent (e.g., mg/L). Since water is the major constituent of blood

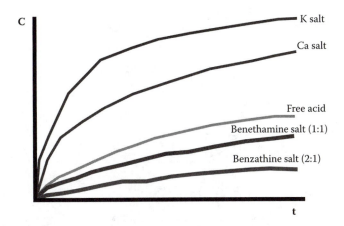

Figure 5.1   Concentration vs. time for various salts of penicillin G.

plasma and cell mass in general, water solubility of drugs is a very important factor during drug development and when choosing a route of administration; it will affect how fast a drug may be absorbed into the systemic circulation. Salts of weak acids and weak bases generally have much higher aqueous solubility than the free acid or base does; therefore, if the drug can be given as a salt, the solubility can be increased and dissolution rates should greatly improve. One example is penicillin G.

Figure 5.1 shows typical dissolution curves for various salts of penicillin G. The shapes of these curves indicate that there is faster dissolution at lower time points (higher slopes), and as time progresses the solution approaches saturation (lower slopes at higher time points). At any given time point, the concentrations of penicillin salts follow the order: K salt > Ca salt > free acid > benethamine salt > benzathine salt. It follows from this analysis that the potassium salt is the most soluble of the penicillin salts mentioned and the benzathine salt is the least soluble. This fact can be correlated to the chemical composition of the various salts, as shown in Figure 5.2.

It is clear from the structural formulas of the salts shown in Figure 5.2, that the molecular size of penicillin benzathine is the largest of all. This form of penicillin also contains large, hydrophobic groups (phenyl rings), which explains the lower water solubility of this salt, compared to the inorganic cation salts preceding it. The calcium salt contains two of the organic anion moieties, vs. one for the sodium salt, which explains the lower water solubility of the calcium salt.

Quite different graphs of plasma concentration versus time can be obtained, as can be seen in Figure 5.3, and peak plasma concentrations usually show good correlation with water solubility. The potassium salt

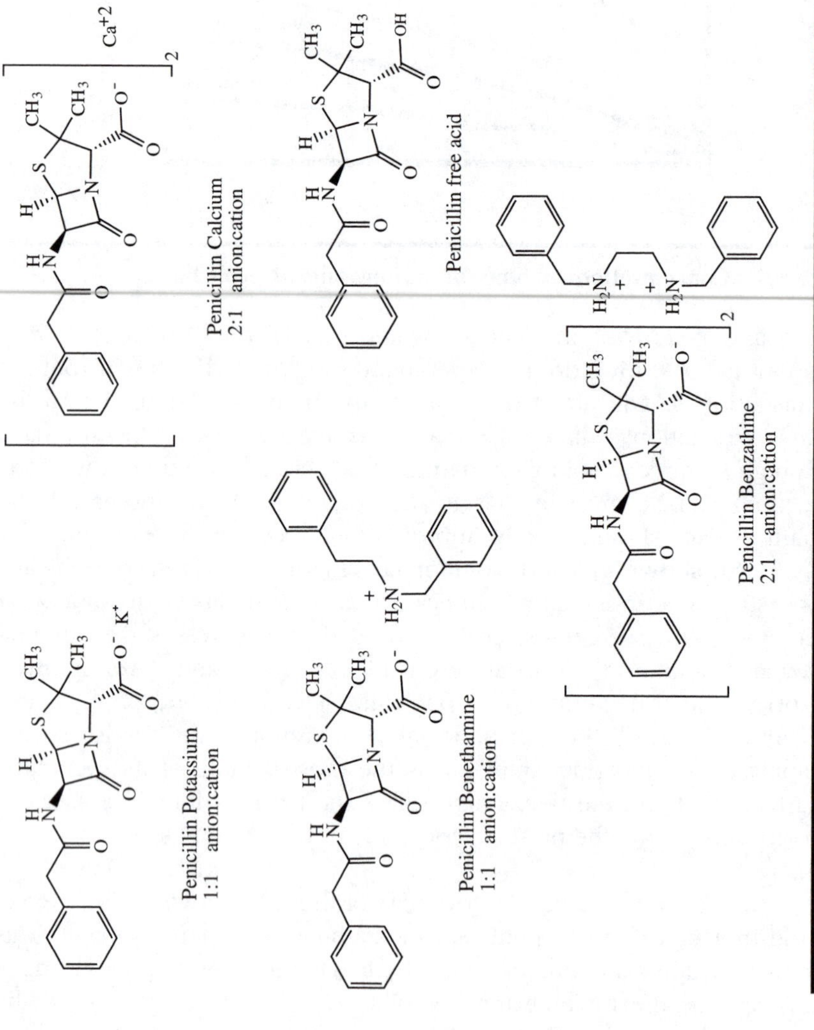

Figure 5.2 Structural formulas of penicillin salts.

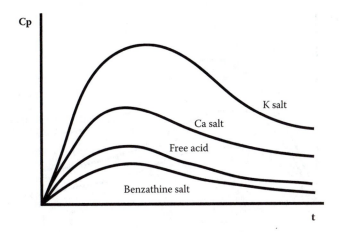

Figure 5.3 Plasma concentration (Cp) of penicillin salts vs. time.

is better for oral absorption, where the drug must dissolve in the aqueous medium of the stomach. The benzathine salt is better for the intramuscular route, where affinity with lipid structures would facilitate absorption.

Polymorphism

Some drugs exist in a number of crystal forms or *polymorphs*. These different forms may well have different solubility properties and thus different dissolution characteristics. This is very important for the extent of drug absorption, especially of solid dosage forms. Chloramphenicol palmitate is one example: it exists in at least two polymorphs. Cortisone acetate can crystallize in five (5) different polymorphic crystals. The existence of different polymorphs of a drug molecule explains differences in bioavailability among commercial products. Depending on the crystal-line form used in the formulation, the drug product of two manufacturers may differ in stability and therapeutic effect.

Figure 5.4 shows plasma concentrations vs. time for three formulations of the antifungal drug fluconazole, with different proportions of two polymorphs. Three polymorphs can be obtained in the manufacturing process of fluconazole but only polymorph III is suitable for the final drug product. Polymorph III is obtained by recrystallization in isopropanol and has very small but detectable differences in the infrared and differential scanning calorimetry spectra compared to polymorphs II and I. Polymorph III of fluconazole was found to have the best dissolution profile and the best bioavailabilty of the three polymorphs or any combination thereof. It is important to note that the differences among polymorphs are significant

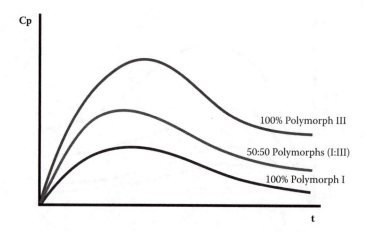

Figure 5.4 Plasma concentration vs. time for three formulations of fluconazole.

only in the solid state. Once the drug is dissolved in body fluids, its molecules are indistinguishable from one another. For this reason, *polymorphism is not important for a drug that is given as an IV solution.* Polymorphism is important, however, for oral dosage forms, where the active ingredient must dissolve in the aqueous medium prior to absorption.

Particle Size

The therapeutic efficacy of a dosage form may be affected by the particle size. As the particles of the drug are reduced in size there is an increase in specific surface area. Since the solution of a given weight of a drug is proportional to the exposed surface, greater solution can be attained with an increase in surface area, and greater amounts of drug can be absorbed from the site of administration. Figure 5.5 shows the effect of particle size on plasma levels of the antidepressant sertraline.

Very small particles may clump together; therefore a wetting agent such as Tween 80 (polysorbate 80) can have a beneficial effect on the overall absorption. The role of wetting agents is to separate the small particles of drug and facilitate wetting during disintegration of oral dosage forms. The intestinal fluids usually contain some materials that can act as wetting agents.

pK_a

For a drug to cross a membrane barrier it must dissolve in the lipid material of the membrane to get into the membrane; also, it has to be soluble in the aqueous phase as well to get out of the membrane. Most

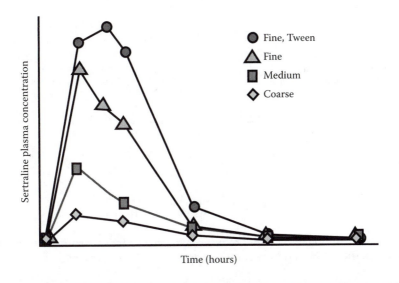

Figure 5.5   Effect of particle size on drug absorption.

drugs have polar and nonpolar characteristics or are weak acids or bases. For drugs that are weak acids or bases, the pK_a of the drug and the pH of the physiological fluids are important in determining the solubility of the drug and the rate of absorption through the membranes. The partition coefficient also plays a key role in determining the absorption of a drug since a drug must have enough lipophilic nature to cross the various membranes in the body en route to the pharmacological target.

In the late 1950s Brodie et al. proposed the pH partition theory to explain the influence of gastrointestinal pH and drug pK_a on the extent of drug transfer or drug absorption. Brodie reasoned that when a drug is ionized it would not be able to get through the lipid membrane; but only when it is nonionized and therefore has higher lipid solubility would it be able to get through. Weak acids can be absorbed readily from the stomach. The high H^+ concentration in the stomach forces the dissociation equilibrium toward the neutral form of the drug, which can cross membranes more readily. Weak bases would be easily protonated at the low pH of the stomach, where they will exist as positively charged ions that do not readily cross cell membranes. Weak bases are better absorbed in the intestines where the pH is higher. The relationship between compartment pH and the drug's pK_a is expressed by the Henderson–Hasselbach equation. The derivation of this equation can be found in Chapter 2:

For acids: $pK_a = pH + \log [HA]/[A^-]$
For bases: $pK_a = pH + \log [BH^+]/[B]$

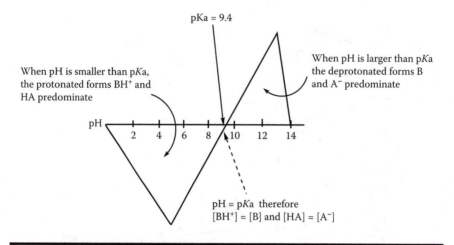

Figure 5.6   Relationship between compartment pH and drug pK_a.

The diagram in Figure 5.6 shows the relationship between compartment pH and drug pK_a.

Weak (HA) acids are better absorbed at pHs lower than their pK_a values. *Example:* aspirin is better absorbed from the stomach, at a pH of 1.8. Weak (B) bases are better absorbed at pHs higher than their pK_a values. *Example:* ephedrine is better absorbed from the small intestine, at a pH close to 8.0.

Therapeutic Objective

Onset of Action

It may be desirable to administer a drug for its fast action in an emergency situation (e.g., digoxin in cardiac failure; diazepam in epileptic seizures) or to induce a physical state in the patient (anesthesia). On the other hand, fast onset of action may not be the desired outcome in many clinical situations, as shown in Figure 5.7.

Use of sodium tolbutamide results in very fast absorption and onset of action, with blood sugar levels lowering so fast that there is risk of a hypoglycemic shock. A more gradual reduction in blood sugar by tolbutamide is better attained by using a form of the drug that is released more slowly into the blood stream, i.e., the free acid rather than the sodium salt.

Long-Term Administration

In chronic disease states it may be necessary to administer a drug for a long time. It also may be necessary to sustain drug activity; therefore, the route of administration should facilitate slow absorption or release of the

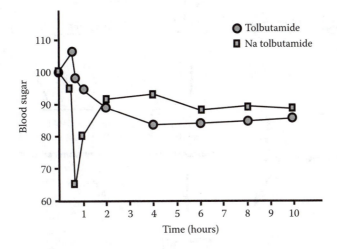

Figure 5.7 Effect of dissolution rate on absorption and biological response.

drug from the dosage form. An example is the use of Procardia XL®
(nifedipine) in the treatment of hypertension. The special "osmotic" formulation of this drug in a laser-drilled Gastro-Intestinal Therapeutic System
(GITS) tablet allows for a very efficient sustained release of the drug.

Restriction to a Local Site

Localized treatment may be desirable to avoid systemic side effects or to
maximize therapeutic effect. Examples are local anesthetics and glucocor-
ticoids in the treatment of asthma. Another important example involves
the use of Premarin® (conjugated estrogens) vaginal cream, rather than
the tablets, to enhance the estrogenic effects of the medication in the
vagina. Using the cream locally instead of the tablets avoids the risk of
hormone replacement therapy intrinsic in the oral formulations.

DRUG ABSORPTION

Absorption is the process of incorporation of drug into the bloodstream.
This process takes place after administration of the drug, which is then
found solubilized in the bloodstream, ready to reach its target. There is
an absorption process for every route of administration except the intravenous route, where the drug is placed directly into the bloodstream. As
mentioned previously, the most common route of drug administration is
the oral route, which includes such dosage forms as tablets, capsules, and
suspensions. Considering the case of a tablet, which contains not only
the active ingredient but also other excipients as adjuncts in a compressed,

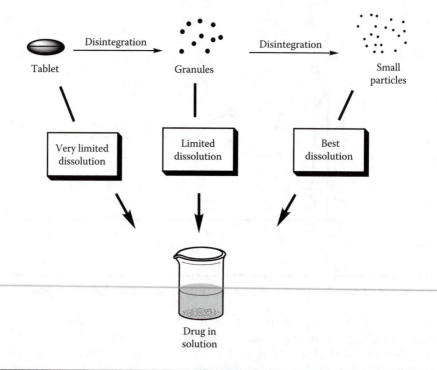

Figure 5.8 Steps preceding absorption for tablets.

molded shape, we can envision the drug going through the steps of disintegration and dissolution before it can be absorbed. This is shown schematically in Figure 5.8.

Once dissolved, the drug molecules must cross a number of membrane barriers on their route to the bloodstream and must also traverse out of the bloodstream and through the membranes leading to the cell targets. Biological membranes are mainly lipid in nature but also contain small aqueous channels or pores. Membranes in different parts of the body have somewhat different characteristics that affect not only absorption but also distribution and elimination. Pore size and pore distribution are not uniform among membranes from different parts of the body. Some membrane types of special significance include the blood–brain barrier, the blood capillaries, and the renal membranes of the tubules and the glomerula. In terms of their porosity they can be described and grouped together in the following manner:

- *Blood–brain barrier.* The membranes between the blood and brain have effectively no pores. This prevents many polar and often toxic materials from entering the brain. However, smaller lipid materials or lipid-soluble materials, such as diethyl ether or halothane, can easily enter the brain. These compounds are used as general anesthetics.

- *Renal tubules.* In the kidney there are a number of regions important for drug elimination. Drugs may be reabsorbed in the tubules; however, because the membranes are relatively nonporous, only lipid compounds or nonionized species (dependent on pH and pK_a) are reabsorbed.
- *Blood capillaries and renal glomerular membranes.* These membranes are quite porous, allowing passage of nonpolar and polar molecules of fairly large size. This is especially useful in the kidneys since it allows excretion of polar substances, both drugs and waste compounds.

PHYSIOLOGICAL AND PHYSICOCHEMICAL FACTORS IN DRUG ABSORPTION

Drug Transport across Membranes

Passive Diffusion

Most drugs cross biological membranes by passive diffusion. Diffusion occurs when the drug concentration on one side of the membrane is higher (C_h) than on the other side (C_l). Drug diffuses across the membrane in an attempt to equalize the drug concentration on both sides of the membrane. If the drug partitions into the lipid membrane, a concentration gradient can be established.

Fick's first law of diffusion, described by Equation (5.1), can describe the rate of transport of drug across the membrane.

$$\frac{dM}{dt} = \frac{D*A*(C_h - C_l)}{X}$$

Equation 5.1   Fick's first law of diffusion.

The variables in Equation (5.1) are as follows:

- *Rate of diffusion: dM/dt*
- *D: Diffusion coefficient.* This parameter is related to the size and lipid solubility of the drug and the viscosity of the diffusion medium, the membrane. As lipid solubility increases or molecular size decreases, then D increases and thus dM/dt also increases.
- *A: Surface area.* As the surface area increases, the rate of diffusion also increases. The surface of the intestinal lining is much larger than that of the stomach. This is one reason absorption from the intestine is generally faster compared with absorption from the stomach.

- *X: Membrane thickness.* The smaller the membrane thickness, the quicker the diffusion process. As one example, the membrane in the lung is quite thin; thus, inhalation absorption can be quite rapid.
- *(Ch – Cl): Concentration difference.* The drug concentration in blood or plasma is usually quite low compared with the concentration in the gastrointestinal tract. It is this concentration gradient that allows the rapid and complete absorption of many drug substances given orally. In this case Cl is much lower than Ch, and Equation (5.1) can be reduced to the expression of a first-order rate constant, as shown in Equation (5.2).

$$\frac{dM}{dt} = \frac{D*A*C_h}{X} = \frac{D*A*X_g}{X*V_g} = k_a * X_g$$

a constant · · · Dose

Equation 5.2 Simplified equation for oral dosage forms.

This explains why the absorption of many drugs from the gastrointestinal often appears to be first order, i.e., to depend only on the amount of drug present in the gut (X_g).

Active Transport

The body has a number of specialized mechanisms for transporting endogenous substances such as glucose and amino acids. Sometimes drugs can participate in this process; 5-fluorouracil is an example. Active transport involves:

- A specific carrier protein
- A form of energy (ATP hydrolysis)
- A process that can be competitively inhibited
- A process that can be saturated
- Transport that proceeds against a concentration gradient

Examples include the transport of Na^+, K^+, I^-, Fe^{+2}, Ca^{+2}, monosaccharides, pyrimidine bases, amino acids, cardiac glycosides, some B vitamins, testosterone, and estradiol.

Facilitated Transport

In this type of transport, a drug carrier is required but no energy is necessary. This is the case with vitamin B_{12} transport. This type of transport:

- Is saturable if not enough carrier is present for the demand
- May show competitive inhibition of carrier
- Does not proceed against a concentration gradient

Ion Pair Transport

This type of transport involves a complex of drug a organic anion with a medium or membrane cation. Examples include the transport of quaternary ammonium compounds, doxorubicin, ampicillin, quinine HCl, and sulfonic acids.

Endocytosis, Pinocytosis, Phagocytosis, and Exocytosis

Endocytosis is the internal uptake of materials (including foreign substances or microorganisms) or solutions by the cell in a process that involves invagination of the plasma membrane and formation of vesicle-like structures. Endocytosis includes both processes of pinocytosis (cell drinking) and phagocytosis (cell eating). Exocytosis is the reverse of endocytosis, whereby substances are secreted from the cell. Although this type of cellular transport is more common in cellular homeostasis and the immune response, it plays an important role in the cellular transport of vitamin D.

pH of Body Compartments

The extent of ionization of weak acids and bases will depend on the pH of the body compartment. These values determine the extent of absorption (and also distribution and elimination) of the drug. The Henderson–Hasselbach equation is useful in determining how much drug will be found on either side of a membrane that separates two compartments that differ in pH, i.e., the stomach (pH 1.0 to 1.5) and blood plasma (pH 7.4). This was shown in Figure 5.6 for the absorption of a drug.

The lipid solubility of the nonionized drug directly determines its rate of equilibration across both sides of any given membrane. One way to measure the lipid solubility of a drug is through its partition coefficient, described in Equation (5.3), as the ratio of the concentration of drug in *n*-octanol (a lipophilic solvent) and the drug concentration in water. *N*-octanol is a convenient choice to use in a biphasic system with water, and together these two solvents resemble the biphasic (lipid:aqueous) system present in biological membranes.

$$P = \frac{[\text{Drug}]_{n\text{-octanol}}}{[\text{Drug}]_{H20}}$$

Equation 5.3   Partition coefficient.

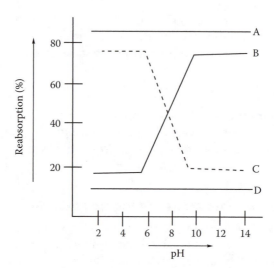

Figure 5.9

Example 5.1

The graph in Figure 5.9 shows the passive reabsorption of four drugs (see structures in Figure 5.10) in the kidneys as a function of urine pH. For each drug choose the appropriate graph A, B, C, or D, that best describes the dependence of its reabsorption on urine pH.

Answer: The problem statement specifically refers to a passive diffusion process. As mentioned in the description of Fick's first law of diffusion, the diffusion coefficient is larger when the lipid solubility is higher. A large organic molecule without any ionizable group would be more lipid soluble than an organic molecule of similar size but containing an ionizable and/or an ionic group. The more lipid-soluble molecule will diffuse better through the lipid environment of the cell membrane. Obviously, the pH of the compartment will affect the degree of ionization and therefore the rate of diffusion. Comparing the four drug molecules shown above, we look for the functional groups present in each to evaluate what effect, if any, pH will have on the molecular species present. Spironolactone is large and hydrophobic (high percent reabsorption), and does not have a functional group that can ionize; therefore, it will not be affected

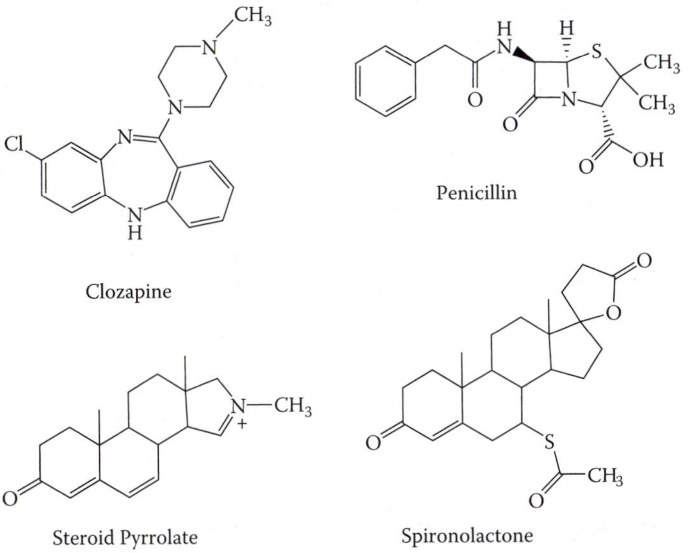

Clozapine

Penicillin

Steroid Pyrrolate

Spironolactone

Figure 5.10

in its distribution pattern by changes in compartment pH (straight line). *Graph "A" corresponds to spironolactone.* Steroid pyrrolate is a quaternary amine and therefore it is fully charged (not lipid soluble = low percent reabsorption) and not affected by compartment pH (straight line). *Graph "D" corresponds to steroid pyrrolate.* The other two drugs have ionizable groups that would be affected in opposite ways by compartment pH: clozapine has basic functional groups (amines) that will be protonated and therefore ionized at low pHs. This ionized form of the drug (not lipid soluble) will show low percent reabsorption. *Graph "B" corresponds to Clozapine (low pH = low % reabsorption).* Penicillin has a carboxylic acid group that at low pH will also be protonated, but this form of the drug is unionized and lipid soluble. *Graph "C" corresponds to penicillin (low pH = high % reabsorption).*

Other Factors That Affect Absorption

Blood Flow to the Absorption Site

Blood flow to the intestines is much greater than flow to the stomach. For this reason, absorption from the intestines is favored over that from the stomach.

Surface Area Available for Absorption

The intestines have a surface rich in microvilli that gives them a total surface area 1000 times that of the stomach; thus, absorption from the intestine is more efficient.

Contact Time at the Absorption Surface

If the drug moves across the gastrointestinal tract very quickly, as in severe diarrhea, it is not well absorbed. Conversely, anything that delays the transport of the drug from the stomach to the intestine delays the rate of absorption of the drug. Exercise or stressful emotions prolong gastric emptying, which in turn results in slower absorption. The presence of food in the stomach dilutes the drug and slows gastric emptying and absorption.

DRUG ABSORPTION, BIOAVAILABILITY, AND FIRST-PASS METABOLISM

Bioavailability refers to the rate and extent of drug absorption into the bloodstream and depends on the physiology of the patient, the physico-chemical properties of the drug, and the formulation of the pharmaceutical product. The pharmaceutical product is the actual dosage form, such as the tablet, capsule, or transdermal patch, containing the active pharma-ceutical ingredient (drug molecules) and other additives that act as dilu-ents, stabilizers, or lubricants. The type and amount of additives and the degree of compression affect how quickly a tablet disintegrates and dissolves. Drug manufacturers adjust these variables to optimize the bio-availability of their oral dosage forms. Tablets that dissolve and release the drug too quickly may produce an excessive response, as was seen in the tolbutamide case discussed earlier in this chapter. On the other hand, tablets that do not dissolve quickly enough may pass into the feces without being absorbed. Food, other drugs, and disease states can also influence drug bioavailability. Reduced bioavailability also occurs in many oral dosage forms because of a process known as first-pass metabolism. Figure 5.11 shows this process in a schematic way.

Most oral dosage forms are absorbed from the gastrointestinal tract and enter the portal vein, which delivers the materials to the liver prior to reaching the general circulation. In the liver, the main organ for metabolism, a significant amount of an administered dose may be changed into inactive metabolites, therefore limiting the efficacy of an oral dosage form. First-pass metabolism can also occur in the small intestine. The bioavailability of an oral dosage form will depend not only on how much

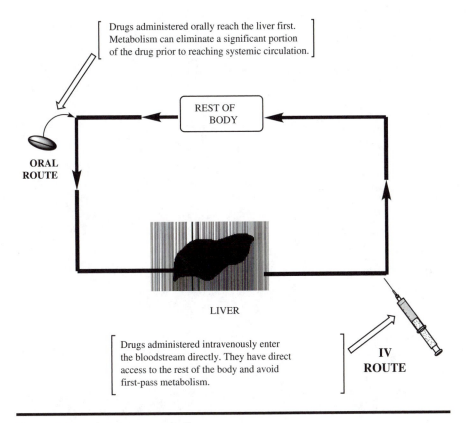

Figure 5.11   First-pass metabolism.

of the dose is absorbed into the portal circulation but also on how much of the actual dose leaves the liver unchanged and can go to its pharmacological target. The equation that describes this important pharmacokinetic variable will be presented in the following chapter, together with the remainder of the key pharmacokinetic variables that determine drug distribution, elimination, and duration of action.

FURTHER READING

1. *Drug Actions: Basic Principles and Therapeutic Aspects* by E. Mutschler (Editor) and H. Derendorf (Editor). Chapters 2.1 and 2.2. CRC Press (1995).

2. *Goodman & Gilman's The Pharmacological Basis of Therapeutics* by Joel Griffith Hardman, Lee E. Limbird, Alfred G. Gilman. Chapter 1. McGraw-Hill Professional; 10th Edition (2001).

3. *Pharmacology — Lippincott's Illustrated Reviews* by M. J. Mycek, R. A. Harvey, and P. C. Champe. Chapter 1. Lippincott Williams & Wilkins; 2nd Edition (2000).

6

DISTRIBUTION AND EXCRETION OF DRUGS

In this chapter we will address the processes of drug distribution and excretion, as well as give an introduction to the pharmacokinetic variables involved in the absorption, distribution, and elimination of drugs. The process of elimination consists of both the metabolism and the excretion of drugs. Drug metabolism is discussed in greater detail in Chapter 7, and drug absorption was discussed in Chapter 5.

After a drug is absorbed into the bloodstream, it circulates throughout the body and has the possibility of entering various organs and tissues. Drugs will penetrate different organs and tissues at different speeds, depending on their ability to cross the various membrane barriers at these locations. Some drugs bind strongly to plasma proteins, such as albumin, and therefore do not quickly leave the blood compartment. Other drugs may pass from the blood into fat tissue, where they may be stored for some time, thereby preventing the drug from reaching its site of action and prolonging the time the drug is in the body. Still other drugs distribute out of the plasma and into the watery parts of tissues such as muscle, while others may have affinity for specific tissues within the liver, the thyroid gland, and the kidneys. The distribution of a drug may also vary among different people, depending on their frame size and fat content. Figure 6.1 shows these interactions that affect drug distribution.

FACTORS IN DRUG DISTRIBUTION

The factors that determine the rate and extent of drug distribution are the following:

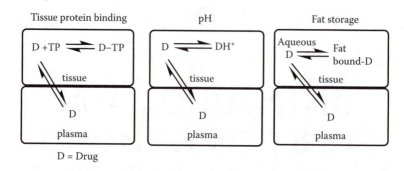

Figure 6.1   Processes affecting drug distribution.

- *Rate of distribution* — Capillary permeability determines how fast a drug can move out of the bloodstream and into body organs and tissues.
- *Extent of distribution* — Drug structure, compartment pH, protein binding, and intracellular binding affect the extent of drug distribution into specific organs or tissues.

Capillary Permeability

Endothelial cells line the inside of the heart, blood vessels, and lymphatic vessels. Capillary permeability to drugs can vary depending on how tight the junctions are between endothelial cells. Capillary endothelium in general has junctions between cells that are discontinuous, which makes capillary walls quite permeable. Lipid-soluble drugs pass through vascular endothelium rapidly, while water-soluble compounds penetrate more slowly, at a rate dependent on their molecular size. Drugs of low molecular weight pass through by simple diffusion.

There are two important deviations from this typical structure of capillary walls that have a profound effect on drug distribution:

1. *Brain capillaries* have essentially no slit junctions and have endothelial cells so close together that they form the so-called blood–brain barrier. Transfer of molecules from blood to brain tissue is highly restricted, a natural consequence of our brains being "central command" for the complex functioning of our bodies. Only lipid-soluble drugs (like the anesthetics) can cross the blood–brain barrier; other drugs can enter the brain by active transport if they resemble an endogenous substance that requires active transport to enter the brain. For example, the large neutral amino acid carrier transfers

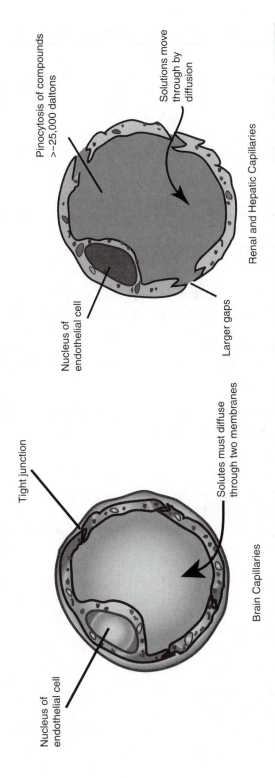

Figure 6.2   Structure of brain, renal and hepatic capillaries.

Table 6.1   Blood Perfusion Rates for Selected Organs

Organ	Perfusion Rate (mL/min/mL of Tissue)	% of Cardiac Output
Skin	0.05	5
Muscle	0.03	15
Fat	0.01	2
Brain	0.55	15
Heart	0.7	4
Liver	0.75	20
Kidneys	4.5	24

levodopa (an anti-Parkinson's drug) into the brain. Other than some special cases, ionized or polar drugs fail to enter the central nervous system.

2. *Renal and hepatic capillaries* (sinusoids) have very permeable capillary walls because their endothelial cells have large gaps in their junctions. This results in more extensive distribution of drugs and proteins out of the capillary bed. This deviation in the capillary structure is specially suited for the organs involved in drug elimination.

Figure 6.2a shows these two deviations in the structure of the capillary walls, which impact drug distribution.

Blood Perfusion

The other major factor that affects the rate of drug distribution is blood perfusion. Blood perfusion is the blood flow (i.e., mL/min) per unit volume of tissue. Table 6.1 shows typical blood perfusion of selected organs. The percent of the cardiac output required by these organs is a measure of their total blood flow.

The organs with highest perfusion rates are the brain, heart, kidneys, and liver. On the other hand, total blood flow is largest to the brain, kidneys, liver, and muscle. Drug concentration is expected to rise most rapidly in these organs.

Perfusion and Permeability

An organ with high perfusion rates has high levels of exposure for drugs circulating in the bloodstream; however, the membranes of the organ may not be very permeable, and therefore drug distribution into the organ will

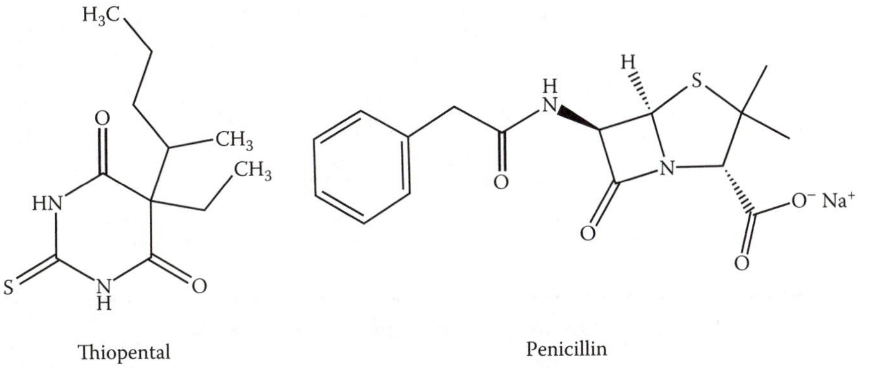

Figure 6.3   Structures of thiopental and penicillin.

be limited. Comparing drug transfer into brain and muscle, for example, it would appear that drug transfer is favored in the brain (high perfusion rate) better than in the muscle (low perfusion rate). However, the brain capillaries are essentially impermeable (blood–brain barrier), while muscle capillaries are much more permeable to drugs. The structure of the drug will play a key role into which of these two organs it distributes. For example, thiopental (pK_a = 7.5) is only partly ionized in the bloodstream (pH = 7.4) and will easily diffuse through membranes. It is not membrane permeability that limits its transport into tissue, but rather organ blood perfusion. Since the brain is more highly perfused than the muscles, thiopental can transfer into the brain faster than into the muscle. This is called "perfusion-limited" transport. On the other hand, penicillin (pK_a = 2.8) is much more ionized at blood pH and therefore does not cross membranes easily. Its transport will be limited by membrane permeability. Since the muscle capillaries are less restrictive, penicillin can penetrate muscles faster than the brain; this is called "permeability-limited" transport. The structures of thiopental and penicillin are shown in Figure 6.3.

Example 6.1

Compare the structures of ipratropium bromide and propranolol (Figure 6.4) and explain which of these drugs will penetrate the brain faster and which will penetrate the muscle faster.

Answer: Ipratropium bromide is a quaternary amine salt and therefore will diffuse extremely slowly. Permeability-limited transport allows this drug to diffuse faster into the muscles than

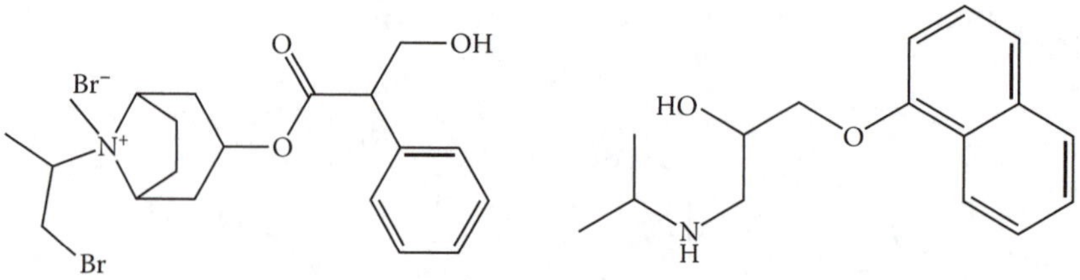

Figure 6.4 Structures of ipratropium bromide and propranolol.

into the brain. Propranolol (pK_a = 9.5), on the other hand, is only partly ionized at the pH of the blood and can diffuse more readily through membranes. Its distribution is limited by organ perfusion, which is higher in the brain than in the muscles. Propranolol distributes in the brain faster than in muscles.

We will now consider the factors that affect the extent of drug distribution. These factors include:

- Drug structure (pK_a, lipid solubility)
- Compartment pH
- Plasma protein binding
- Intracellular binding

Drug Structure and Compartment pH

The lipid solubility of a drug gives an indication of *how fast it will equilibrate* across the membrane barriers, but it is the pK_a and compartment pH that will determine the amount of the drug (extent) that will distribute into a given compartment or organ. Examples of this interrelationship between a drug's structure, its pK_a, and the compartment pH were discussed in Chapter 2, when the acid–base nature of drugs and the Henderson–Hasselbach equation were discussed.

Plasma Protein Binding

Binding to plasma proteins can cause a drug to remain largely in the blood compartment. The most common protein involved in this type of interaction is albumin, which comprises about 50% of the total protein in blood. Acidic drugs, such as warfarin, commonly bind to albumin, while basic drugs (i.e., chlorpropamide) bind to glycoproteins and lipoproteins.

Intracellular Binding

Drugs not only bind to plasma proteins, they may bind to intracellular molecules, some of which may be the actual drug receptors. Therefore, the interaction that occurs may represent the molecular basis of their pharmacological effect.

The affinity of a drug for a tissue may be due to several interactions, including binding to tissue proteins, binding to nucleic acids, or dissolution into the lipid material. For example, chloroquine binds to DNA in the liver; therefore, high levels of this drug distribute into the liver tissues. Barbiturates are highly lipid soluble and therefore distribute extensively into fat tissue. Tetracyclines bind to bone and developing teeth and for this reason can cause discoloration of permanent teeth in young children.

The nature of the binding forces between drugs and macromolecules in the blood and tissues have been encountered before: electrostatic interactions, hydrogen bonding, and Van der Waals forces. These concepts were reviewed in Chapter 1.

Groups in protein molecules that are responsible for electrostatic interactions with drugs include:

- The $-NH_3^+$ of lysine and N-terminal amino acids
- The $-NH_2^+-$ of histidine's imidazole ring nitrogens
- The $-S^-$ of cysteine
- The $-COO^-$ of aspartic and glutamic acids

Hydrogen bonding occurs between an electronegative atom containing nonbonding electrons (i.e., O, N) and a hydrogen atom attached to an electronegative element by a covalent bond. Van der Waals forces are weak but can be very numerous and therefore significant.

Often there may be competition between drugs for the binding sites of macromolecules. For example, coumarin anticoagulants (i.e., warfarin) can displace less tightly bound compounds from albumin.

PATTERNS OF DISTRIBUTION

The distribution of drugs can be thought of as following one of four patterns, as shown in Figure 6.5. Drugs that are highly bound to plasma proteins remain largely in the blood compartment. This is shown in Figure 6.5 as pattern #1. Many low-molecular-weight, water-soluble compounds (e.g., ethanol, some sulfonamides) distribute uniformly throughout body water. This is shown in Figure 6.5 as pattern #2. Some drugs concentrate in tissues that may or may not be their sites of action. As mentioned previously, chloroquine binds to liver DNA and tetracycline binds to bone

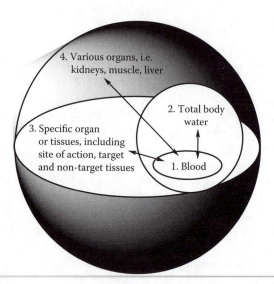

Figure 6.5 Patterns of drug distribution.

and developing teeth. Iodine concentrates in the thyroid gland. This is shown in Figure 6.5 as pattern #3. Most drugs exhibit a combination of all of these patterns, shown in Figure 6.5 as pattern #4. This nonuniform distribution pattern is the result of variations in the ability of drugs to cross membranes, as well as all the other factors discussed under rate and extent of distribution. A useful indicator of the type of distribution pattern of a drug is its "apparent volume of distribution." This is an important pharmacokinetic variable that is not a real volume but rather a hypothetical volume of fluid into which the drug distributes. Equation (6.1a) is the mathematical expression of the volume of distribution (V_d); it expresses the relation between total amount of drug in the body and the plasma concentration of the drug.

$$V_d = \frac{\text{Total amount of drug in the body (A)}}{\text{Plasma drug concentration (C}_P)}$$

Equation 6.1a Volume of distribution of a drug.

The major determinant of the volume of distribution is the relative strength of the binding of drug to plasma proteins vs. binding to tissue components.

Although the volume of distribution is not a real physiological fluid, it is sometimes useful to compare the distribution of a drug with the volumes of various water compartments in the average 70-kg individual. Figure 6.6 and Table 6.2 show these distribution volumes.

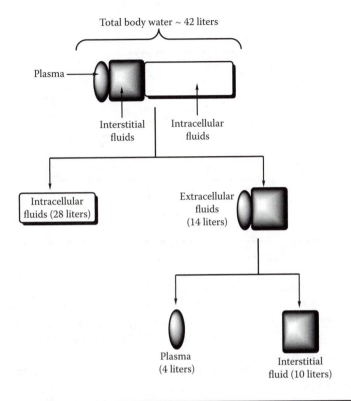

Figure 6.6   Water volumes of several body compartments.

Table 6.2   Body Compartment Volumes[a]

Compartment	Volume (L)
Plasma	3 to 4
Interstitial fluids	10 to 13
Extracellular fluid	13 to 16
Intracellular fluids	25 to 28
Total body water	40 to 46

[a] Approximate values

A value of Vd in the vicinity of 4 liters would be comparable to distribution pattern #1 (Figure 6.5) and indicates that the drug most likely distributes in the plasma compartment (Figure 6.6). This is the case for tolbutamide or furosemide. On the other hand, a Vd of 40 L for enalapril indicates that it distributes according to pattern #2 (Figure 6.5) in total

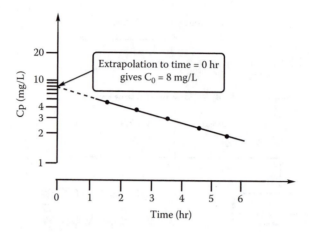

Figure 6.7   Determination of Vd.

body water (Figure 6.6). Very large volumes of distribution such as that of fluoxetine or chloroquine indicate that the drug is being sequestered in some tissue, making the plasma concentration very low. A very small number in the denominator of Equation (6.1d) makes the resulting Vd a very large number.

Drugs that follow distribution pattern #4 may have Vd within a wide range of values.

DETERMINATION OF THE VOLUME OF DISTRIBUTION

A common method for determining Vd is illustrated in Figure 6.7, which shows a linear relationship between the logarithm of plasma drug concentration and time.

Let us assume a dose of 240 mg of drug X is given to a patient, and blood samples are collected every hour, starting at 1.5 hours after administration. Plasma drug concentrations (Cp) can then be measured and their logarithms plotted against the time values for blood sampling. Extrapolation back to time = 0 hr gives the plasma drug concentration when the whole 240 mg dose is still in the body and prior to elimination. In this case, the intercept on the y-axis gives a Cp of 8 mg/L (see Figure 6.7). Substituting these values in Equation (6.1a) gives a Vd of 30 L (see Equation 6.1b).

$$V = \frac{\text{Dose}}{C_0} = \frac{240 \text{ mg}}{8 \text{ mg/L}} = 30 \text{ L}$$

Equation 6.1b   Determination of Vd.

Table 6.3   Apparent Volumes of Distribution

Drug	L/kg	L/70 kg
Tolbutamide	0.1	7
Furosemide	0.11	8
Enalapril	0.57	40
Ciprofloxacin	1.86	130
Morphine	3.29	230
Fluoxetine	35.7	2500
Chloroquine	94–250	6600–17,500

In order to achieve a target plasma drug concentration we need to know the volume of distribution of the drug so we may administer a suitable loading dose. Equation (6.2) expresses this.

$$\text{Loading dose} = V_d * \text{target } C_p$$

Equation 6.2   Loading dose of a drug.

Example 6.2

Calculate the loading dose of theophylline at the start of a theophylline infusion if Vd= 0.5 L/kg (35 L for a 70 kg person) and the desired Cp = 10 mg/L.

Answer: The desired Cp and the value of Vd are given. Using this data in Equation (6.2) gives Equation (6.3):

$$\text{Loading dose} = 0.5\,\frac{L}{kg} * 70\,kg * 10\,\frac{mg}{L} = 350\,mg$$

Equation 6.3   Calculation of theophylline loading dose (Example 6.2).

Result: Loading dose = 350 mg

Table 6.3 gives the apparent volumes of distribution for selected drugs.

Aside from volume of distribution, the other primary pharmacokinetic parameter is clearance (CL). Clearance is defined as the volume of blood cleared of drug per unit time. Clearance describes the efficiency of "irreversible" drug elimination, which includes:

- Excretion of unchanged drug in urine, sweat, expired air, feces, etc.
- Biotransformation into a different chemical

Uptake of the drug into various tissues is not clearance (as long as it remains the same chemical entity administered) since the drug can eventually come back out of the tissue.

CLEARANCE AND ELIMINATION RATE

Clearance is also the constant relating the rate of elimination of a drug to its plasma concentration, as shown in Equation (6.4).

$$\underset{\text{(mg/h)}}{\text{Elimination rate}} = \underset{\text{(L/h)}}{\text{CL}} \times \underset{\text{(mg/L)}}{C_{plasma}}$$

Equation 6.4   Elimination rate.

From Equation (6.4) it is evident that for a given clearance, which is a constant for a particular drug and a specific patient, the elimination rate varies directly with the plasma drug concentration.

CLEARANCE AND THE MAINTENANCE DOSE RATE

Clearance is a key parameter that allows the pharmacist to determine the maintenance dose rate required to achieve a target plasma concentration at steady state. *At "steady-state" the rate of drug administration equals the rate of drug elimination,* so the amount of drug in the body, and therefore Cp, remains constant. Equation (6.5) expresses this relationship.

$$\text{Elimination rate} = \text{Maintenance dose rate (DR)}$$

Equation 6.5   Maintenance dose rate.

Combining Equation (6.4) and Equation (6.5), it follows that the maintenance dose rate required to achieve the steady-state plasma drug concentration (Css) can be calculated by Equation (6.6).

$$\underset{\text{(mg/hr)}}{\text{Maintenance Dose Rate (DR)}} = \underset{\text{(L/hr)}}{\text{Clearance (CL)}} * \underset{\text{(mg/L)}}{\text{Css}}$$

Equation 6.6   Clearance and maintenance dose rate.

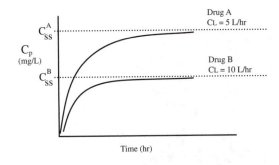

Figure 6.8 Clearance and steady state plasma concentration in IV infusion.

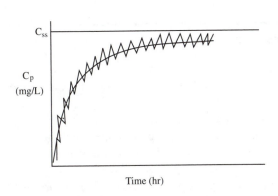

Figure 6.9 Clearance and steady-state plasma concentration with oral dosing.

This is illustrated in Figure 6.8 for two drugs, A and B, administered as continuous intravenous infusions.

Drug B has a clearance double that of Drug A. In both cases, the plasma drug concentrations rise steadily until a plateau is reached, which is the steady state. It is clear from Equation (6.4) that the plasma concentration is inversely related to clearance, and for this reason Drug B, with twice the clearance of A, gives a Css that is only half of the clearance that can be achieved by Drug A. The situation is more complex for oral dosing, since the drug concentrations fluctuate during the dosing intervals due to absorption and elimination. This is shown in Figure 6.9.

Eventually, however, the amount of drug eliminated during the dosing interval equals the dose administered. At this point, Cp fluctuates over the same range every dosing interval, steady state has been reached, and the average Cp over the dosing interval equals Css of the constant IV

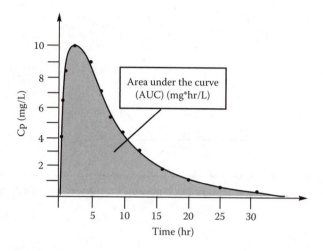

Figure 6.10 Measurement of clearance.

infusion. The effect of clearance will be the same as described above, i.e., if clearance is reduced by half, the steady-state concentration (Css) will double.

Clearance can be determined by measuring plasma drug concentration at several time intervals following a single, intravenous dose. This is illustrated in Figure 6.10, which shows the exponential decay of Cp over time.

The area under the curve (AUC) and the dose administered can then be used to calculate clearance, as seen in Equation (6.7).

$$\frac{\text{Clearance}}{\text{(L/hr)}} = \frac{\text{Dose}}{\text{AUC}} \left(\frac{\text{mg}}{\text{mg} * \text{hr/L}} \right)$$

Equation 6.7 Clearance and AUC.

Clearance can also be measured using Equation (6.8) if we know when to measure the steady state concentration (Css). (Compare with Equation 6.6.)

$$\text{Clearance} = \frac{\text{Infusion rate}}{C_{ss}}$$

Equation 6.8 Clearance and steady state.

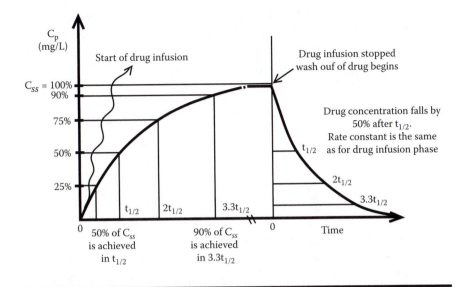

Figure 6.11   Half-life and steady state.

This brings us to the discussion of another pharmacokinetic variable, namely, half-life ($t_{1/2}$).

HALF-LIFE AND THE STEADY STATE

Drug concentration rises from zero at the start of the infusion until it reaches the steady-state level at the constant infusion rate. Half-life ($t_{1/2}$) is the time required for the drug concentration to change by 50%. Figure 6.11 shows the relationship between the half-life and steady state.

For convenience, it is frequently assumed that the steady state is reached after four $t_{1/2}$. The rate of approach to steady state, as shown in Figure 6.11, is a first-order process. When drug infusion is stopped, its plasma concentration declines (washes out) to zero with the same kinetic profile as the approach to steady state. Equation (6.9) gives the rate expression for first-order elimination after drug infusion is stopped.

$$Ct = C_o e^{-kt}$$
Drug elimination

Equation 6.9   Drug elimination.

C_t is the concentration of the drug at various times, C_o is the initial concentration at time zero, and k is the elimination rate constant.

Solving Equation (6.9) when $C_t = 0.5\ C_0$, that is, when drug concentration has changed by 50%, gives Equation (6.10).

$$0.5C_o = C_o e^{-kt}$$

$$0.5 = e^{-kt}$$

$$\ln(1/2) = -kt$$

$$\ln 1 - \ln 2 = -kt$$

$$-0.693 = -kt_{1/2}$$

$$t_{1/2} = \frac{0.7}{k}$$

1st Order elimination

Equation 6.10   Half-life for first-order drug elimination.

The rate constant (k) in Equation (6.10) depends on clearance and volume of distribution as shown in Equation (6.11).

$$k = \frac{CL}{Vd}$$

Equation 6.11   Elimination rate constant.

Substituting Equation (6.11) into Equation (6.10) gives Equation (6.12).

$$t_{1/2} = \frac{0.7\,Vd}{CL}$$

Equation 6.12   Half-life.

Half-life is decreased by an increase in clearance or a decrease in volume of distribution, and vice versa. The effects of Vd and CL on half-life are illustrated in Table 6.4 for several common drugs.

Chloroquine has a high clearance but very long $t_{1/2}$ because of the large volume of distribution. On the other hand, erythromycin and lithium

Table 6.4   Interrelationships of Vd, CL, and t$_{1/2}$

Drug	Vd	CL	t$_{1/2}$
Chloroquine	13,000	45	214
Erythromycin	55	38.4	1.6
Lithium	55	1.5	22
Acyclovir	48	19.8	2.4
Amikacin	19	5.46	2.3

have approximately the same volume of distribution, but erythromycin has a clearance about 25 times larger than that of lithium. For that reason lithium has a t$_{1/2}$ ~14 times longer than that of erythromycin. Acyclovir and amikacin have the same t$_{1/2}$, however, acyclovir has the larger of the two Vd values, as well as the larger clearance, with the two values canceling out to give approximately the same fraction (t$_{1/2}$) as amikacin.

In summary, half-life is used to determine:

■ Time required to reach steady state
■ The duration of action after a single dose
■ The frequency of drug administration

The last of the pharmacokinetic parameters to be discussed in this chapter is bioavailability, which was mentioned in Chapter 5 since it relates to the process of drug absorption. It is discussed here in the context of presenting the mathematical expressions for all the pharmacokinetic variables.

BIOAVAILABILITY

Bioavailability (F) is the fraction of *unchanged* drug reaching systemic circulation by any route. It is equal to 1 (one) for intravenous dosing, but for other routes, bioavailability will depend on how well the drug is absorbed (f$_g$) and how much can escape elimination by the liver in the first pass (f$_h$). First-pass metabolism of a drug is expressed by the hepatic extraction ratio (E$_h$). The expression for bioavailability is given by Equation (6.13).

$$F = f_g * f_H$$

Bioavailability (F) = fraction absorbed * fraction escaping first-pass elimination

---

Equation 6.13   Bioavailability.

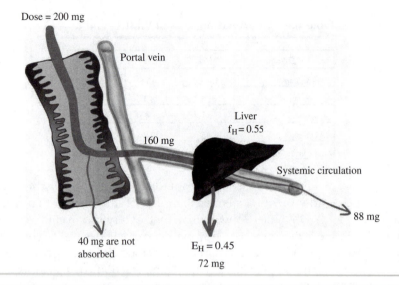

Dose = 200 mg

Portal vein

Liver
$f_H = 0.55$

160 mg

Systemic circulation

88 mg

40 mg are not
absorbed

$E_H = 0.45$

72 mg

Figure 6.12   Bioavailability exercise.

Example 6.3

A drug is administered in a 200 mg dose, is 80% absorbed, and has a hepatic extraction ratio of 0.45. What is its bioavailability?

Answer: 44%. Figure 6.12 shows the problem in schematic form. Since the drug is 80% absorbed into the portal circulation, 0.8×200 mg = 160 mg enter the liver and 40 mg (the remainder of the dose) is excreted in the feces. The 160 mg entering the liver is metabolized (first-pass effect) by 45% (0.45 hepatic extraction ratio) and only 55% of it escapes metabolism and enters systemic circulation. Substituting appropriate values in the bioavailability equation (Equation 6.13) gives the following result (Equation 6.14):

$$F = 0.8 * 0.55 = 0.44 \text{ or } 44\%$$

Equation 6.14   Calculation of bioavailability (Example 6.3).

Some drugs are so highly extracted by the liver during first pass that their oral bioavailability is negligible. This is the case for glyceryl trinitrate, which must be administered by the sublingual or transdermal route in order to avoid first-pass effect.

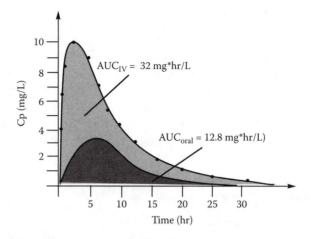

Figure 6.13   Area under the curve (AUC) and absolute bioavailability.

Bioavailability can be measured by comparing the area under the curve (AUC) for a dose given orally with the AUC for the same dose administered by intravenous infusion. This is shown in Equation (6.15) and Figure 6.13.

$$F = \frac{AUC_{oral}}{AUC_{iv}} = \text{Absolute bioavailability}$$

Equation 6.15   Absolute bioavailability.

The area under the curve for the oral dose (AUC_{oral}) is 40% of the area under the curve for the intravenous dose (AUC_{iv}). The absolute bioavailability for the oral formulation is in this case 40%.

Relative bioavailability is used to compare a new oral formulation of a drug against a reference oral formulation of the drug, as seen in Equation (6.16).

$$\text{Relative bioavailability} = \frac{AUC_{test}}{AUC_{ref}}$$

Equation 6.16   Relative Bioavailability.

The two formulations are bioequivalent if the ratio of their AUCs is in the range 0.8 to 1.25.

DRUG ELIMINATION

Drugs can be eliminated from the body either by physical removal, through the process of excretion, or by change into a different chemical entity, through metabolism. The biotransformation reactions of metabolism are explained in Chapter 7, so we can focus on the process of drug excretion for the remainder of the present chapter.

Drugs may be removed from the body through the lungs, the intestines, the bile, or the milk (in nursing mothers), but most importantly through the kidneys.

The Enterohepatic Cycle

Many drugs are excreted from the liver into the bile, and from the bile they reach the small intestines. However, many of the drugs that reach the intestines in this way do not end up in the feces but are reabsorbed into the superior mesenteric vein, entering the liver again through the portal vein. This recycling process is called the enterohepatic cycle, and is shown in Figure 6.14.

Enterohepatic cycling is responsible for the extended presence in the body of drugs such as the hypnotic glutethimide, digitoxin in the therapy of heart failure, and the contraceptive ethinyl estradiol. Eventually, the drug will be removed from the body by a combination of metabolism and excretion, but the effect of enterohepatic cycling can be detrimental in some cases, as the concentration of the drug in the body will increase with every additional dose, leading to possible toxic side effects. This is seen in the therapy of acute gout attacks with colchicine. Erythromycin also exhibits enterohepatic cycling but does not have as many toxicity problems as colchicine does.

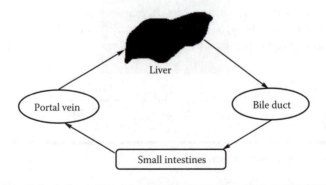

Figure 6.14 Enterohepatic cycle.

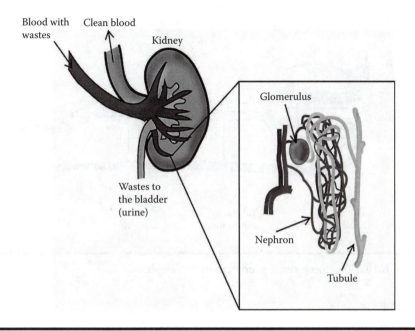

Figure 6.15   Functional elements of the kidneys.

Renal Excretion

The kidney is the most important organ for drug excretion. Within the kidney, the nephrons are the cellular units responsible for the kidney's filtering activities, processing a constant flow of blood full of waste, and able to sort out fluids, proteins, and nutrients. The latter are returned to the bloodstream, while toxic and unnecessary substances are collected in the urine and forwarded to the bladder for removal from the body.

Figure 6.15 shows the two key structural elements of the nephron: the tubule and the glomerulus. The tubule is a long tube that at one point extends into a bulb-like section called "Bowman's capsule." The glomerulus is contained within this capsule and consists of capillaries originating in branches of the renal artery, where blood is received for filtration. The blood at this point carries many waste materials but also other valuable components that must be retained in the body, such as water, glucose, and amino acids. The fluid resulting from blood filtration at the glomerulus passes into the tubule, which itself is surrounded by many thousands of capillaries. In a very complicated process, water and valuable materials are reabsorbed into the bloodstream during passage of this fluid through the renal tubules. The waste materials continue down the tubule and end up as urine in the bladder.

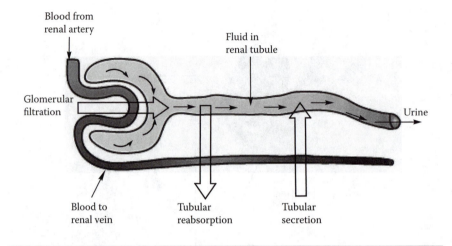

Figure 6.16   The three renal processes at the nephron.

Renal Processes

The three key processes involved in renal excretion are as follows:

1. *Glomerular filtration*: Blood is filtered into the tubule, forming the primitive urine.
2. *Tubular reabsorption*: Substances needed by the body, such as water, minerals and amino acids, are absorbed from the tubules back into the bloodstream. For most drugs, reabsorption is a passive diffusion process, depending on drug solubility, pK_a of the drug, and urine pH. It is possible to alter the urinary pH to enhance excretion of a drug; this was discussed in Chapter 2 under the acid–base properties of drugs.
3. *Tubular secretion*: As the primitive urine travels down the tubule, some substances, including drugs and excess ions, are secreted from the capillaries surrounding the tubule and into the fluid that is flowing toward the bladder. This is an energy-requiring, carrier-mediated process (active transport). There are carrier systems in the tubules capable of transporting numerous acids (e.g., penicillin) and bases (e.g., ranitidine) against a concentration gradient.

The excretion rate for any given substance will be a combination of these three processes, as shown in Equation (6.17) and Figure 6.16, which shows these three processes in a single nephron.

$$\text{Excretion Rate} = \text{Filtration} - \text{Reabsorption} + \text{Secretion}$$

Equation 6.17   Rate of renal excretion.

FURTHER READING

1. *Drug Actions: Basic Principles and Therapeutic Aspects* by E. Mutschler (Editor) and H. Derendorf (Editor). Chapters 2.3 and 2.5. CRC Press (1995).
2. *Basic and Clinical Pharmacology* by Bertram G. Katzung (Editor). Chapter 3. Lange Medical Books/McGraw-Hill; 9th Edition (2004).
3. *Pharmacokinetics Made Easy* by D. J. Birkett. McGraw-Hill Book Company Australia (2002).

7

METABOLIC CHANGES
OF DRUGS

Metabolism is a fundamental process in the body that transforms drugs and other foreign substances (xenobiotics), as well as endogenous substances, into entities that can be excreted or sometimes recycled. The body, when presented with the challenge of a chemical from the outside, will compensate by changing it, in a series of reactions, into a substance that can be more readily eliminated from the body. Otherwise, drugs and other xenobiotics would remain indefinitely in the body eliciting their biological effects, whether beneficial or detrimental, a situation that is not to be desired if most of the biological effects of the xenobiotic are toxic.

Metabolism transforms drugs and xenobiotics into more polar, water-soluble products that can be excreted in the urine, for example, and the products are generally (but not always) less toxic and less pharmacologically active. However, many drugs are metabolized into substances that have greater or different pharmacological effects than those of the parent compound. The enzymes and cofactors required to carry out the task of metabolism can be found in most cell types but are present in especially large concentrations in the liver.

Pharmaceutical manufacturers usually anticipate and evaluate the pharmacological actions of all major metabolites of a drug before obtaining approval by the Food and Drug Administration (FDA) for a New Drug Application. Indeed, the science of metabolic reactions has advanced to the point where the enzymes responsible for the biotransformations are commercially available and can be used to study the metabolic changes of a drug in the laboratory.

Metabolic reactions of drugs are categorized as Phase I, or functionalization reactions, and Phase II, or conjugation reactions. In Phase I reactions a functional group is "uncovered" in the drug molecule; this functional group will later act as a handle for the conjugation (Phase II) reaction. Phase I reactions include oxidations, reductions, and hydrolysis of certain functional groups in drug molecules. Phase II reactions include the conjugation of the Phase I reaction product (metabolite) with endogenous substances such as glucuronic acid, glutathione, amino acids, sulfate, and acetate. The sequence of metabolic reactions most frequently follows the path shown in Equation (7.1).

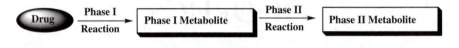

Equation 7.1   The sequence of metabolic reactions.

Later in this chapter we will discuss each reaction type, but we must focus first on a key player of metabolic reactions, the cytochrome P450 enzyme system. Most of the oxidations in Phase I reactions involve this oxidase enzyme, which is part of a multicomponent electron-transfer chain that transfers a *single* oxygen atom from O_2 into the drug molecule, while the second oxygen atom from O_2 ends up in water. For this reason, the cytochrome P450 enzymes are called "mixed-function oxygenase" or "monooxygenase" enzymes, in order to describe their function. But much of the individual enzyme nomenclature has a genetic origin, as will be seen in the following paragraphs.

CYTOCHROMES P450

The cytochromes P450 are families of heme proteins present in a large number of cell types and are also very widespread in nature. They are present in large amounts in the liver, which is the main organ for drug metabolism, but are also present in kidneys, gastrointestinal tract, and lungs.

Designation of a protein as cytochrome P450 was made on the basis of its spectral properties, before the catalytic functions of these proteins were understood. This family of proteins has a unique absorbance spectrum that is obtained by adding a reducing agent to a suspension of microsomes from the endoplasmic reticulum followed by bubbling of carbon monoxide gas into the solution. Carbon monoxide binds to the reduced heme protein and produces an absorbance spectrum with a maximum at approximately 450 nm. The name "P450," then, refers to the "pigment" with a peak at "450" nm. The various forms of cytochrome P450 have slightly different absorbance peaks, but they are usually in the range of 446 to 452 nm. The many forms of cytochrome P450 that exist are classified based on their sequence homologies into gene families and subfamilies. The term CYP is used as a preface and is composed of the first two letters in cytochrome and the first letter in P450. CYP450 nomenclature follows these guidelines:

- A *family* is denoted by CYP plus an Arabic numeral. All enzymes in a given family must have >40% homology in amino acid sequence. Examples: CYP1, CYP2, CYP3, etc.
- A *subfamily* is denoted by adding an Arabic letter and numeral to the family name of the enzyme. To belong to the same subfamily, enzymes must share greater than 55% homology in their amino acid sequences. Examples: CYP1A2, CYP3A4.

Because there are many different genes and therefore many different enzymes, we give the name of "isoforms" to the different CYP450 enzymes. Specific genes for the various CYP450 enzymes are distinguished from the actual isoforms by using italics for the gene (i.e., *CYP2D6*) and normal case for the enzyme (CYP2D6). A CYP450 isoform may be capable of metabolizing many different drugs, but a single enzyme may primarily metabolize a given drug. Several isoforms may also be involved in different metabolic reactions of any given drug molecule; for example, CYP1A2 and CYP2C19 are both involved in the metabolism of imipramine.

The majority of drug metabolic reactions in humans involve six isoforms within the CYP1, CYP2, and CYP3 families. Isoforms in the remaining 14 CYP families are involved in the biosynthesis and degradation of steroids, fatty acids, prostaglandins, and other endogenous compounds. This substrate specificity is depicted in Table 7.1.

The importance of the cytochrome P450 system is highlighted by the following facts:

1. It is the major system for xenobiotics and drug metabolism.
2. It explains many drug interactions.
3. It explains some toxic effects of drugs.
4. It is a source of variability in drug metabolism in different populations.

In the following paragraphs we will use specific examples to illustrate these statements.

Table 7.1 Substrates for Some CYP450 Families

CYP450 Family	Substrates
CYP1, CYP2, CYP3	Drugs and xenobiotics
CYP4 through CYP17	Steroids, fatty acids, vitamins, prostaglandins

Inhibition of Drug Metabolism

The six major CYP450 isoforms for drug metabolism in humans are: CYP1A2, CYP2C9, CYP2C19, CYP2D6, CYP3A4, and CYP2E1. CYP1A2, for example, metabolizes such drugs as clozapine, theophylline and warfarin. It also metabolizes ciprofloxacin and cimetidine, but more importantly, the latter drugs fit the active site of the enzyme better and they block the metabolism of theophylline, clozapine and warfarin (or any other CYP1A2 substrate), leading to *drug interactions*. CYP2C9 substrates include phenytoin and S-warfarin while inhibitors include fluconazole and isoniazid. CYP2C19 substrates include omeprazole and diazepam, and coadministration of a CYP2C19 inhibitor like fluoxetine would also lead to adverse drug interactions.

Many xenobiotics, including drugs, can inhibit metabolic enzymes. The result is decreased metabolic capacity and metabolic rate, not only of the inhibitor, but also of other drugs, xenobiotics, and endogenous compounds.

Consequences of enzyme inhibition in drug therapy include:

■ Increase in plasma levels with time in long-term medication
■ Prolonged pharmacological effects of parent drug
■ Enhancement of drug-induced toxicity

Induction of Drug Metabolism

Drug interactions can also arise when one drug administered to a patient *induces* the metabolism of a second drug taken concomitantly.

Many xenobiotics, including drugs, can induce increased levels of metabolic enzymes. The result is increased metabolic capacity and metabolic rate, not only of the inducer, but also of other drugs, xenobiotics, and endogenous compounds.

Consequences of enzyme induction in drug therapy include:

■ Decreased plasma levels with time in long-term medication
■ Decreased drug activity with time if metabolites are less active
■ Increased drug activity with time if metabolites are more active
■ Fall in plasma levels of endogenous compounds to below-normal levels

Table 7.2 shows the six major CYP450 isoforms with some of their substrates and inhibitors.

Example 7.1

Metronidazole is just one example of a drug that can significantly affect warfarin (anticoagulant) metabolism, causing marked elevations of prothrombin time and potential for serious bleeding. Select the best statement below about this drug interaction.

a. Metronidazole inhibits the P450 isoform responsible for warfarin metabolism and decreases its plasma levels.
b. Metronidazole inhibits the P450 isoform responsible for warfarin metabolism and increases its clearance.
c. Metronidazole binds strongly to the P450 isoform that metabolizes warfarin, causing an increase in plasma warfarin levels.
d. Metronidazole inhibits warfarin metabolism and decreases warfarin $t^{1/2}$.

Example 7.2

Administration of prednisone to a patient taking the anticonvulsant phenytoin can result in decreased $t_{1/2}$ and the need to adjust the dose of phenytoin. This drug interaction most likely involves the following two features:

a. Inhibition of phenytoin metabolism by CYP450
b. Induction of phenytoin metabolism by CYP450
c. Decreased plasma levels of phenytoin
d. Increased plasma levels of phenytoin

(Answers: 7.1, c; 7.2, b and c)

In vitro experiments on drug–drug interactions are now a routine part of the development of new drugs.

Different CYP450 isoforms are readily available; their ability to metabolize new drug molecules is easily investigated in the laboratory. Thus, the P450 isoform responsible for metabolism of most new drugs is known at an early stage, and likely drug interactions can be predicted.

Environmental and Genetic Factors in Metabolism by CYP450

There are often major differences between individuals in the rate at which they dispose of drugs; this is one important reason why dose requirements often differ between patients. For example, some patients will have their hypertension controlled by 40 mg propranolol twice a day while others will need 160 mg twice a day.

Table 7.2 Substrates, Inhibitors, and Inducers of Human Cytochrome P_{450} Isoforms

Substrates

1A2	2C19	2C9	2D6	2E1	3A4
Caffeine	Amitriptyline; Clomipramine	Celecoxib; Diclofenac	Amitriptyline; Flecainide	Acetaminophen	Alprazolam; cerivastatin; Verapamil
Clozapine	Diazepam; Lansoprazole	Irbesartan; naproxen	Carvedilol; Haloperidol	Ethanol	Amlodipine; Astemizole
Cyclobenzaprine	Cyclophosphamide	Fluvastatin; Glipizide	Clomipramine; Tamoxifen		Chlorpheniramine; diazepam
Imipramine	Omeprazole; Pantoprazole	Sulfamethoxazole	Codeine; Ondansetron		Buspirone; Clarithromycin; Diltiazem
Naproxen	Phenobarbitone; Phenytoin	Ibuprofen; Losartan	Desipramine; Imipramine		Cyclosporine; lovastatin; methadone
Propranolol	Progesterone; Triazolam	Phenytoin; Piroxicam	Dextromethorphan		Erythromycin; Midazolam; Indinavir
Theophylline		Tamoxifen; tolbutamide	Paroxetine; S-Metoprolol		Haloperidol; Nifedipine; Ritonavir
Warfarin - R		Torsemide; Warfarin - S	Risperidone; Timolol		Quinidine; Saquinavir; simvastatin
			Thioridazine; Tramadol		Quinine; Sildenafil; Triazolam
					Tacrolimus; tamoxifen; Vincristine
					Atorvastatin; Trazodone

Inhibitors

1A2	2C19	2C9	2D6	2E1	3A4
Cimetidine	Cimetidine	Amiodarone	Amiodarone	Disulfiram	Amiodarone; Ritonavir
Ciprofloxacin	Fluoxetine	Fluconazole	Chlorpheniramine	Acute Ethanol	Cimetidine; Saquinavir
Citalopram	Fluvoxamine	Fluoxetine	Cimetidine	Isoniazid	Diltiazem; Verapamil
Fluvoxamine	Ketoconazole	Fluvastatin	Clomipramine		Erythromycin
Ofloxacin	Lansoprazole	Isoniazid	Fluoxetine		Fluconazole
Ticlopidine	Omeprazole	Paroxetine	Haloperidol		Fluvoxamine
	Ticlopidine	Ticlopidine	Indinavir; sertraline		Fluoxetine
			Quinine; Ticlopidine		Grapefruit juice
			Ritonavir		Indinavir
			Methadone		Itraconazole
			Paroxetine		Ketoconazole
			Quinidine		Nelfinavir
					Clarithromycin

			Inducers		
1A2	**2C19**	**2C9**	**2D6**	**2E1**	**3A4**
Broccoli; tobacco	Carbamezipine; Prednisone	Rifampin	Tobacco - cigarette	Isoniazid	Barbiturates; Griseofulvin; Rifampin
Cabbage; burned meat	Norethindrone; Rifampin	Secobarbital		Chronic Ethanol	Carbamazepine; phenytoin
Carbamazepine	Phenobarbital				Glucocorticoids; St. John's Wort

In terms of CYP450 metabolism, both environmental and genetic factors control the rate of drug disposition in the individual patient. Several examples of CYP450 isoforms will be used next to illustrate their regulation by the environment and genetics, and also along the way, to illustrate how they can cause drug interactions.

Clozapine and CYP1A2 Activity

The antipsychotic drug clozapine is subject both to drug interactions and environmental control of its metabolism. The antidepressant drug fluvoxamine can act as an inhibitor of the metabolism of clozapine. It does this by binding avidly to the actual CYP1A2 enzyme in the liver and preventing it from metabolizing clozapine. The result is that plasma clozapine levels may rise to inappropriately high levels by the time steady state is reached. Clozapine is known to have its half-life decreased and steady-state plasma levels reduced by smoking. Many of the polycyclic aromatic hydrocarbons in cigarette smoke are potent inducers of CYP450 gene transcription; their actions result in an increased amount of CYP enzyme, which metabolizes clozapine more rapidly. This interaction is via the promoter region at the 5' end of the gene. These inducers selectively turn on CYP1A2 and may affect a range of drugs metabolized by the isoform (e.g., theophylline, caffeine).

Genetic Polymorphism and *CYP2D6*

CYP2D6 was the first isoform for which a polymorphism was demonstrated. This was seen with the metabolism of debrisoquine and sparteine in the 1980s. Essentially, if one looks at the ability of individuals in a population to metabolize a drug, they can be divided into two distinct groups. These are called *phenotypes* and for these drugs they are called *extensive metabolizers (EM)* or *poor metabolizers (PM)*. The genetic basis for these two phenotypes has recently been shown to be due to one or more point mutations in the *CYP2D6* gene or to a deletion of a number of bases. Thus we have identified different genotypes that correspond to the observed phenotypes. Specific genes *CYP2D6A, B, C,* and *D* have been identified; these result in an individual with PM status. The individual with the normal or nonmutated *CYP2D6* gene is called the *wild type*; this produces the EM phenotype.

The *CYP2D6* polymorphism shows up in different racial/ethnic groups: 7% of Caucasians and only 1% of Chinese are PMs. The balance is EM phenotype. The 2D6 polymorphism affects a wide range of drugs.

CYP2D6 and Codeine

The metabolism of codeine reveals the consequences of being a poor metabolizer (PM). Codeine is metabolized to a number of different metabolites, but its action in preventing pain is due to CYP2D6 metabolism to morphine. PM subjects who do not have an active *2D6* isoform of P450 do not make any morphine and thus fail to get any pain relief from codeine. Morphine itself will still works in these subjects as it is their metabolism that is different, not their opioid receptors.

Genetic Polymorphism and *CYP2C19*

CYP2C19 also shows an ethnic race-dependent polymorphism in the metabolism of a small range of drugs including diazepam and omeprazole. It has been found that 16% of Orientals but only 5% of Caucasians are PMs.

The cause of the PM phenotype is a single base pair mutation in the *CYP2C19* gene. This produces a defective CYP2C19 protein that does not metabolize drugs. Again, this polymorphism leads to variability in drug disposition, changes in steady-state levels, and corresponding variability in drug response.

Drug Interactions Via the *CYP2C19* Isoform: Omeprazole–Diazepam Interaction

Drug interactions via this isoform are also possible, as illustrated by the fact that omeprazole blocks the metabolism of diazepam at the level of the CYP2C19 protein. This is reflected *in vivo* in a decreased clearance of diazepam and an increased half-life. Only the pathway of diazepam metabolism to form nordiazepam is affected.

CYP3A Family

CYP3A4 is the most abundant of the P450 enzymes in the liver. There are also significant amounts in the intestinal wall. At present there is no evidence for polymorphism in this P450 family, although there is a significant interindividual variability in 3A4 levels and rates of drug metabolism between individuals. This suggests environmental control by some as yet unidentified means or alternately may just mean that we have not detected an important mutation of the gene.

A wide range of drugs is metabolized by CYP3A4. Potent inhibitors and potent inducers also exist. A common inducer of this isoform is carbamazepine, which can lower the steady-state levels of other drugs that are substrates for the same isoform of CYP450. Inhibition of metabolism and higher steady-state levels of theophylline result when patients also take ketoconazole, ciprofloxacin, or erythromycin.

Not all interactions are necessarily unwanted. For example the interaction between ketoconazole or diltiazem and cyclosporine is used clinically as a means of dose reduction for the very expensive immunosuppressant cyclosporine.

CYP3A4 and Grapefruit Juice

The metabolism of several drugs is inhibited in patients who also drink grapefruit juice. Examples are nifedipine and felodipine. If one looks at the number of drugs where the grapefruit juice interaction has been investigated, it is apparent that its significance varies between different drugs. Several studies have identified a flavinoid component which is peculiar to grapefruit (narangin or narangenin) as the substance that blocks CYP3A4 metabolism at the enzyme level. A careful look at these studies reveals that the interaction occurs only with oral administration and not when the drug and inhibitor are given intravenously. The effect is also lower if the dose of juice is delayed or reduced in size. This means that the interaction occurs by inhibition of P450 enzymes in the intestinal wall, which normally contribute to first-pass metabolism of drugs like felodipine and nifedipine.

REDOX REACTIONS AND THE CYP450 ENZYME COMPLEX

We now turn our attention to the biochemical aspects of the CYP450 enzyme complex, where the specific P450 isoforms function as oxidase enzymes in a multicomponent electron transfer chain. Within the oxidase family of enzymes, the CYP450 isoforms are functionally called "monooxygenases" because they introduce a single atom of molecular oxygen (O_2) into the substrate undergoing metabolism. The other oxygen atom ends up in water.

Before proceeding with our discussion we must review some concepts from general chemistry:

1. Reduction involves addition of electrons to a compound.
2. Oxidation involves removal of electrons from a compound.

In biological systems, the loss or gain of electrons from a compound often takes the form of addition or loss of hydride ion, or $:H^-$, and therefore:

1. Reduction is the addition of hydride to a compound.
2. Oxidation is the removal of hydride from a compound. Sometimes this is accompanied by the addition of oxygen to the compound.

Oxidation and reduction reactions are coupled, and in drug metabolism this means that if a drug is being oxidized by CYP450, some other component of the enzyme complex will be reduced. There are three primary oxidizing agents in biological systems:

1. The "oxene" ion, which is supplied by the CYP450 of the liver microsomal fraction. Note that the CYP450 enzyme system is also referred to as the mixed function oxidase system in some textbooks.
2. NAD$^+$ (nicotinamide adenine dinucleotide).
3. FAD (flavin adenine dinucleotide).

The oxidized and reduced forms of adenine dinucleotides of nicotinamide and flavin are shown in the next paragraphs.

NAD$^+$/NADH SYSTEM

The chemical structure of nicotinamide adenine dinucleotide (NAD, Figure 7.1) is shown in Figure 7.2 in its reduced (NADH) and oxidized forms (NAD$^+$):

■ NADH can donate a hydride ion (can donate electrons) — it is a reducing agent.
■ NADH acting as a reducing agent becomes oxidized to NAD$^+$.
■ NAD$^+$ can accept a hydride ion (can accept electrons) — it is an oxidizing agent.
■ The driving force for hydride addition to NAD$^+$ is the neutralization of positive charge. This is shown in Figure 7.2.

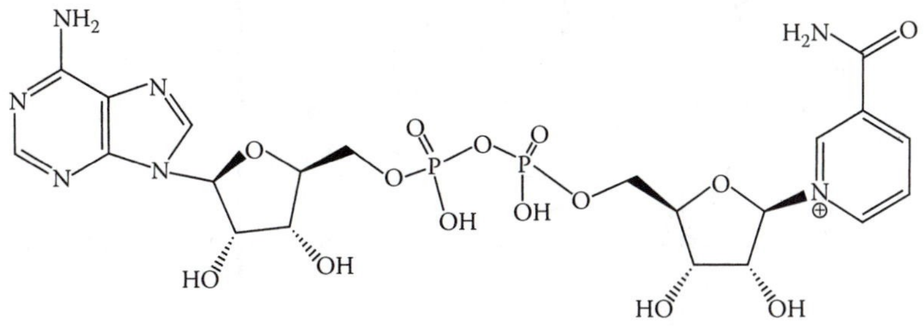

Nicotinamide Adenine Dinucleotide

Figure 7.1

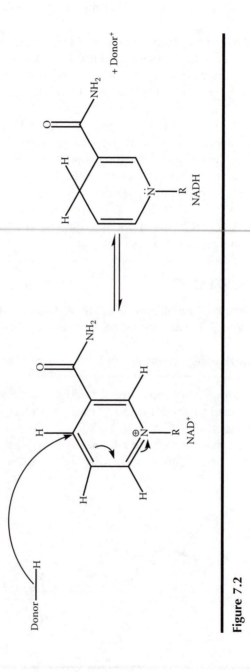

Figure 7.2

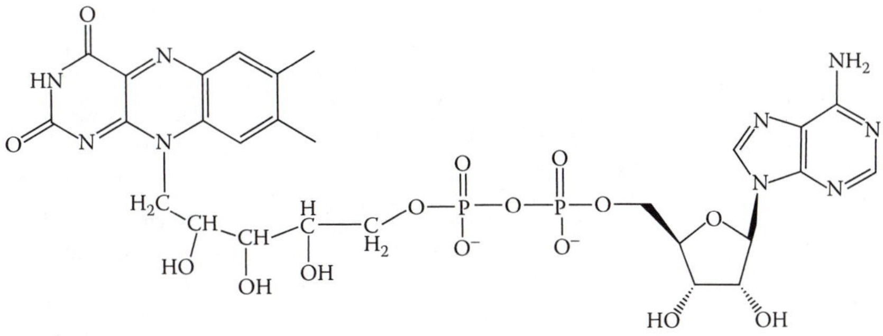

Flavin Adenine Dinucleotide

Figure 7.3

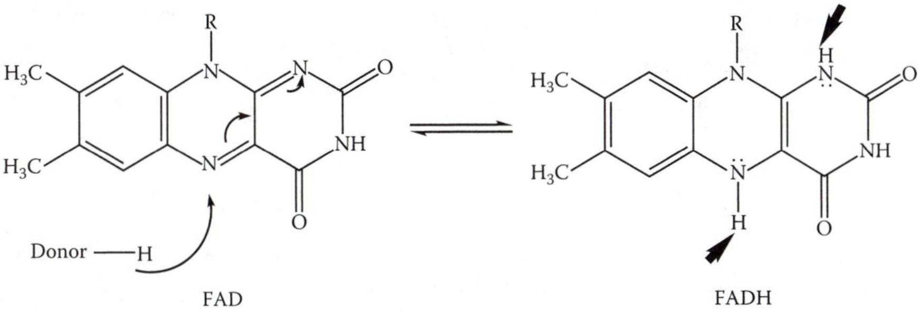

FAD   FADH

Figure 7.4

FAD/FADH SYSTEM

The structure of FAD is shown in Figure 7.3. In electron transport, the crucial part of the molecule is the tricyclic flavin ring system. The flavin ring system can accept a hydride ion (become reduced) in the process of oxidizing a drug molecule. FAD is reduced to FADH. This is shown in Figure 7.4.

THE CYTOCHROME P450 CYCLE

A simplified representation of the CYP450 oxidation reaction is shown in Equation (7.2).

$$\text{Drug} - \text{H} + O_2 + \text{NADH} + \text{H}^+ \longrightarrow \text{Drug}-\text{OH} + H_2O + \text{NAD}^+$$

Equation 7.2 The CYP450 redox reaction.

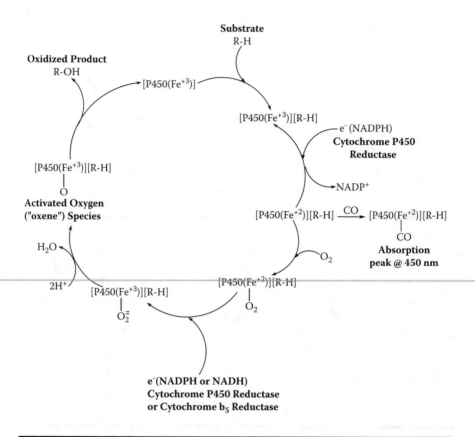

Figure 7.5   Proposed catalytic cycle in the oxidation of drugs by CYP450.

The mechanistic details of this complex reaction are summarized in Figure 7.5.

The active sites of the CYP450 enzymes contain a porphyrin ring system with iron (Fe) as the central ligand (very similar the heme group of hemoglobin). Diatomic oxygen binds to the central iron, which is in the Fe^{+2} oxidation state. Two electrons are then added to the oxygen molecule; one of the electrons is provided by NADH (or its phosphorylated form NADPH), and the other electron is provided by iron, leaving the iron atom in its Fe^{+3} oxidation state. After the addition of the two electrons to diatomic oxygen, one of the oxygen atoms is split off from the complex as O^{2-}, and this oxygen is then combined with two protons to form water. The oxygen atom remaining bound to iron (it is in a form known as "oxene") does not have the full complement (octet) of electrons surrounding it, and this, in addition to the strong electron-withdrawing nature of Fe^{+3} to which it is bound, renders the oxene atom highly electron deficient, and hence in need of electrons. The oxene can directly interact with the π electrons (as found in multiple bonds or aromatic rings) of the drug to form an epoxide, or else strip a hydride ion from the substrate (drug). Note that the drug is always bound in the immediate vicinity of the iron–oxygen complex. In stripping a hydride ion, the oxene atom is converted to hydroxyl (OH⁻) ion. Once the extraction of electrons (in the form of hydride ion) from the drug is complete, the hydroxyl ion can be recombined with (be inserted into) the drug, and the oxidized (hydroxylated) drug is released from the complex. NADH (or NADPH) then reduces the porphyrin Fe^{+3} to Fe^{+2}, the Fe^{+2} can now bind diatomic oxygen once again, and the cycle is repeated for the next drug molecule.

PHASE I AND PHASE II REACTIONS OF DRUG METABOLISM

The purpose of metabolism is to transform drugs and xenobiotics into substances that are more polar. Metabolic reactions are divided into two groups: Phase I and Phase II. Table 7.3 shows these two major categories, and the individual reaction names as subcategories. We will cover each reaction type and give examples from the drug literature. It is left to the student to apply this knowledge in predicting the metabolic reactions that can take place in other drug molecules with similar functional groups.

Phase I Reactions

In the functionalization phase of metabolism, selected parts of drug molecules are oxidized, reduced, or hydrolyzed in order to uncover or create a suitable functional group to undergo Phase II. As can be seen form Table 7.3, the majority of Phase I reactions are oxidations, and most of these are mediated by the CYP450 system. In most cases, Phase I metabolism results in loss of pharmacological activity. One notable exception to this is found in prodrugs, which are metabolized by Phase I to the active species.

Oxidations Using CYP450 Enzymes

The cycle shown in Figure 7.5 is used by the different CYP450 isoforms. The substrate RH and the product R–OH are generic structures in the cycle. We now study in greater detail the nature of these substrates and products.

Aromatic Oxidation

Oxidation of aromatic rings occurs through an intermediate epoxide. The active "oxene" intermediate in Figure 7.5 inserts itself in between the two

Table 7.3   Classification of Metabolic Reactions

Phase I Reactions (Functionalization)

Oxidation using CYP450 Enzymes

Aromatic oxidation
Aliphatic oxidation
N-, O-, and S-Dealkylation
Oxidative deamination
N-Oxidation
Sulfoxide/sulfone formation
Desulfuration
Dehalogenation

Oxidation using Other Enzymes

Alcohol and aldehyde oxidation
Oxidative deamination

Reduction

Ketone and aldehyde reduction
Nitro and azo group reduction

Hydrolysis

Ester and amide hydrolysis
Peptide bond hydrolysis
Epoxide hydration

Phase II Reactions (Conjugation)

Glucuronidation
Acetylation
Glutathione conjugation
N-, O-, and S-methylation
Sulfate conjugation

carbon atoms sharing a π bond. Several alternatives are available to epoxides, as is shown in Figure 7.6:

1. Reaction with water using the enzyme "epoxide hydrolase" to yield a vicinal diol.
2. Conjugation (Phase II) with glutathione.

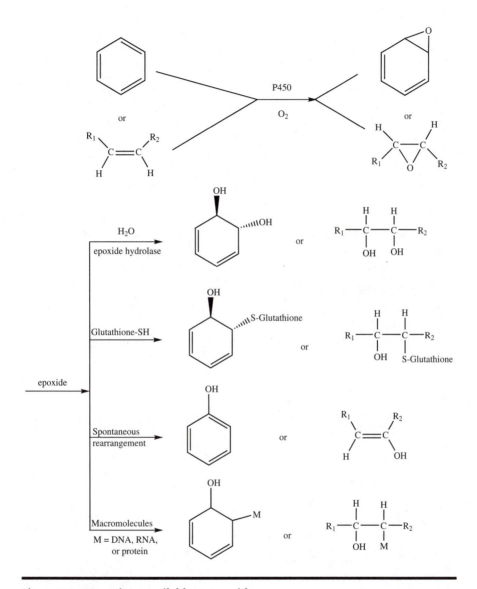

Figure 7.6 Reactions available to epoxides.

3. Spontaneous (nonenzymatic) rearrangement to the alcohol or phenol.
4. Reaction with nucleophilic centers in DNA, RNA, or proteins. This causes *toxicity*.

Epoxides are reactive chemical species, electron deficient and avid to react with any available nucleophile. With a good supply of the enzyme "epoxide hydrolase" and/or the endogenous nucleophile glutathione, the toxicity of these reactive intermediates is averted.

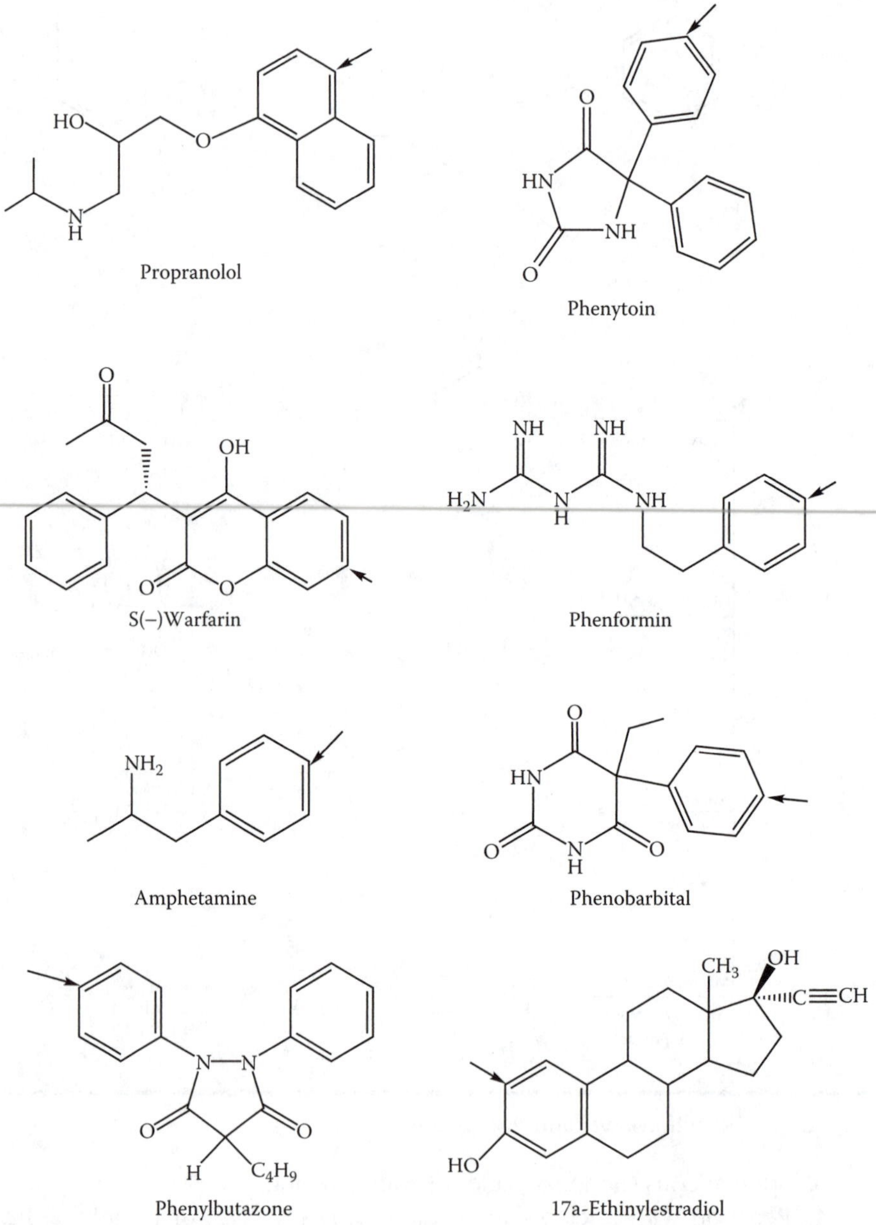

Propranolol

Phenytoin

S(−)Warfarin

Phenformin

Amphetamine

Phenobarbital

Phenylbutazone

17a-Ethinylestradiol

Figure 7.7 Aromatic hydroxylation of some common drugs.

Epoxides can also form in other double bonds present in the drug molecule, other than those in an aromatic ring. The most common end products of aromatic oxidations are phenols (one –OH) or diols (two

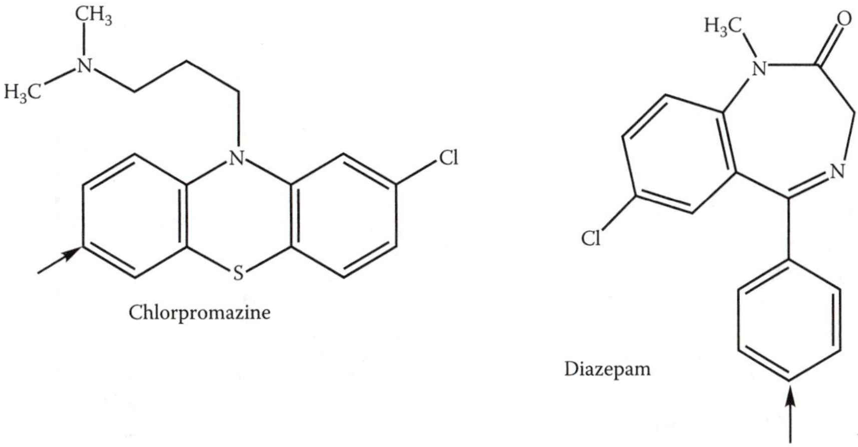

Figure 7.8 Ring selectivity in aromatic hydroxylation.

–OH), and for this reason this reaction is also commonly known as aromatic hydroxylation.

The drugs shown in Figure 7.7 undergo aromatic hydroxylation at the positions indicated by the arrows. Aromatic hydroxylation takes place in the most electron-rich, least hindered position of the ring. This most frequently coincides with the *para*-position, as can be seen for the drugs in Figure 7.7, except for 17α-ethinyl estradiol, in which case hydroxylation takes place *ortho* to the –OH group. Ring selectivity when there is more than one aromatic ring is seen in the aromatic hydroxylation of chlorpromazine and diazepam, as shown in Figure 7.8. Since the halogen, Cl, is an electron-withdrawing group, hydroxylation will take place in the adjacent ring, which has greater electron density to offer to the ["oxene" –Fe^{+3}] intermediate in the CYP450 enzyme complex.

The toxicity of the epoxide intermediates is exemplified in the oxidation metabolism of polycyclic aromatic hydrocarbons. These are common pollutants, derived from industrial processes, cigarette smoke, auto emissions, and other combustion processes. Figure 7.9 shows the formation of the ultimate carcinogen derived from the metabolism of benzo[a]pyrene.

Aliphatic Oxidation

Oxidation of aliphatic chains in drug molecules leads to hydroxylated products that *do not* involve the intermediate formation of epoxides. Examples of drug molecules undergoing aliphatic hydroxylation are shown in Figure 7.10. The most common products are either the terminal alcohol (ω-oxidation), or the alcohol at the carbon adjacent to the last one of the chain (ω – 1 oxidation), as can be seen in Figure 7.11 for pentobarbital.

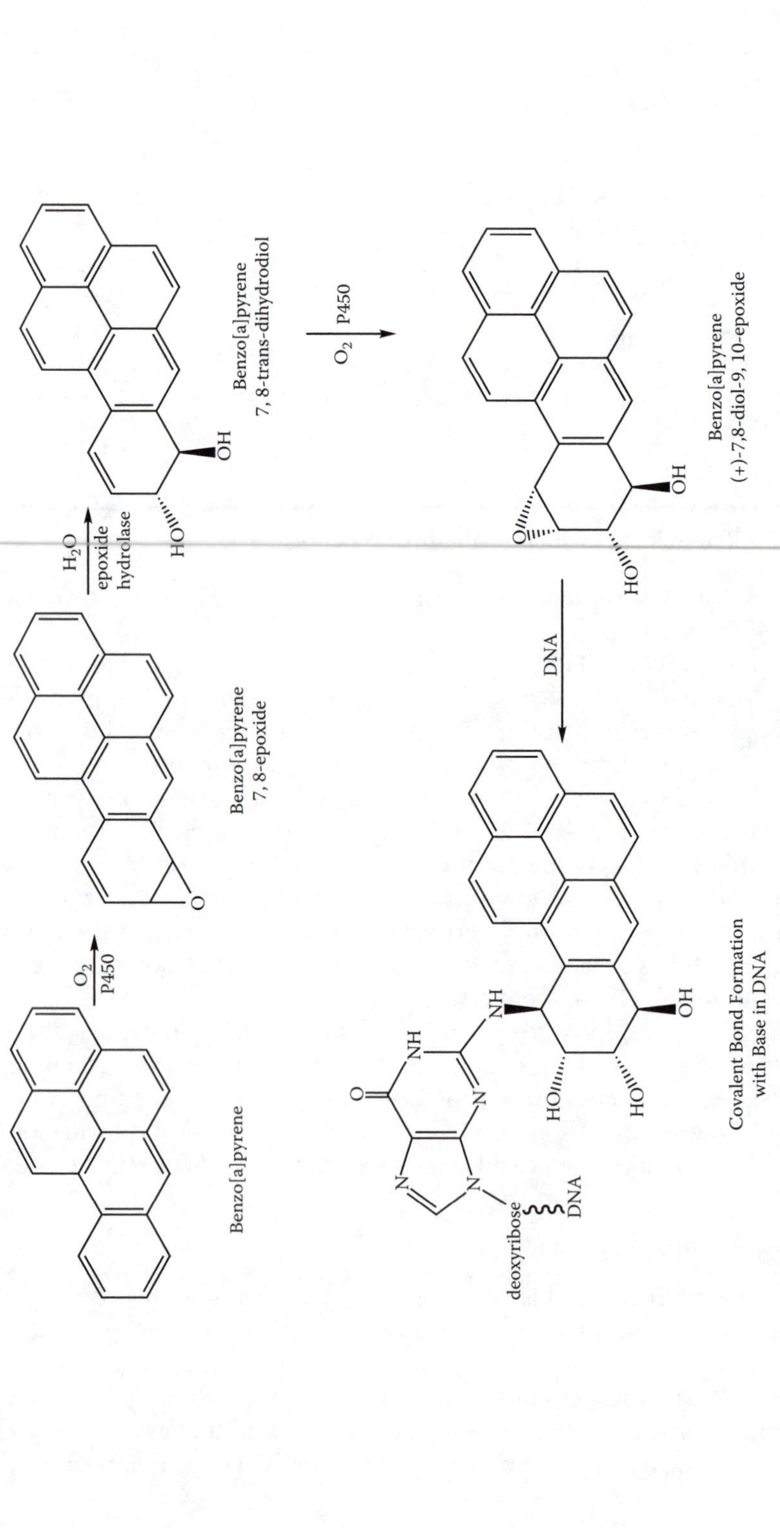

Figure 7.9   The ultimate carcinogen in benzo[a]pyrene metabolism.

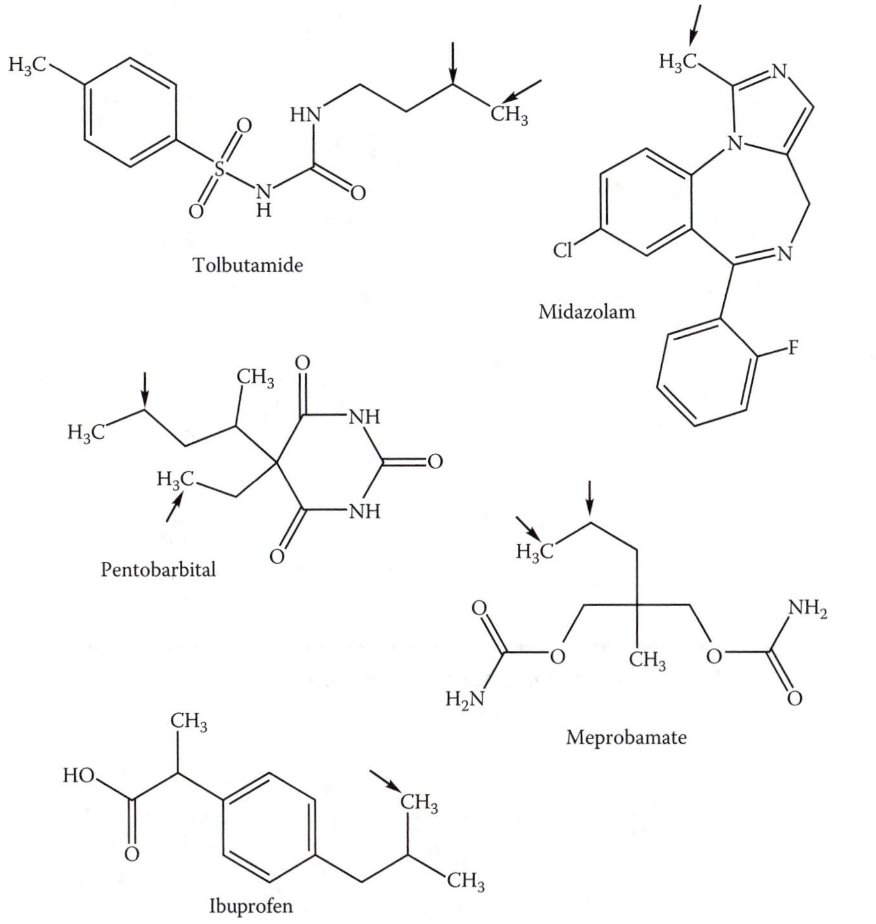

Figure 7.10   Site of aliphatic hydroxylation in some common drugs.

Other enzymes different from the P450 isoforms can further oxidize aliphatic alcohols. These are called alcohol dehydrogenase and aldehyde dehydrogenase and are present in the soluble fraction of the cell. Sequential oxidation of the ω-oxidation product shown in Figure 7.11 will yield the corresponding carboxylic acid, as shown in Figure 7.12.

A similar pathway for the ω – 1 oxidation product will yield a ketone (Figure 7.13) but cannot proceed to the carboxylic acid because there are no additional hydrogen atoms at the reactive center to lose in an oxidation reaction. Due to valence considerations, i.e., the lack of hydrogen atoms to lose in an oxidation reaction, tertiary alcohols cannot be further oxidized by the cytosolic oxidases mentioned above (Figure 7.14).

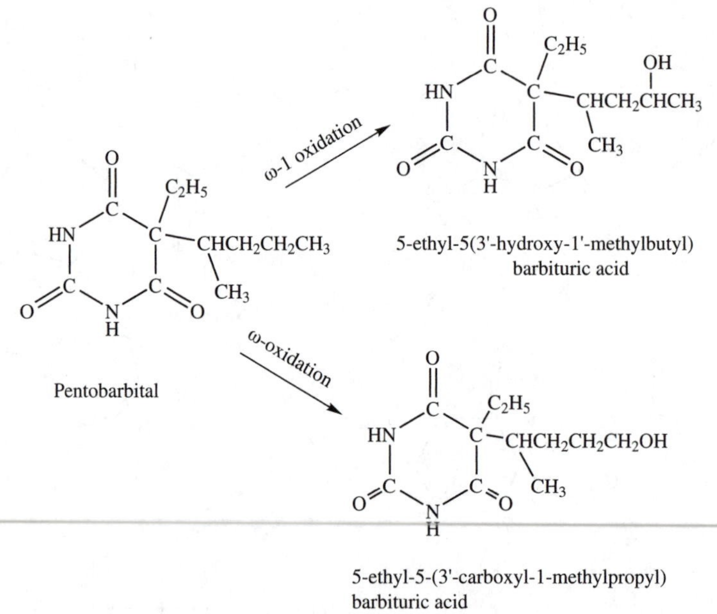

Figure 7.11   **Aliphatic oxidation options for pentobarbital.**

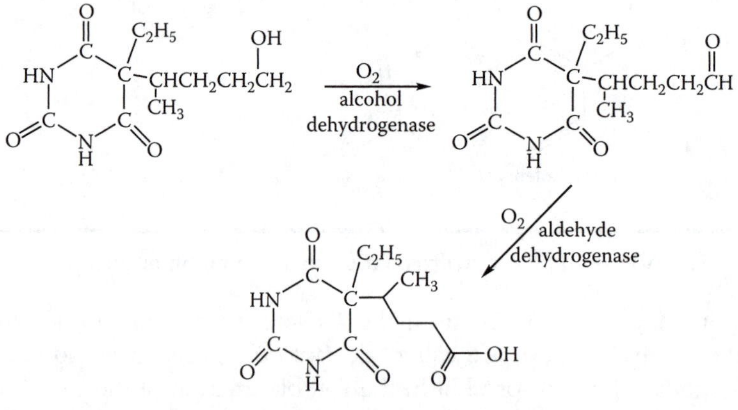

Figure 7.12   **Further oxidation of p450 hydroxylation products.**

N-, O-, and S-Dealkylation

Nitrogen and oxygen functional groups occur frequently in drugs, while sulfur groups are not as common. Nonetheless, these three heteroatoms share a common P450-mediated oxidation pathway that involves the sequence shown in Figure 7.15.

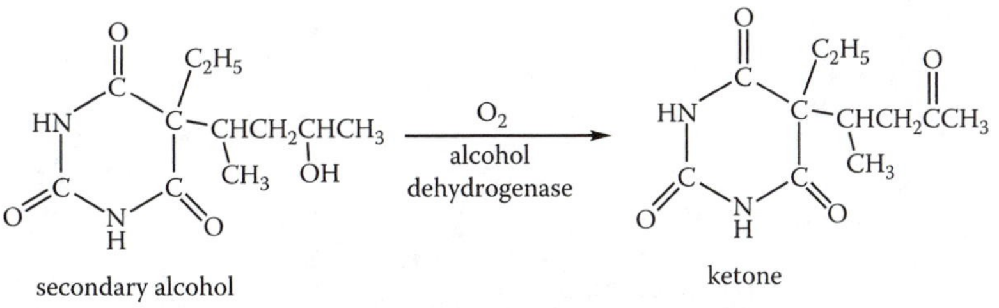

Figure 7.13 Oxidation of secondary alcohols to ketones.

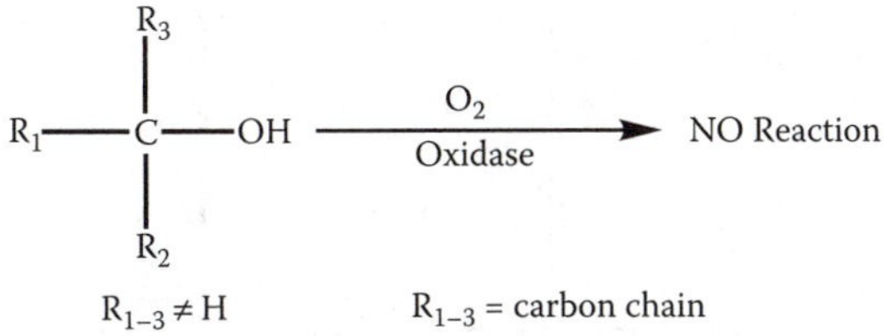

$R_{1-3} \neq H$ R_{1-3} = carbon chain

Figure 7.14 Lack of reactivity of tertiary alcohols toward oxidation.

As can be seen from the reaction pathway shown in Figure 7.15, insertion of the "oxene" oxygen atom occurs at the carbon α to the heteroatom. The resulting intermediate is unstable and breaks down into the carbonyl compound of the alkyl chain, and the rest of the drug molecule ends with an –YH group. Figure 7.16 shows examples of drug molecules undergoing dealkylation reactions, with dealkylation sites indicated by an arrow. Smaller alkyl chains react faster in dealkylation reactions than longer alkyl chains do. Dealkylation of tertiary alkyl chains is not possible since α-hydroxylation cannot take place. This is shown in Figure 7.17.

Oxidative Deamination

Drugs and their metabolites that contain primary amine groups can undergo oxidative loss of the $-NH_2$ group by a pathway similar to N, O, and S dealkylation reactions. The carbon α to the amine group is hydroxylated to form the unstable carbinolamine intermediate, followed by cleavage of the C–N bond and formation of the carbonyl compound and ammonia. The reaction sequence is shown in Figure 7.18.

As indicated in Figure 7.18, at least one of the atoms in the α–C must be hydrogen, i.e., a tertiary α–C cannot undergo an oxidative deamination

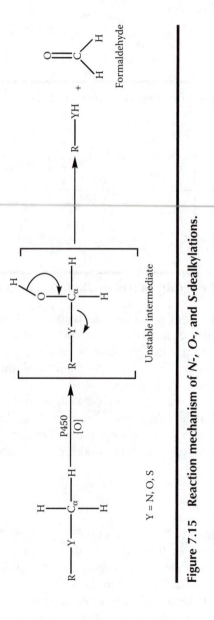

Figure 7.15   Reaction mechanism of *N*-, *O*-, and *S*-dealkylations.

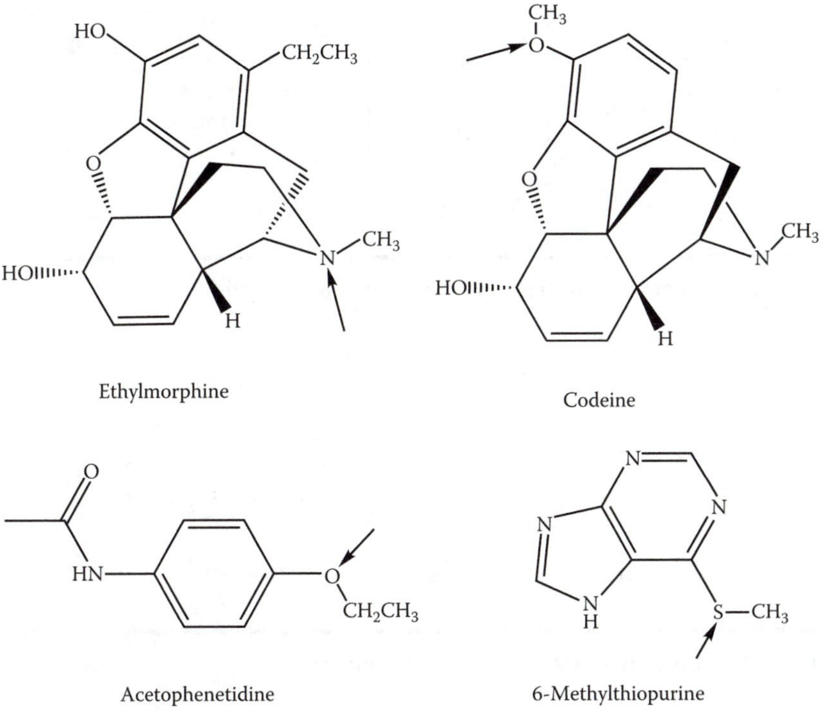

Ethylmorphine

Codeine

Acetophenetidine

6-Methylthiopurine

Figure 7.16 N-, O-, and S-dealkylations in selected drug molecules.

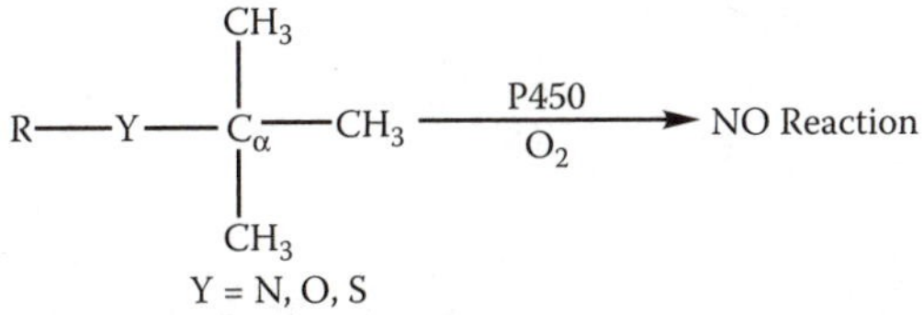

$$R\!-\!Y\!-\!\overset{\displaystyle CH_3}{\underset{\displaystyle CH_3}{\overset{|}{\underset{|}{C_\alpha}}}}\!-\!CH_3 \xrightarrow[O_2]{P450} \text{NO Reaction}$$

Y = N, O, S

Figure 7.17 Lack of reactivity of tertiary alkyl groups in N-, O-, and S-dealkylations.

for the same reasons discussed for dealkylation reactions. Amphetamine is an example of a drug undergoing oxidative deamination, as shown in Figure 7.19.

Many primary amine groups are generated by N-dealkylation reactions. These metabolites can then undergo oxidative deamination. The metabolic sequence is shown in Figure 7.20 for propranolol. The drugs methamphetamine and ketamine undergo similar sequential N-dealkylation/oxidative deamination.

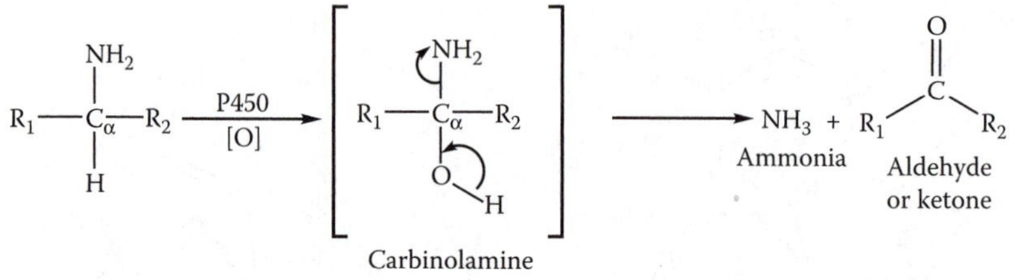

Figure 7.18 Reaction mechanism of oxidative deamination.

Amphetamine   Phenylacetone

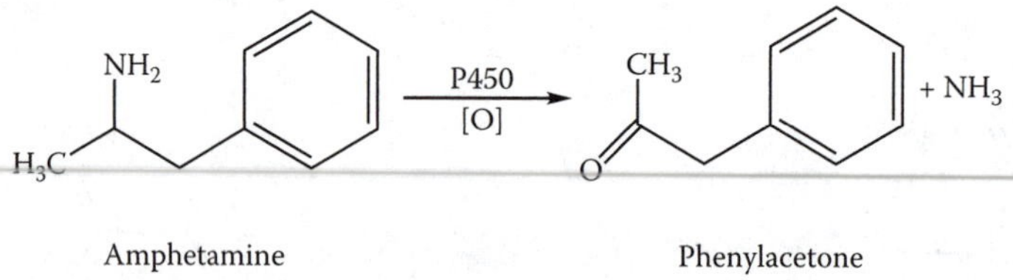

Figure 7.19 Oxidative deamination of amphetamine.

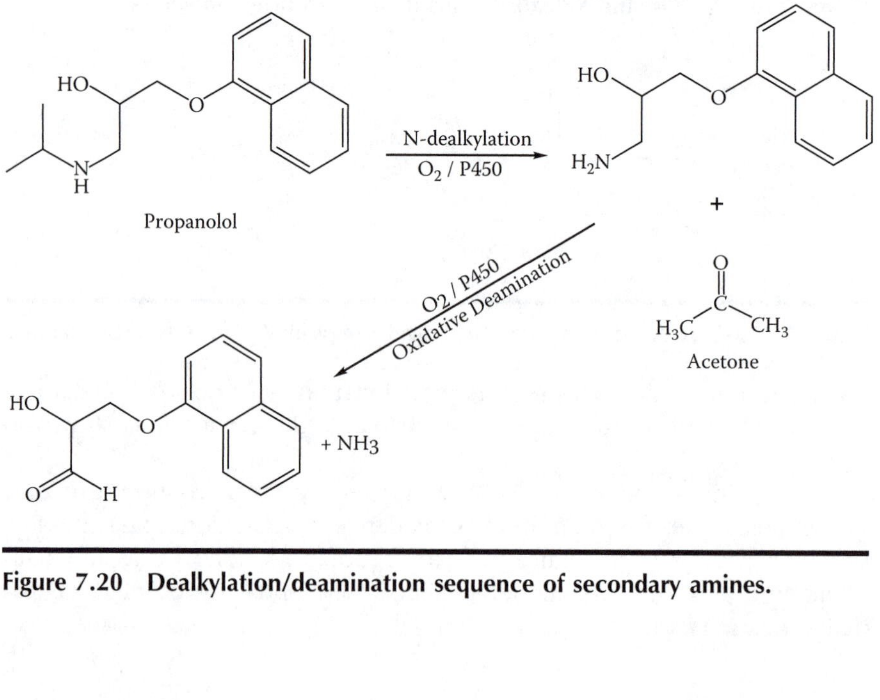

Figure 7.20 Dealkylation/deamination sequence of secondary amines.

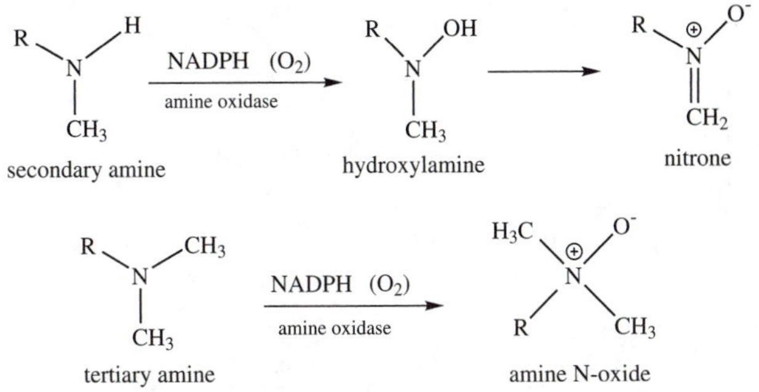

Figure 7.21 **N-Oxidation of secondary and tertiary amines by non-P450 amine oxidase.**

N-Oxidation

Secondary and tertiary amines are oxidized at the nitrogen atom by P450 enzymes but also by other oxidases that do not contain the P450 enzyme. These amine oxidases require Nicotinamide Adenine dinucleotide phosphate (NADPH) and molecular oxygen to carry out the N-oxidation. The reaction sequence for a secondary and a tertiary amine is shown in Figure 7.21.

N-Oxidation is an important metabolic pathway for drugs that cannot undergo oxidation at the carbon α to the amine, i.e., cannot undergo P450-mediated oxidative deamination or N-dealkylation. An example is found in the drug phentermine, which has one more methyl (CH_3) group than amphetamine does. As shown in Figure 7.22, p-hydroxylation and N-oxidation are the main metabolic pathways of phentermine. The intermediate N-hydroxylamines are unstable compounds and undergo further oxidation to the nitroso (−NO) and nitro(−NO_2) products.

Chlorphentermine and amantadine undergo similar oxidative metabolism. N-Oxidation of aromatic amines yields N-hydroxylamines that can lead to reactive intermediates, capable of covalent bonding to protein, DNA, and RNA. However, the most common metabolic pathways for aromatic amines are aromatic hydroxylation and N-acetylation.

Sulfoxide/Sulfone Formation

Oxidation at the sulfur atom of a thioether (sulfide) yields the sulfoxide. The sulfoxide can be oxidized further to the sulfone. This is shown in Figure 7.23 for chlorpromazine. Similar oxidation reactions at sulfur take place in the drug molecules of thioridazine, cimetidine and oxisuran.

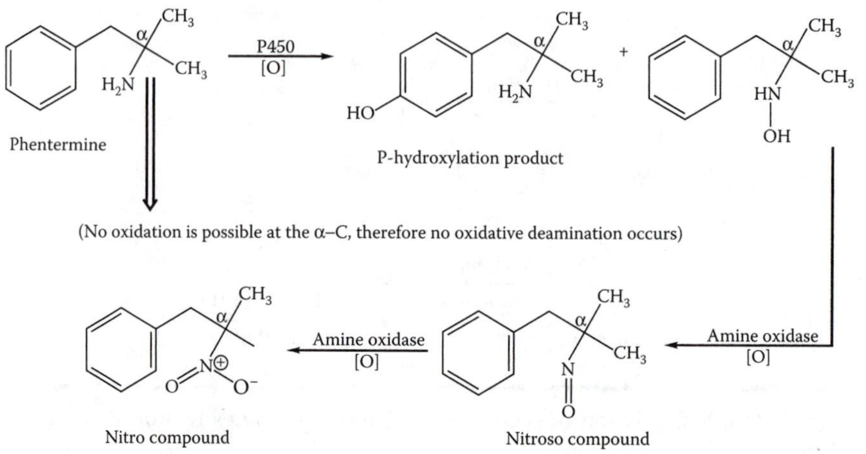

Figure 7.22 N-Oxidation of phentermine.

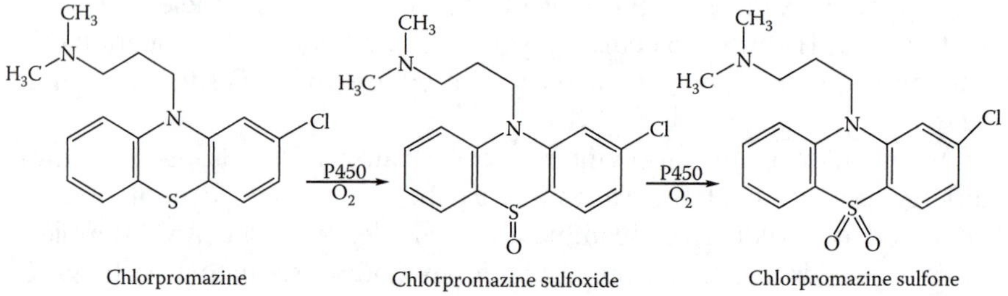

Figure 7.23 Sulfur oxidation in the metabolism of chlorpromazine.

Desulfuration

The oxidative conversion of carbon–sulfur double bonds (C=S) to the corresponding carbon–oxygen double bond (C=O) is called "desulfuration." A well-known example of this reaction is the conversion of thiopental to pentobarbital. Phosphorus-sulfur (P=S) double bonds undergo similar desulfuration reactions. This is shown in Figure 7.24.

Dehalogenation

Many halogen-containing drugs and xenobiotics can lose halogen atoms through an oxidative process. This is shown for the volatile anesthetic

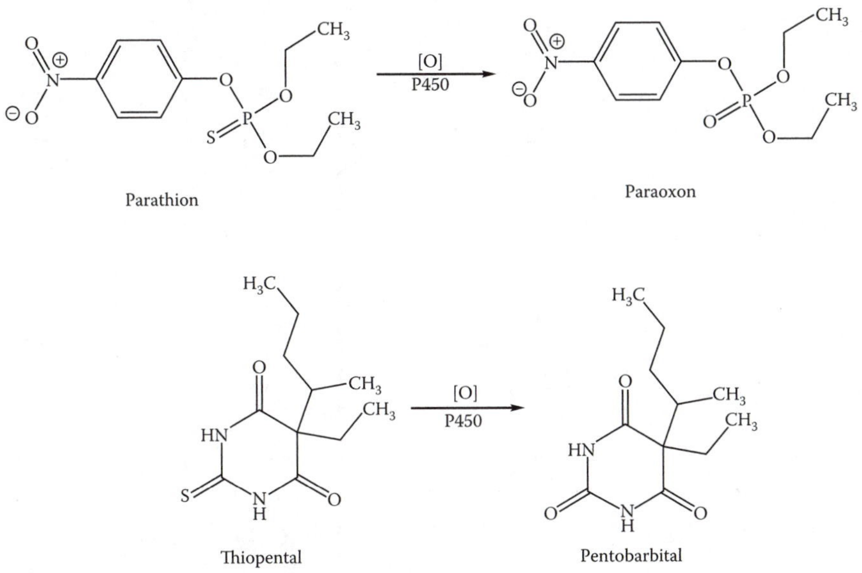

Figure 7.24 Desulfuration reactions in some drug molecules.

halothane in Figure 7.25. The acyl halide intermediate (a) is very reactive and is hydrolyzed quickly to the carboxylic acid. The reactive intermediate (a) could also acylate tissue nucleophiles and therefore has toxic effects. A similar dehalogenation pathway is involved in the metabolism of chloroform ($CHCl_3$). The intermediate acyl halide, phosgene, is most likely responsible for the liver and kidney toxicity associated with chloroform inhalation.

Oxidation using Other Enzymes

Alcohol and Aldehyde Oxidation

Many of the oxidations discussed so far generate alcohol intermediates. If they do not undergo Phase II (conjugation), the hydroxyl group can be further oxidized to an aldehyde (if primary alcohol) or ketone (if secondary alcohol). A tertiary alcohol cannot undergo further oxidation, as discussed previously. The oxidase enzymes involved in these reactions are found in the soluble fraction of the liver and are rather nonspecific. They are called alcohol dehydrogenase and aldehyde dehydrogenase, and they require $NAD^+/NADH$ as a cofactor. A well-known example of this reaction is the oxidation of ethanol all the way to acetic acid, as shown in Figure 7.26.

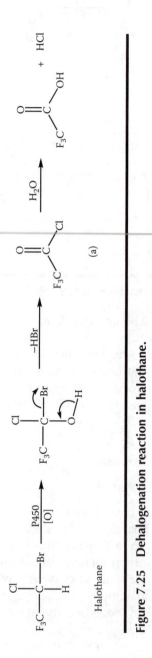

Figure 7.25 Dehalogenation reaction in halothane.

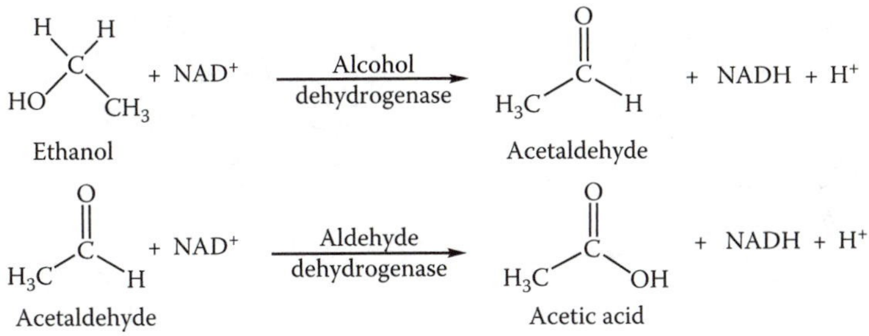

Figure 7.26   Oxidation of ethanol by oxidases other than P450.

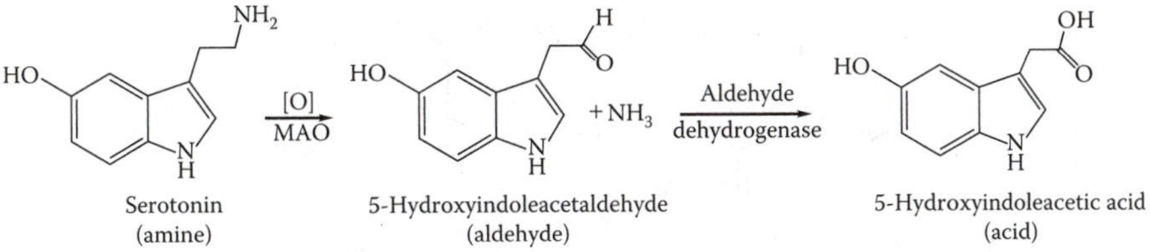

Figure 7.27   Oxidative deamination of serotonin by MAO.

Oxidative Deamination

Naturally occurring amines and many drugs can lose the amino group in an oxidative process involving the enzymes "monoamine oxidase" (MAO) and "diamine oxidase" (DAO). The products are aldehydes, which are usually oxidized further by aldehyde dehydrogenase into the carboxylic acid. A typical example is the oxidative deamination of serotonin, as shown in Figure 7.27.

MAO is a mitochondrial enzyme especially abundant in the liver, kidneys, intestines, and neurons. MAO substrates include tyramine, phenylethylamine, the catecholamine neurotransmitters (epinephrine, norepinephrine, dopamine, and tryptophan derivatives (tryptamine, serotonin). MAO is relatively nonspecific and will accept a variety of amines; however, sterically hindered amines such as amphetamine and other phenylethylamines with branched carbon chains next to the amino group are not good substrates. DAO's substrate specificity overlaps that of MAO, and it can also convert amines to aldehydes in the presence of oxygen. DAO is localized in the soluble cell fractions of the intestines, the placenta, and the liver. The best substrates for DAO are polymethylene diamines like putrescine, $H_2N-(CH_2)_2-NH_2$, and cadaverine, $H_2N-(CH_2)_5-NH_2$.

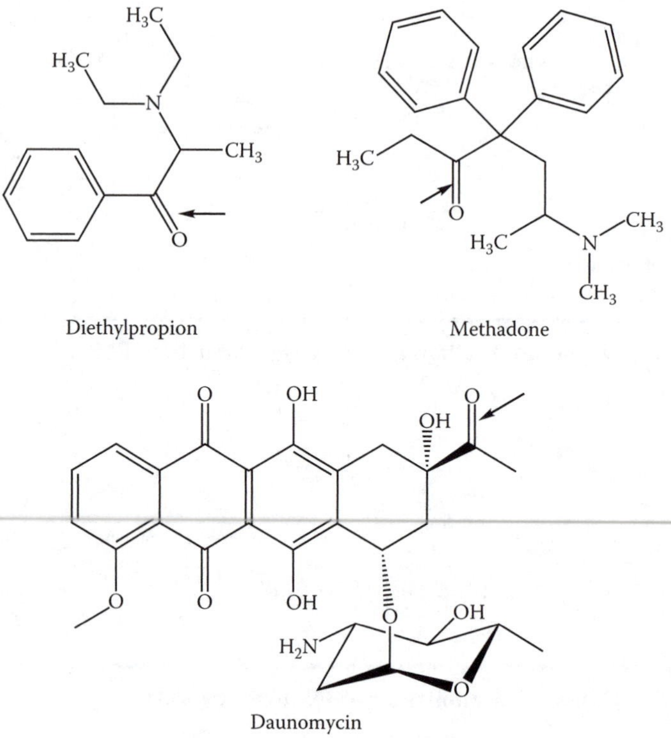

Diethylpropion

Methadone

Daunomycin

Figure 7.28 Ketone reduction in drug metabolism.

Reduction

Ketone and Aldehyde Reduction

Although it is metabolically possible to convert a secondary alcohol to a ketone, the reverse reaction usually happens more frequently: reduction of ketones to secondary alcohols. Reduction of other functional groups such as nitro and azo also occurs in drug metabolism.

Reduction of carbonyl compounds generates alcohols, while azo and nitro reduction generates amino groups. The resulting functional groups can be conjugated in Phase II reactions more readily than their precursors can. Soluble enzymes called "aldo-keto reductases" carry out the reduction of aldehydes and ketones and require NADPH as a cofactor. Examples of carbonyl reductions in drug metabolism are shown in Figure 7.28. It can be noticed that reduction of ketones will generate a chiral center in the molecule; usually one stereoisomer predominates, as can be seen for warfarin in Figure 7.29. Bioreduction of aldehydes does not generate a chiral center, as can be seen in Figure 7.30 for chlorpheniramine.

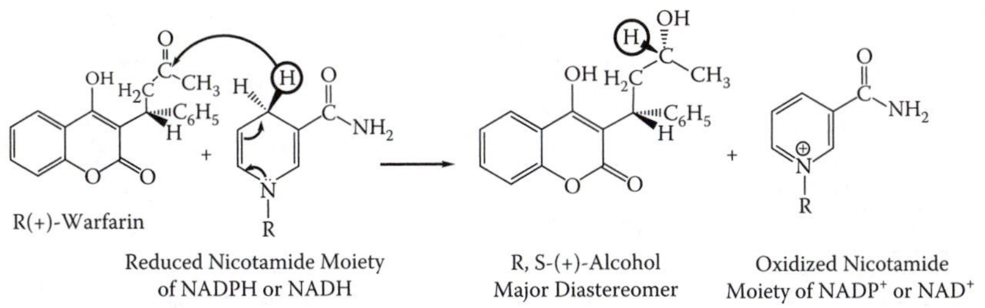

Figure 7.29 Stereoselectivity in the metabolic reduction of warfarin.

Nitro and Azo Group Reduction

Nitro and azo group bioreduction is carried out by NADPH-dependent reductases in the microsomes but can also be carried out by bacterial reductases in the intestine. Examples of nitro and azo bioreduction in drug metabolism are shown in Figure 7.31. Prontosil is a "prodrug"; its metabolite sulfanilamide is the actual antibacterial agent.

Hydrolysis Reactions

Ester and Amide Hydrolysis

Hydrolysis is a major Phase I reaction for drugs containing an ester group. Classic examples are the conversion of acetylsalicylic acid (aspirin) to salicylic acid and hydrolysis of the methyl ester in cocaine. These reactions are shown in Figure 7.32.

The presence of esterases in many tissues and plasma makes ester derivatives the "prodrugs" of choice whenever a drug needs to be modified to overcome some difficulty such as bitter taste or poor bioavailability. Such is the case with chloramphenicol, for example, which is converted into its palmitate ester to reduce the bitter taste and therefore improve palatability of pediatric oral suspensions. The enzymes responsible for ester hydrolysis include acetylcholinesterases, plasma cholinesterase, and carbonic anhydrase. Ester hydrolysis yields an acid and an alcohol as the two major products of the reaction. Likewise, amide hydrolysis yields an amine and an acid. Amides are hydrolyzed more slowly than esters are. For example, hydrolysis of the amide bond in procainamide is slow compared to ester hydrolysis in its analog procaine. This is shown in Figure 7.33.

Drugs in which amide hydrolysis has been reported include carbamazepine, lidocaine, indomethacin, hexobarbital, 5-phenylhydantoin, and phensuximide.

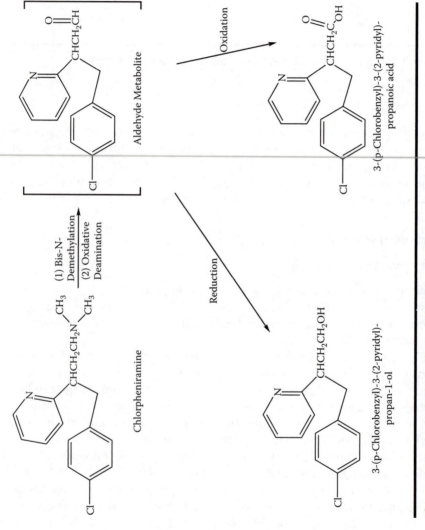

Figure 7.30 Major metabolites of chlorpheniramine.

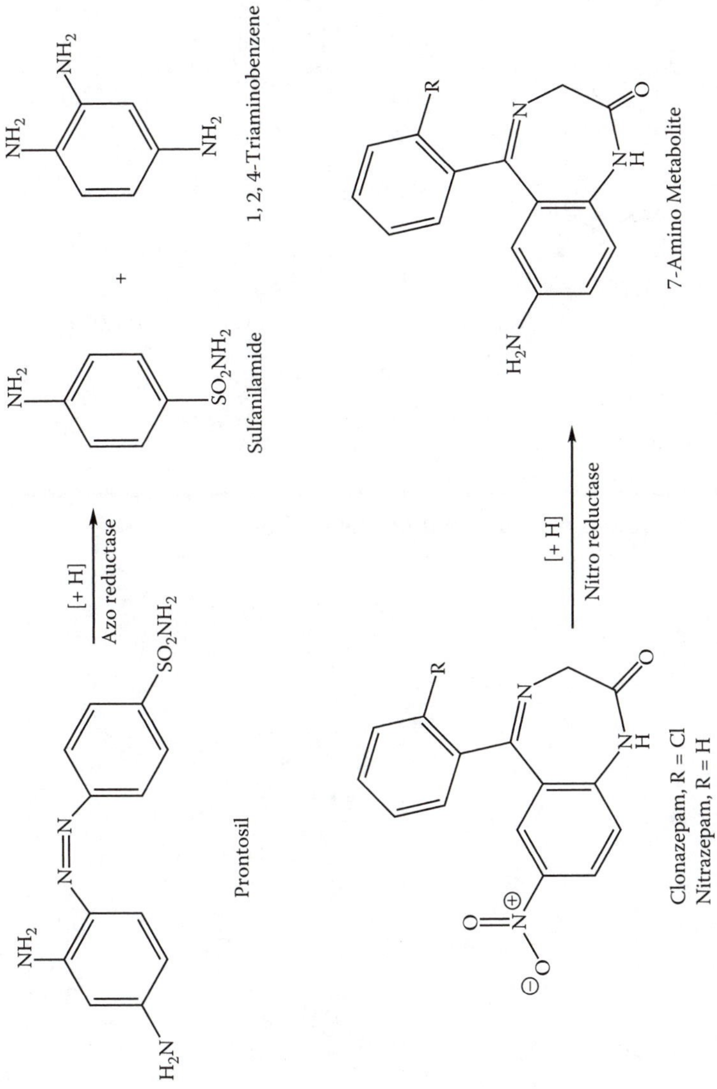

Figure 7.31 Nitro and azo reduction in drug metabolism.

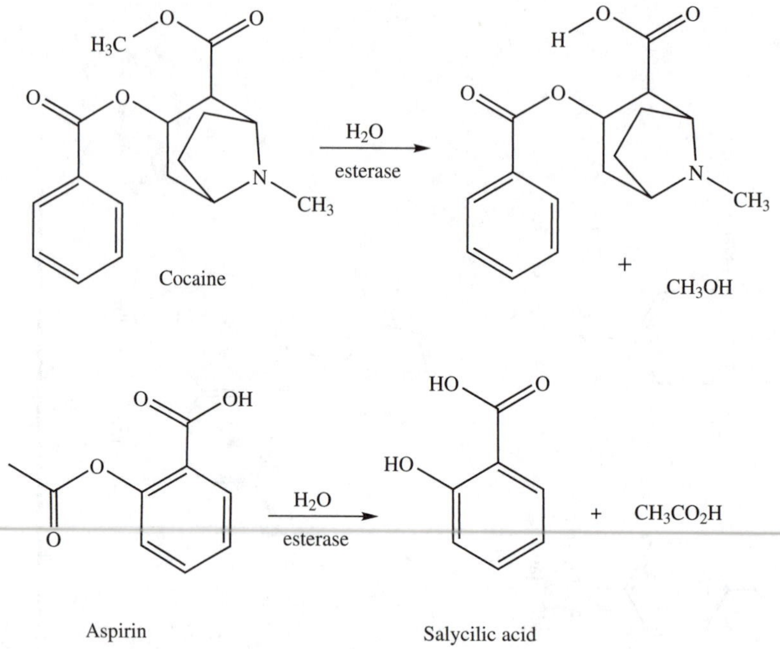

Figure 7.32 Hydrolysis reactions in drug metabolism.

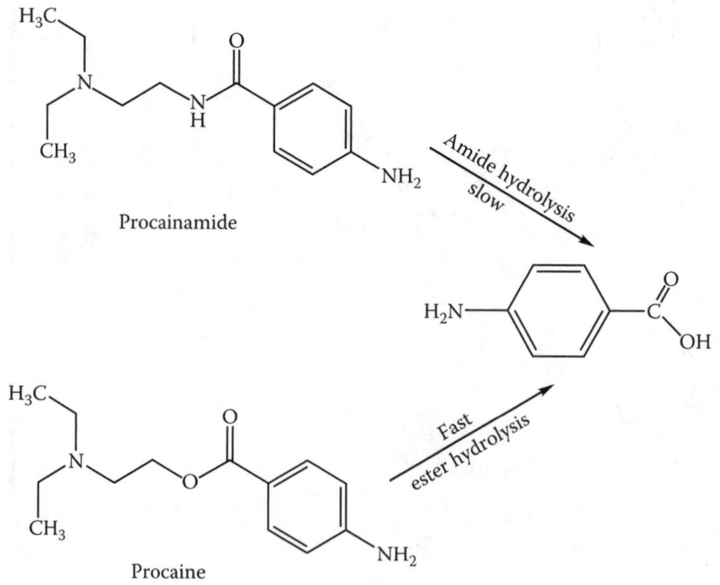

Figure 7.33 Procaine and procainamide hydrolysis.

Peptide Bond Hydrolysis

Peptide drugs and protein hormones can undergo hydrolysis at the N– or C–terminal amino acid by carboxy- and aminopeptidases, as well as proteases in blood and other tissues. Examples include human insulin, growth hormone, prolactin, and atrial natriuretic factor.

Epoxide Hydration

Epoxides formed from a variety of aromatic compounds and alkenes can undergo a hydrolysis reaction where the molecule of water adds across the epoxide bond without cleavage into two distinct chemical entities. Multiple forms of epoxide hydrolases exist in human liver. A cytosolic form has also been detected. A classic example of epoxide hydration is the formation of a carcinogen from benzo[a]pyrene in cigarette smoke. This was shown in Figure 7.9.

Phase II Reactions (Conjugation)

Phase I reactions do not always terminate activity or produce more hydrophilic metabolites that can be excreted. In order to achieve one or both of these goals, a series of reactions can be performed on the Phase I metabolite and sometimes on the drug or xenobiotic itself. These are called Phase II reactions because they most commonly follow in sequence to Phase I reactions. They are also called "conjugation" reactions because a functional group in the drug or its metabolite "binds" (conjugates) with endogenous molecules, such as glucuronic acid, sulfate, or simple amino acids like glycine. Phase II reactions such as methylation and acetylation do not increase water solubility but take place to diminish biological activity. Another hallmark of Phase II reactions is that either the endogenous molecule or the drug molecule is first "activated" to facilitate even further the ensuing synthesis reaction. The next paragraphs give drug examples of some of the more common Phase II reactions.

Glucuronidation

Enzymes that catalyze the formation of uridine diphosphate glucuronic acid (UDPGA) can be found in the soluble fraction of the liver. UDPGA donates the glucuronic acid portion to various acceptors, a process that is mediated by various enzymes called "transferases." UDPGA is the "activated" form of glucuronic acid; its synthesis is shown in Figure 7.34.

The most common type of products of glucuronidation reactions are called "ether" glucuronides, so called because a hydroxyl group (aromatic or aliphatic) has attacked UDPGA to form an ether linkage. This is shown

α-D-Glucose-1-phosphate   UDP-α-D-Glucose (UDPG)

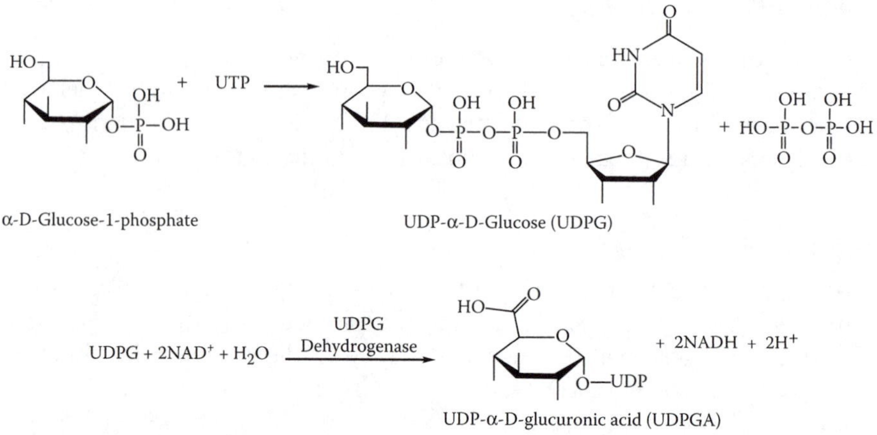

$$\text{UDPG} + 2\text{NAD}^+ + \text{H}_2\text{O} \xrightarrow{\quad \substack{\text{UDPG} \\ \text{Dehydrogenase}} \quad} \text{UDP-α-D-glucuronic acid (UDPGA)} + 2\text{NADH} + 2\text{H}^+$$

UDP-α-D-glucuronic acid (UDPGA)

Figure 7.34 Biosynthesis of UDPGA.

in Figure 7.35 for *p*-hydroxyacetanilid (acetaminophen, Tylenol). The –OH group of a carboxylic acid can also react with UDPGA to form "ester glucuronides." This is shown in Figure 7.36 for benzoic acid.

It must be noted that these reactions take place with inversion of configuration at the –O-UDP bond, that is, the electron-rich oxygen atom displaces the good leaving group (UDP) in a bimolecular nucleophilic substitution reaction.

Other examples of hydroxyl-containing drugs undergoing this reaction include morphine, chloramphenicol, and propranolol. Other carboxylic acids undergoing glucuronidation include such drugs as salicylic acid, naproxen and fenoprofen.

Glucuronidation of drugs or metabolites containing –NH$_2$ and/or –SH groups is also possible. Examples for –NH$_2$-containing drugs are desipramine, sulfisoxazole, and 7-amino-5-nitro indazole. Examples of –SH-containing drugs are methimazole and propylthiouracil.

Acetylation

Incorporation of an acetyl group into a primary amino group is a major metabolic route for primary aromatic amines (Ar–NH$_2$), primary aliphatic amines (Alkyl–NH$_2$), hydrazines (–NHNH$_2$), hydrazides (–CONHNH$_2$), and sulfonamides (Ar–SO$_2$NH$_2$). *N*-Acetyltransferase enzymes present in the liver and other tissues (lung, spleen, lymphocytes, red blood cells, gastric mucosa) transfer the acetyl group from acetyl–CoA. Acetyl–CoA is the cofactor in this reaction and the "activated" form of the acetyl group. The reaction is shown in Figure 7.37 for sulfanilamide, and although acetylation

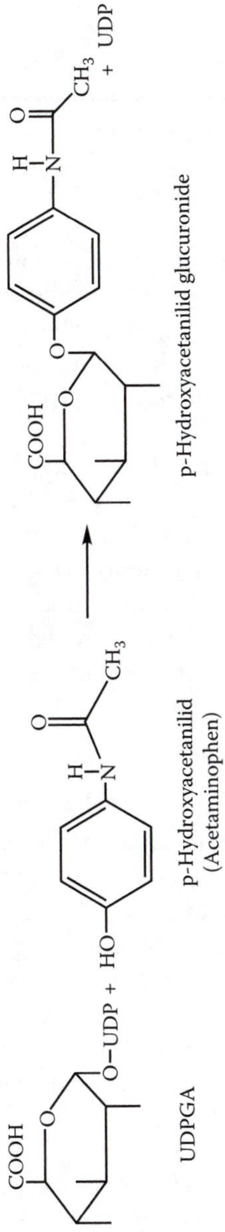

Figure 7.35 Ether glucuronide of acetaminophen.

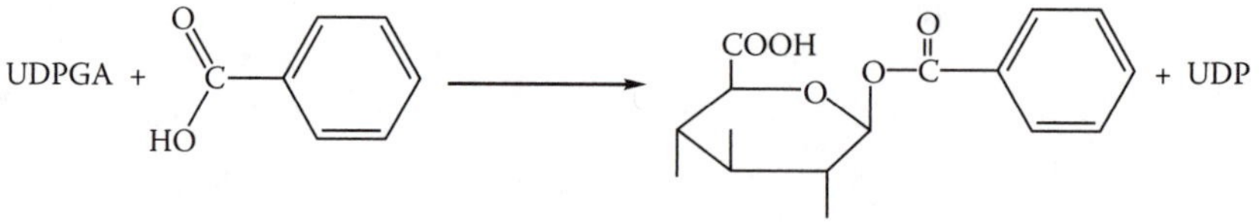

Figure 7.36   Ester glucuronide of benzoic acid.

at the amino group is the major product, the sulfonamide group is also acetylated.

Drug examples of acetylation at Ar–NH$_2$ groups include: p-aminobenzoic acid, dapsone, procainamide, sulfisoxazole, sulfamethoxazole, sulfamethazine, and sulfapyridine. Drug examples of acetylation at hydrazine and hydrazide groups include hydralazine, phenelzine, and isoniazid. Examples of aliphatic amines undergoing acetylation include mescaline and histamine.

Different ethnic groups around the world show different acetylating ability due to genetic polymorphism of the N-acetyltransferase enzyme. This causes the population to be classified as either slow or fast acetylators and has consequences for the therapeutic response and adverse effects of some drugs, such as isoniazid (an anti-tuberculosis drug). Slow acetylators are more likely to develop adverse reactions, while fast acetylators are more likely to show an inadequate therapeutic response.

Glutathione Conjugation

Glutathione (GSH) is a nucleophilic tripeptide (α-glutamyl-cysteinylglycine) that provides an important detoxification pathway for chemically reactive electrophilic compounds. The products of glutathione (GSH) conjugation undergo further metabolism to yield mercapturic acid derivatives as the final products. The reaction sequence is shown in Figure 7.38 for naphthalene epoxide, an electrophic metabolite of the xenobiotic naphthalene.

The process shown in Figure 7.38 involves sequential cleavage of glutamic acid and glycine from the GSH adduct, with N-acetylation of the remaining S-substituted cysteine residue. The cytosolic liver and kidney enzymes, which carry out the GSH conjugation, are called glutathione S-transferases. Microsomal enzymes carry out degradation of the GSH conjugate. There is no need to activate the coenzyme or the substrate prior to the GSH conjugation, which distinguishes this reaction from other Phase II reactions. GSH is sufficiently reactive toward a large variety of electrophilic substrates, which provides sufficient driving force for the reaction. Two different mechanisms are possible for GSH conjugation:

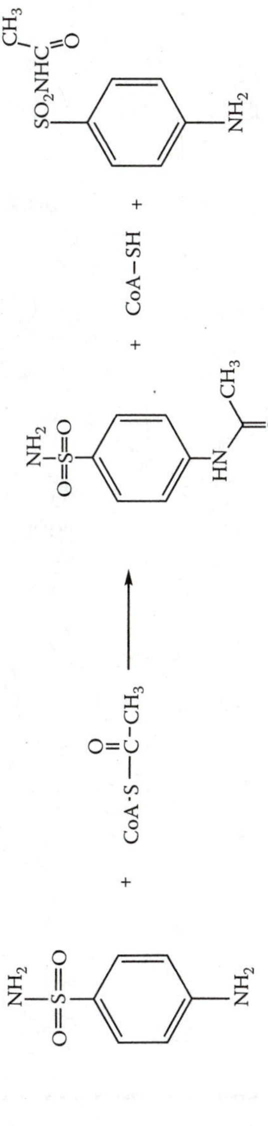

Sulfanilamide

N4-acetylsulfanilamide

Minor

Figure 7.37 Acetylation at amino and sulfonamide groups.

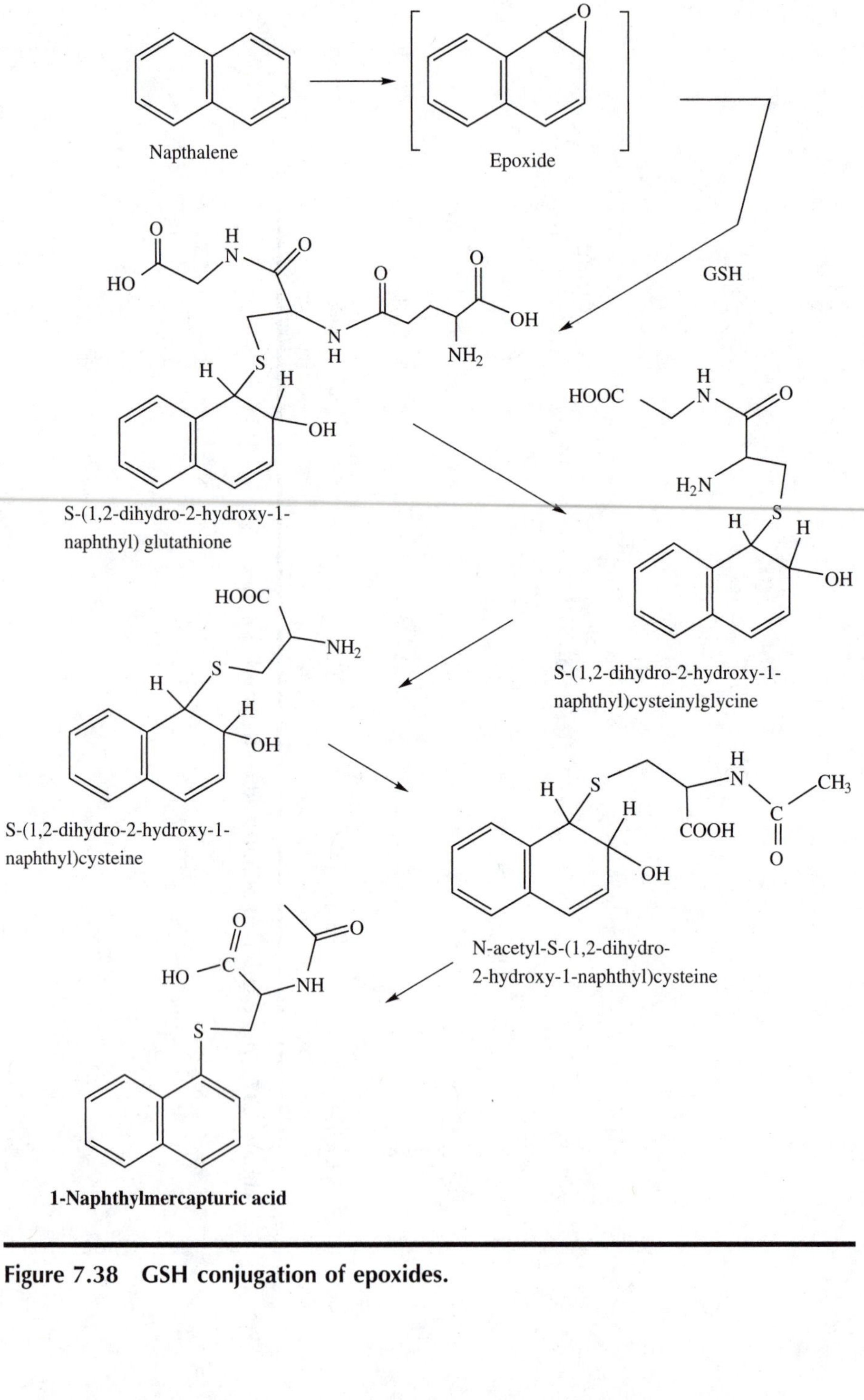

Figure 7.38   GSH conjugation of epoxides.

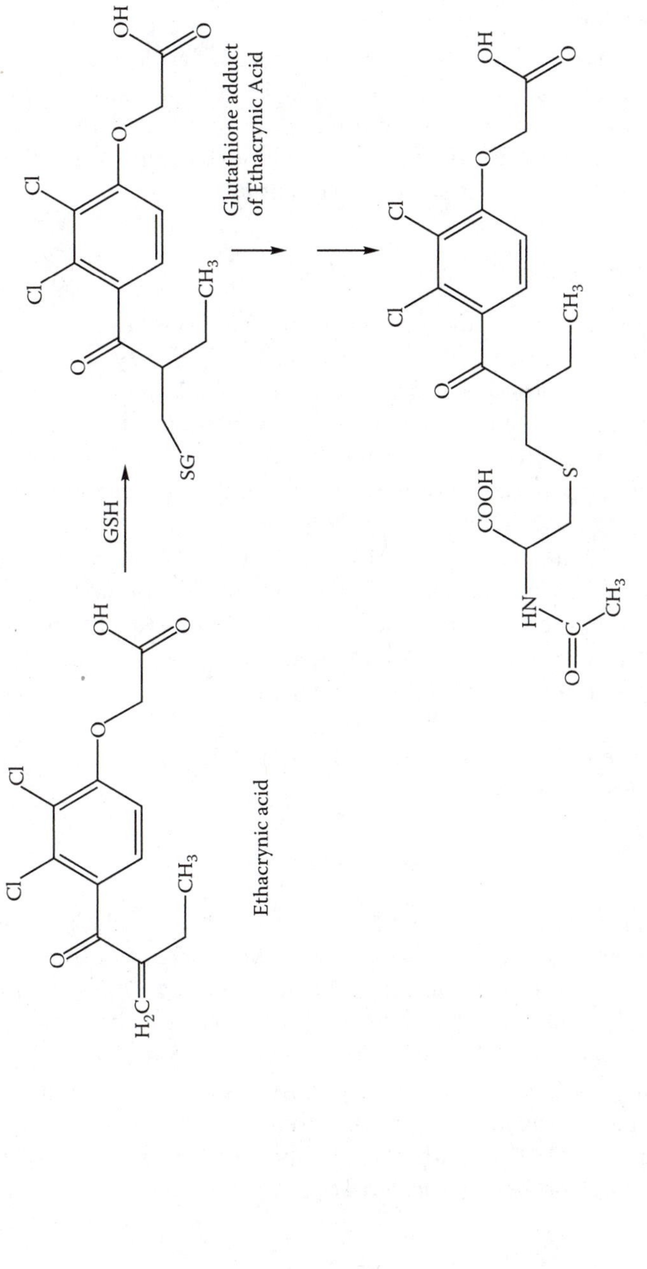

Figure 7.39 GSH conjugation of electron-deficient double bonds.

1. Nucleophilic displacement at an electron-deficient center
2. Nucleophilic addition to an electron-deficient double bond (Michael addition)

The metabolism of the immunosuppressive drug azathioprine is an example of mechanism type 1 (similar to naphthalene epoxide). The metabolism of the diuretic ethacrynic acid is an example of the second mechanism, shown in Figure 7.39.

Other compounds that can react with GSH in a similar Michael addition include diethylmaleate, acrolein, crotonaldehyde, and arecholine. Many steroidal agents possessing an α,β-unsaturated carbonyl moiety, such as digitoxigenin and prednisone, do not undergo GSH conjugation due to steric factors, susceptibility to metabolic reduction, or both.

N-, O-, and S-Methylation

Methylation takes place by a pathway involving S-adenosylmethionine as the methyl donor and one of several methyltransferase enzymes. Methylation does not lead to more polar or more water-soluble metabolites, but it is an important reaction in the biosynthesis of epinephrine and melatonin. It also plays a key role in the inactivation of biogenic amines such as norepinephrine, dopamine, serotonin, and histamine. the reaction pathway is shown in Figure 7.40 for norepinephrine.

The most abundant enzyme is cathecol-O-methyltransferase; other enzymes used by drugs in this type of reaction include phenyl-O-methyltransferase, N-methyltransferases, and S-methyltransferases. Phenylethanolamine N-methyl transferases (PNMT) methylate phenylethanolamine derivatives such as norepinephrine, as shown in Figure 7.41, to generate epinephrine.

The sites of methylation of some common drugs are indicated by arrows in the structures shown in Figure 7.42.

Sulfate Conjugation

Sulfate conjugation is an important pathway for aromatic alcohols but can also take place with aliphatic alcohols and N-hydroxy compounds. The enzymes are called sulfotransferases, and the sulfate donor is 3'-phosphoadenosyl-5'-phosphate (PAPS). This activated form of the sulfate group is formed from inorganic sulfate by a process shown in Figure 7.43. A classic example of sulfate conjugation of a drug by PAPS is shown in Figure 7.44 for p-hydroxyacetanilid (acetaminophen). Although glucoronidation often represents a major competing pathway, sulfation of the drugs shown in Figure 7.45 occurs at the sites indicated by the arrows.

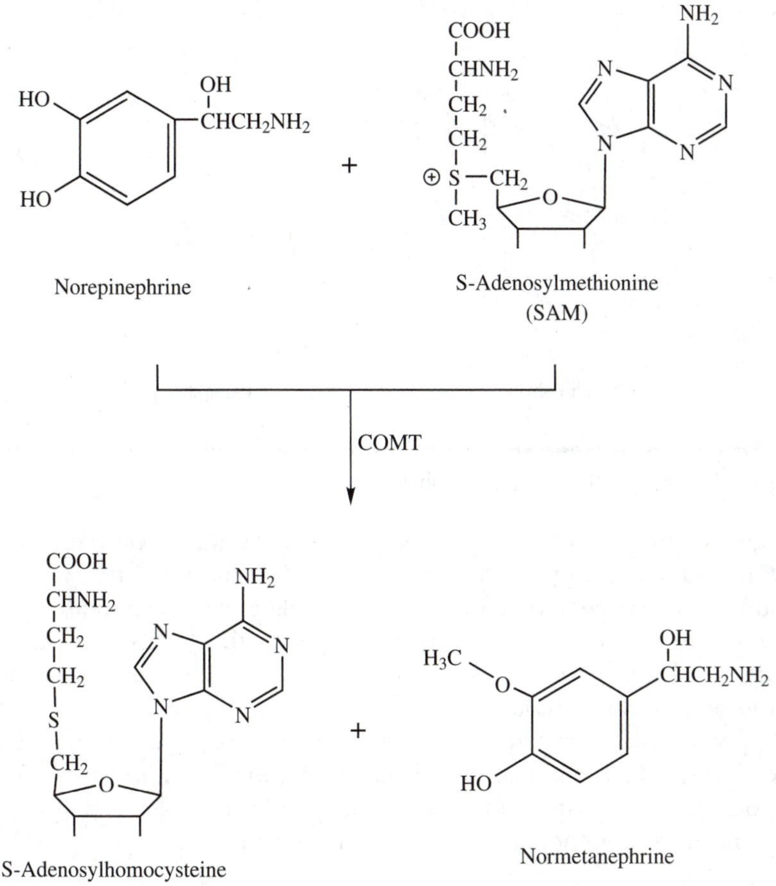

Figure 7.40 Methylation of norepinephrine by catechol-*O*-methyl transferase (COMT).

DOSE-DEPENDENT TOXICITY OF ACETAMINOPHEN

The last example to be discussed in this chapter deals with the metabolism of acetaminophen and the conditions under which it generates toxic metabolites. This is shown in Figure 7.46, and it illustrates the dynamic nature of metabolic processes.

Approximately 96% of a normal dose of acetaminophen is metabolized to nontoxic sulfate and glucuronide derivatives. The remaining 4% is oxidized by CYP450 at the nitrogen atom to generate a toxic metabolite after loss of water from the molecule. This toxic metabolite is called *N*-acetylbenzoquinoneimine, and at normal doses it is expediently detoxified by reaction with glutathione. At levels 7 to 10 times the recommended

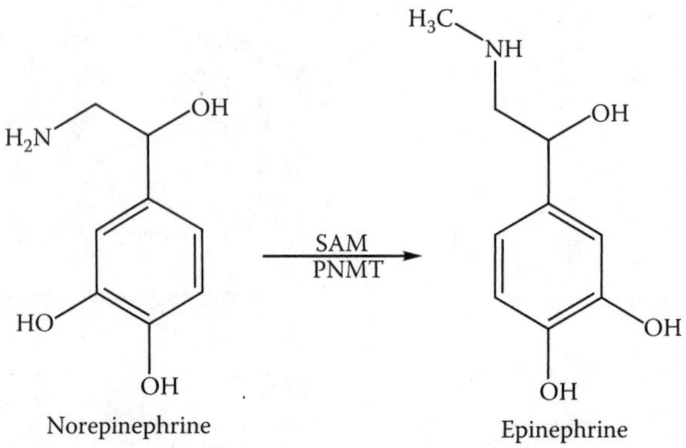

Figure 7.41 Biosynthesis of epinephrine.

dosage, or under conditions that exacerbate P450 induction (i.e., alcoholism), the sulfate and glucuronide pathways become saturated, and larger amounts of toxic metabolite begin to accumulate, which cannot efficiently be eliminated by reaction with glutathione. As the levels of glutathione are depleted, the toxic metabolite causes fatal liver damage by reacting with important macromolecules.

Applying the information presented in this chapter, it is possible to anticipate similar functional group transformations in other drugs. It also provides the healthcare team with the molecular basis for biotransformations and dose-dependent adverse effects of drugs.

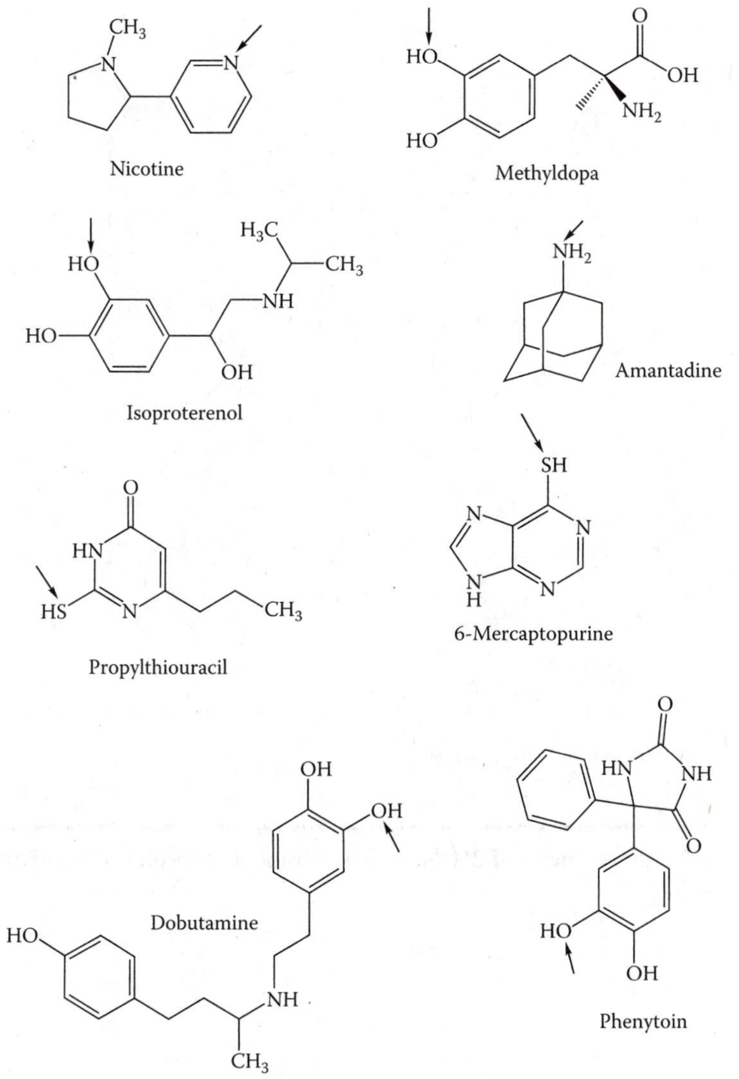

Nicotine

Methyldopa

Isoproterenol

Amantadine

Propylthiouracil

6-Mercaptopurine

Dobutamine

Phenytoin

Figure 7.42   Methylation of some common drugs.

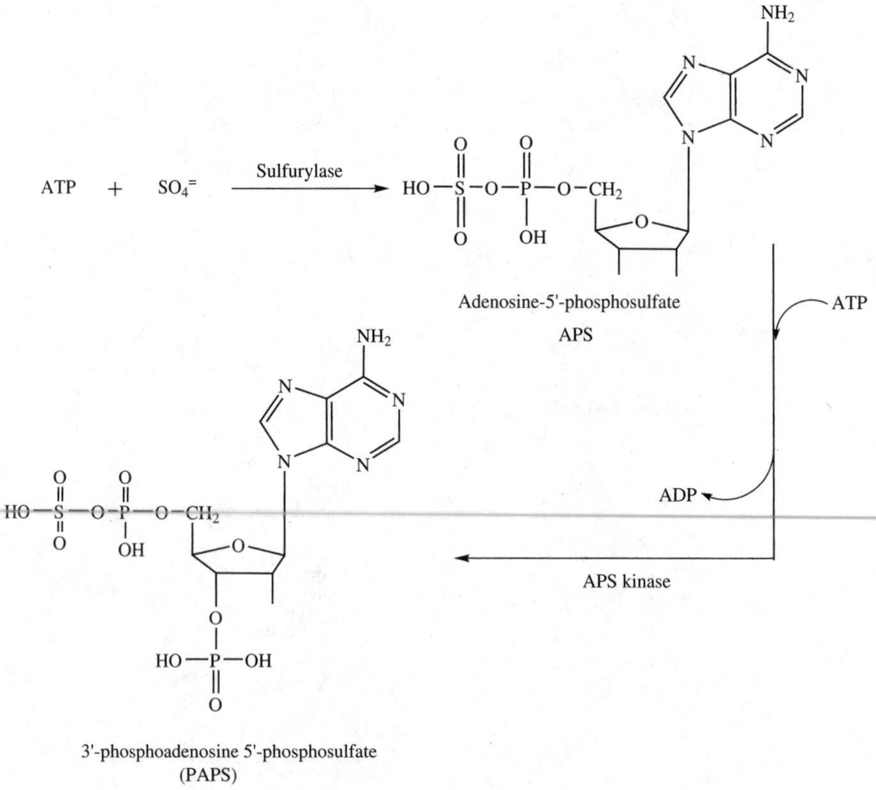

Figure 7.43   Biosynthesis of 3'-phosphoadenosine 5'-phosphosulfate (PAPS).

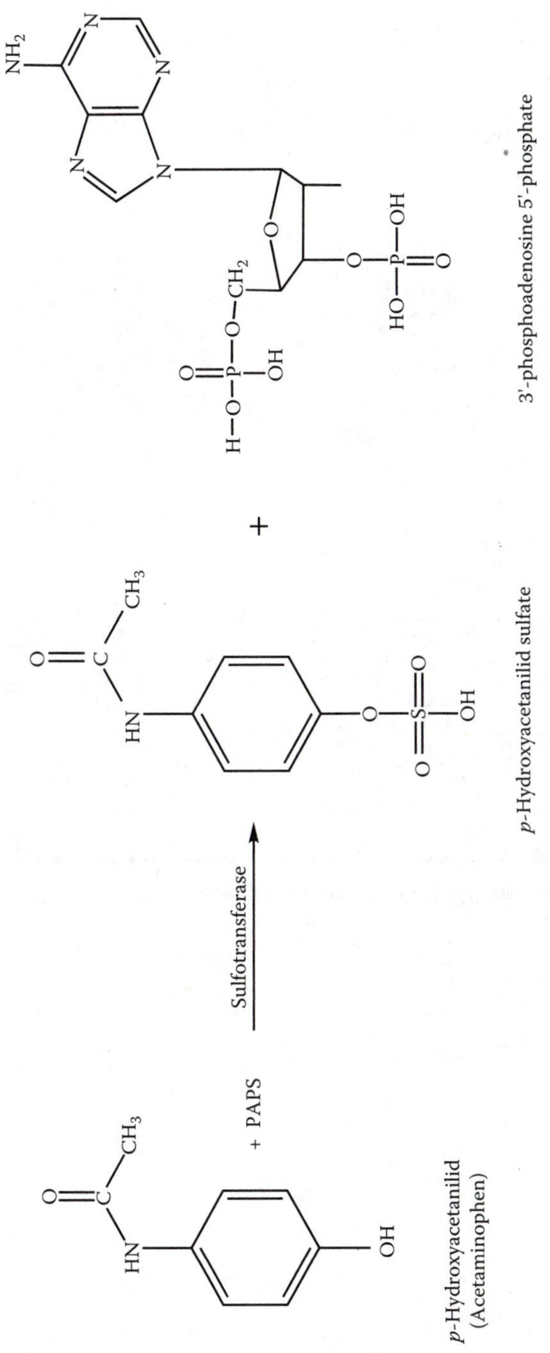

3'-phosphoadenosine 5'-phosphate

+

Sulfotransferase

p-Hydroxyacetanilid (Acetaminophen)

+ PAPS

p-Hydroxyacetanilid sulfate

Figure 7.44 Sulfate conjugation of acetaminophen.

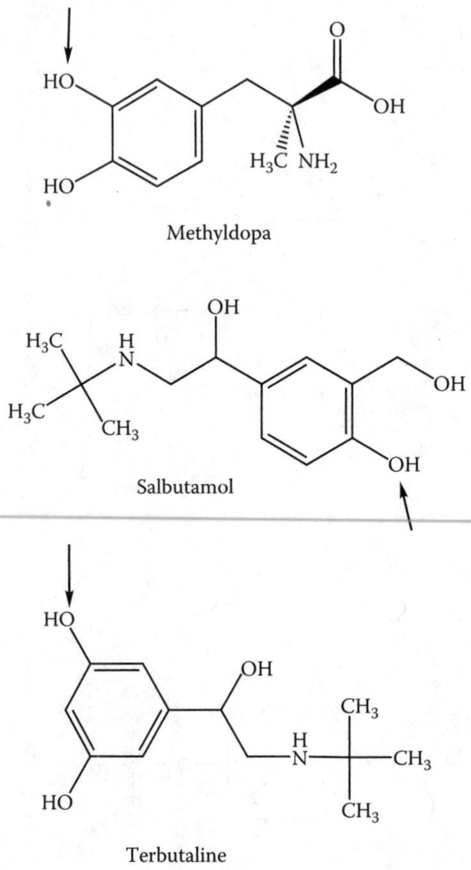

Methyldopa

Salbutamol

Terbutaline

Figure 7.45 Sulfate conjugation of some common drugs.

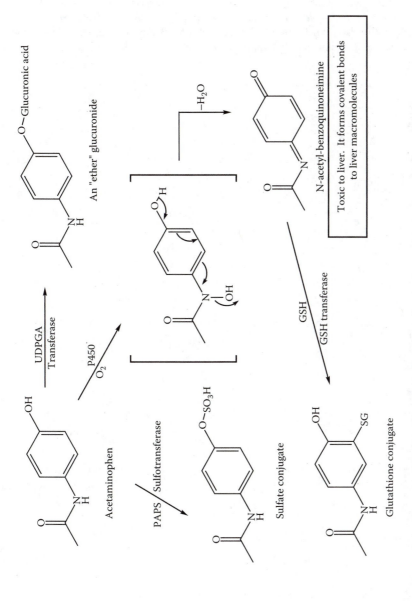

Figure 7.46 Dose-dependent toxicity of acetaminophen.

FURTHER READING

1. *Basic and Clinical Pharmacology* by Bertram G. Katzung (Editor). Chapter 4. Lange Medical Books/McGraw-Hill; 9th Edition (2004).
2. *Principles of Drug Action: The Basis of Pharmacology* by W. B. Pratt (Editor) and P. Taylor (Editor). Chapter 5. Churchill Livingstone; 3rd Edition (1990).
3. *Wilson and Gisvold's Textbook of Organic Medicinal and Pharmaceutical Chemistry* by John H. Block (Editor), John M. Beale, Jr. Chapter 4. Lippincott Williams & Wilkins; 11th Edition (2004).

III

PRINCIPLES
OF DRUG–RECEPTOR
AND DRUG–ENZYME
INTERACTIONS

8

DRUG RECEPTORS AND PHARMACODYNAMICS

MECHANISMS OF DRUG ACTION

A drug can be taken through different routes — oral (PO), intravenous (IV), intraperitoneal (IP), intramuscular (IM), etc. Once the drug enters the body, before it is metabolized into an inactive form through one of many different pathways and excreted from the body, it produces a desired pharmacological effect. The pharmacological as well as toxicological effects of most drugs result from their interaction with cellular components such as DNA, RNA, or proteins of a target organism (Figure 8.1). The interactions between drug molecules and the macromolecules of the body eventually initiate biochemical and physiological changes that are very characteristic of the drugs.

Drug interactions occur through different forms of macromolecules that may have specific functions. For example, the protein molecules interacting with drugs may be *receptors, enzymes, transporters,* or just a *membrane component* of a cell (Figure 8.2). As a result of a drug interaction their function may be either enhanced or decreased. The imposed changes on the macromolecules may act independently or initiate chain reactions that are responsible for the pharmacological effect of the drug.

CHEMICAL SIGNALING AND RECEPTOR FUNCTION

Chemical Signaling

Communication between cells is required to coordinate the activities of different organs within the body. Cells of various organs and tissues interact

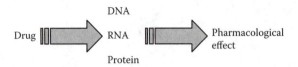

Figure 8.1   The three important macromolecule targets that interact with drug molecules.

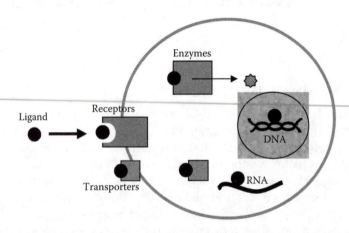

Figure 8.2   The different kinds of intracellular and extracellular macromolecules and receptors that can bind a ligand.

with each other by transmitting chemical signals. Signals activating a cell may come from distant sites or from very close proximity in the form of *hormones, growth factors, neurotransmitters,* or other substances. These signaling molecules are called *first messengers.* The cells present in any organism are thought to communicate in five different ways, as illustrated in Figure 8.3:

1. *Autocrine*: Signaling chemicals coming from a cell act on their own receptors (e.g., norepinephrine acting on the presynaptic receptors and cytokines acting on lymphocytes).
2. *Paracrine*: Signaling chemicals influence the function of neighboring cells and cells present in the close vicinity (e.g., histamine, serotonin).
3. *Endocrine*: Signaling chemicals are carried to the distant sites and act on discrete organs (insulin, estrogen, testosterone, etc.).

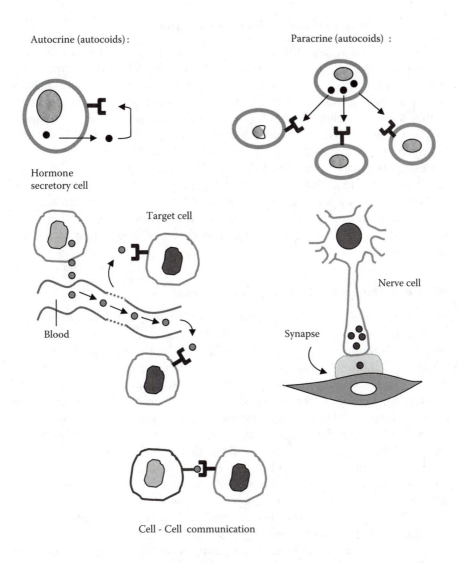

Autocrine (autocoids):

Paracrine (autocoids) :

Hormone
secretory cell

Target cell

Blood

Nerve cell

Synapse

Cell - Cell communication

Figure 8.3   Some examples of signaling molecules.

4. *Neurotransmission*: Signaling chemicals are present in gap junctions and activate postsynaptic neurons or interacting cells (acetylcholine, norepinephrine, etc.).
5. *Cell–cell communication*: Direct communication occurs through interaction of signaling molecules anchored on the cell membranes (T cell–B cell interaction, HIV [gp120]–T cell [CD4] interaction).

Autocrine, Paracrine, and Endocrine Function

The signaling molecules involved in autocrine and paracrine function are the local chemical mediators that are normally referred as *autocoids* (Greek: "self-remedy"). The autocoids could be short-lived biochemicals whose actions are often limited to receptors found on the cells or tissues within a close viscinity from the origin of the autocoids. Some examples of autocoids are lymphokines, histamine, and prostaglandin E_2. On the other hand, hormones that are secreted from glands or glandular tissues generally carry out endocrine functions. Hormones are biochemicals that are stable and are able to reach target receptors located on distant organs and remote tissues. Some good examples of hormones are insulin, adreno-corticotropic hormone, thyroid stimulating hormone, somatropin, and epidermal growth factor. Examples of various types of signaling molecules are given in Table 8.1.

Nature of the Signaling Molecules (Ligands)

Signaling molecules can be either *water soluble* or *lipid soluble*. All known neurotransmitters as well as most hormones and local chemical mediators are water-soluble molecules. The main exceptions are the steroid and thyroid hormones, which are relatively water *insoluble*. These water-insoluble hormones are made soluble for transport in the bloodstream by binding to specific carrier proteins. This difference in solubility gives rise to a fundamental difference in the mechanism by which the two classes of molecules influence target cells. Due to their hydrophilic nature the water-soluble ligands cannot pass through the lipid bilayer, due to the *hydrophylic* nature; hence, they bind to receptor proteins on the *cell surface*. On the other hand, the steroid and thyroid hormones are *hydrophobic* (lipophilic); hence, they can easily pass through the plasma membrane of the target cells. These hormones bind to specific receptor proteins that are located *inside* the cell (Figure 8.4).

In the body all three kinds of signaling molecules may coordinate to produce a desired effect. For example, when the body is suddenly exposed to severe cold temperature, subsequent events leading to the release and hormonal action of thyroxine (T_4), which controls metabolic activity in target cells, involve the action of all three types of signaling molecules — local chemical mediators, neurotansmitters, and hormones. The signaling cascade starts when nerve cells in the hypothalamic regions of the brain are stimulated to secrete local chemical mediators into the blood vessels of the pituitary to activate the pituitary gland. The pituitary in turn stimulates the release of thyroid stimulating hormone (TSH) from the pituitary glands in response. The TSH then acts on the cells in the thyroid gland to initiate the synthesis and secretion of thyroid hormone. The

Table 8.1 Some Examples of Signaling Molecules

Type of Mediator	Site of Secretion	Site of Action
Autocoids		
Autocrine		
Lymphokines (IL-2)	Helper T-cells	IL-2 receptor on helper T-cells
Norepinephrine	Presynaptic neurons	Presynaptic neurons
Paracrine		
Histamine	Mast cells	H_1, H_2, and H_3 receptors on smooth muscle, endothelial cells, cardiac muscle, and nerve cells
Serotonin	Serotonergic neurons and enterochromaffin cells	Brain and GI tract
Endocrine		
Insulin	β-cells of pancreas	Liver, muscle, etc.
Somatotropin	Anterior pituitary	Skeletal muscle and bone
Neurotransmitter		
Acetylcholine	Parasympathetic neurons	Pre- and postsynaptic neurons, neuromuscular junctions, etc.
Norepinephrine	Peripheral sympathetic neurons	Pre- and postsynaptic neurons, neuromuscular junctions etc.
γ-aminobutyric acid (GABA)	Inhibitory neurons	Central nervous system (corpus striatum)
Cell–cell communication	B cell and T cells	Class II MHC (major histocompatibility complex) and TCR (T cell receptor)
	HIV and helper T-cell	Gip_{120} (glycoprotein$_{120}$) and CD_4 (clusters of differentiation$_4$)

thyroid hormone then stimulates a variety of metabolic processes in most cells in the body that eventually maintain the body temperature. This sequence of events is illustrated in Figure 8.5.

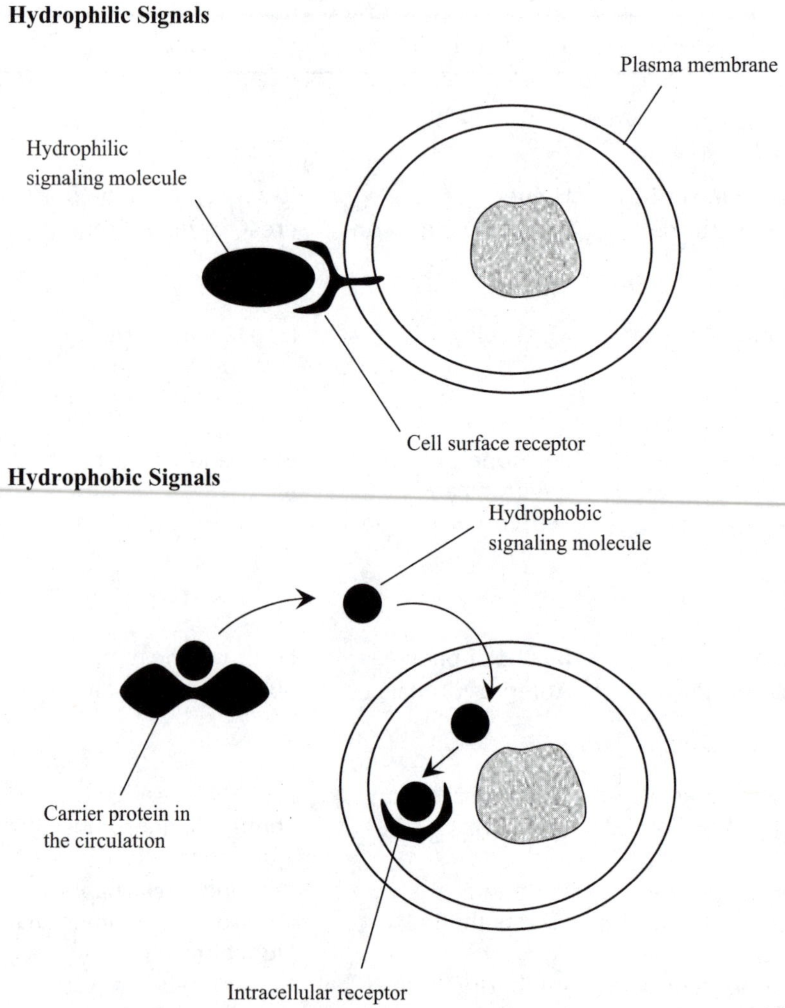

Hydrophilic Signals

Plasma membrane

Hydrophilic
signaling molecule

Cell surface receptor

Hydrophobic Signals

Hydrophobic
signaling molecule

Carrier protein in
the circulation

Intracellular receptor

Figure 8.4 The nature and major classification of signaling molecules.

Different Kinds of Receptors

Receptors in the cell are the receivers of signals coming from another location. In most instances the primary function of receptors is to conduct the signals received by them to an intracellular component and produce necessary biochemical or physiological effects. Receptors can be broadly classified into three categories depending on their location and function (Figure 8.6).

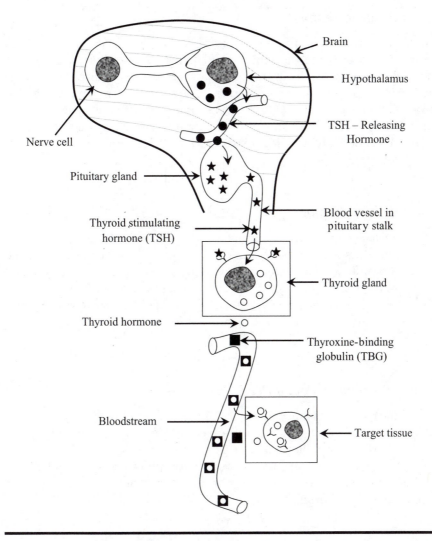

Figure 8.5 A schematic illustration of how different kinds of signal molecules coordinate to produce either a physiologic or metabolic activity in the body.

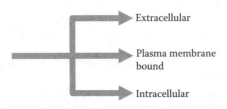

Figure 8.6 Three classes of receptor molecules.

Extracellular Receptors

Extracellular receptors are present as free receptors outside of a cell. They can be found either in the blood circulation or in the fluids surrounding the cells. The extracellular receptors mostly act as transporters or as clearance molecules. Good examples of extracellular receptors are thyroxine binding globulins (TBG), which transport thyroxine; immunoglobulins (IgG), which bind antigens, and atrial natriuretic peptide clearance (ANP-C) receptors, which clear excess ANP (atrial natriuretic peptide) from the circulation.

Intracellular Receptors

Intracellular receptors are typically steroid hormone–binding receptors. These receptors are normally found in the cytoplasm of the cells. Once these intracellular receptors are bound by an appropriate ligand, they might translocate to the nucleus and initiate transcription of a target gene. These receptors are normally bound by ligands that can cross the cell membrane and reach the cytoplasm, such as estrogen, testosterone, and thyroxine.

Plasma Membrane–Bound Receptors

This is the most abundant form of the three classes of receptors, normally attached to the plasma membrane of cells. These receptors are mostly activated by hydrophilic ligands that cannot cross the cell membrane. Therefore, the plasma membrane–bound receptors act as the mediators of the signals that are carried by hormones or other types of signaling molecules coming from distant sites.

Three Types of Plasma Membrane–Bound Receptors

The plasma membrane–associated receptors can be broadly classified into three categories (Figure 8.7):

1. *Peripheral receptors*, which are loosely attached to the cell membrane
2. *Integral receptors*, which are anchored deeply into the lipid bilayer of the cell membrane
3. *Transmembrane receptors*, which traverse the cell membrane one or more times

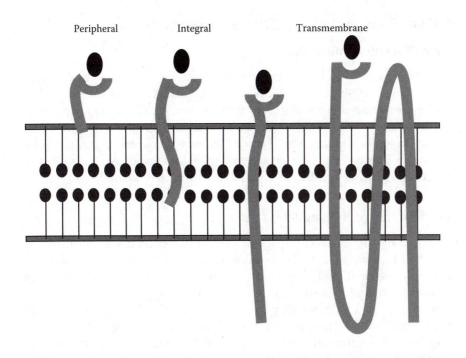

Figure 8.7   Three kinds of membrane receptors: peripheral, integral, and transmembrane receptors.

Membrane-bound receptors perform different functions depending on the type of linkage they have with the cell membrane. Some peripheral receptors such as T-cell receptors simply serve as capturing molecules with no signal-transducing ability. Other peripheral receptors such as atrial natriuretic peptide (ANP-C) or insulin receptors can detach very easily from the cell membrane subsequent to ligand binding and go into the circulation with the bound ligand. The second kind, integral receptors, do not have long cytoplasmic portions and therefore may not have any enzyme activity transmembrane domains physically attached to them. However, the integral receptors might be able to transmit signals via activation of intermediary components such as G proteins. The third kind, transmembrane receptors, are the most common. Some transmembrane receptors span the membrane once; others (e.g., adrenergic) span it several times. Typically, transmembrane receptors conduct the signal to the inside of a cell via activation of a single enzyme or enzyme systems. Therefore, the transmembrane receptors often have an enzyme activity portion in their cytoplasmic domain that becomes activated subsequent to agonist binding.

MODELS OF DRUG–RECEPTOR INTERACTION

Drug–Receptor Interactions

For a drug to be useful either as a therapeutic or scientific tool, it must show a high degree of biological specificity. In other words, it must bind and act only on a particular cell type or tissues. This is determined by the receptors accepting only a certain type of ligans with specific functional groups into its binding site. Hence, ligands are specific for receptors; responses involving any given type of receptors are elicited by a narrow range of chemical substances that have structural similarity.

Key Features of Binding Sites

The binding site of a receptor is the region that contains chemical groups that direct participate in the binding of a ligand. The binding site is a three-dimensional entity formed by groups that come from different parts of the linear amino acid sequence in a receptor molecule. Most of the amino acids in a receptor may not even come in contact with the ligand, but they create the three-dimensional structure of the receptor. The three-dimensional conformation of the receptor molecule is generally required for ligand binding. The specificity of ligand binding to a receptor is also fully dependent on the precise arrangement of atoms in the binding site.

In general, the interactions of drug with receptors resemble the interactions of substrates with enzymes. Generally, there is no great difficulty in measuring the activity of an enzyme but, during the drug receptor interaction, measuring the activation of receptors is very complex and must be performed indirectly. In addition, when a substrate binds to an enzyme it is almost always converted into a product. However, the receptors normally do not modify the ligands that bind to their active site.

Lock-and-Key Fit

The binding of a drug to a receptor molecule is analogous to a *key* (the drug) fitting into a *lock* (the receptor's binding site), and the ability for a ligand to activate a receptor can be compared to the ability of a key to open a compatible lock (Figure 8.8). Therefore, to fit into the binding site, the ligand (drug) must also have a matching or compatible structure and the suitable three-dimensional configuration necessary for the binding. When these requirements are met, the ligand fits into the receptor's binding site like a key fitting into a lock. Hence, this model of interaction is known as *lock and key model* (see Figure 8.8). Though the analogy is crude, it can convey very valid implications and some of them are listed here:

Similar to a key opening a lock, drug "unlocks" the response in a cell.

Lock & Key
Model

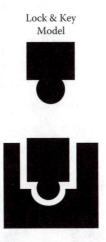

Figure 8.8   The lock-and-key type fitting of a ligand to its receptor.

The lock may be opened by a number of different "keys" (chemically related drugs); hence, a series of chemically related drugs may have same pharmacological action.

Similar to a "master key" opening many rooms in a building, some ligands may be able to activate several subtypes of receptors. Ligands that can activate a few subtypes can be compared to a *submaster* key, and the ligands that are specific for only one subtype of receptors can be compared to a *room-specific key*.

The "lock" (receptor) can be "jammed" by using not-so-completely fitting *blockers*; this inhibits pharmacological responses.

Induced Fit

Another model for ligand receptor interaction is the *induced fit model*. This is because the essential functional groups on the active site of a free receptor may not be in their optimal position for promoting ligand binding when the binding site is unoccupied. When a suitable ligand molecule approaches the receptor, the binding affinity forces the receptor molecule into a conformation in which the active groups assume a favorable conformation that is optimal for ligand binding (Figure 8.9). This is known as *induced fit*. A poor ligand with low affinity would have much difficulty in forcing the receptor molecule into a suitable configuration for optimal binding, while a high-affinity ligand would be able to force these changes easily. For example, many receptors cannot bind the smaller homologs of their ligands; glucose transporters are a good example. Glucose transporters can transport hexoses, yet they cannot transport lower homologs of glucose such as glyceraldehyde. Even though glyceraldehyde is a

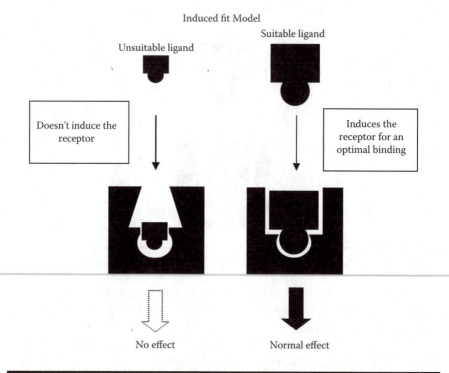

Figure 8.9 The induction of the receptor molecule's binding site structure is changed by a suitable ligand that facilitates appropriate binding.

smaller molecule, because of the presence of similar functional groups (aldehyde, hydroxyl, and carboxylic) it would be expected to penetrate readily to the binding site and function as a very effective ligand. However, in reality glyeraldehyde does not activate the glucose transporter.

AFFINITY AND INTRINSIC ACTIVITY

Affinity

The affinity of a drug is the tenacity or persistent ability with which the drug binds to the specific receptors on the cell membrane. In statistical terms, the *affinity* is the probability of a drug molecule binding to *free drug receptors* at any given instant.

Intrinsic Activity

The *intrinsic* activity of a drug is the inherent property of the drug to impart biological signals (structural changes or changes in the three-dimensional configuration that result in the activation of the receptor-linked enzymes) on the receptor molecules that result in biological response. Therefore, an immediate consequence of intrinsic activity is the activation of a second messenger system. Thus, affinity gets the drug to the receptors, and the intrinsic activity determines what the drug can do when it gets to the receptors. The intrinsic activity is normally a property of the drug, not the tissues.

AGONISTS, ANTAGONISTS, AND PARTIAL AGONISTS

Agonists

By simple definition, a drug that produces stimulation of the receptor is labeled as an *agonist*. Powerful drugs that can produce the maximal response in any given tissue are termed *full agonists*. Endogenous chemicals such as hormones and neurotransmitters naturally have full affinity and intrinsic activity to stimulate a specific receptor molecule as a result of binding and therefore are considered full agonists. To explain it simply, full agonists are expected to have 1.0 (full) affinity and 1.0 (full) intrinsic activity.

Antagonists

Pharmacological antagonists have no or very little intrinsic activity; however, they can bind to receptors with more-or-less the same affinity as agonists. By simple definition, a drug that blocks the stimulation of an agonist is called an *antagonist*. Therefore, antagonists can have full (1.0) affinity, but their intrinsic activity is always zero (0).

Partial Agonist

A *partial agonist* (Figure 8.10) can bind with full affinity, the same as a full agonist, but can produce only a partial effect. The ability to produce the partial effect is generally attributed to the partial *intrinsic activity* that resides with the partial agonist. For easy understanding the partial agonists can be considered as drugs with full (1.0) affinity but with an intrinsic activity greater than 0 (zero) but less than 1.0 (full).

Ligand Structure and Activity Relationship

The affinity and intrinsic activity of a ligand for a receptor are largely determined by its chemical structure. Therefore, even minor modifications in drug molecules may result in major changes in their pharmacological properties. Sometimes, structural modification of agonists has resulted in the development of therapeutically useful antagonists as well.

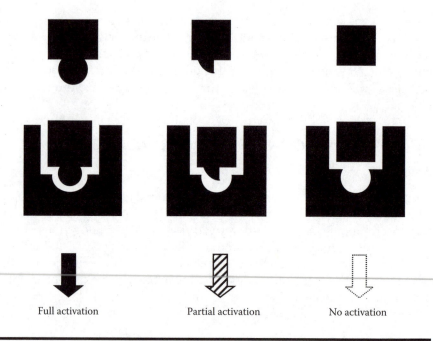

Figure 8.10 The structural difference between an agonist, a partial agonist, and an antagonist.

Why is the Receptor Concept Important?

The receptor concept is important for understanding the consequences of drug action and also for making therapeutic decisions in clinical practice, as follows:

1. *Receptors largely determine the quantitative relationships between dose or concentration of a drug and pharmacological effects.* The receptor's affinity for binding to a drug determines the concentration of a drug needed to form a significant number of drug–receptor complexes.
2. *Receptors are responsible for the selectivity of drug action.* The molecular size, shape, and electrical charges of a drug determines with what affinity ligands will bind to the receptors.
3. *Receptors mediate the actions of pharmacological antagonists.*

DIFFERENTIAL EFFECTS OF AGONISTS

Differential Effects of Epinephrine

Different target cells may respond in different ways to the same agonist because different organs may express different subtypes of a particular

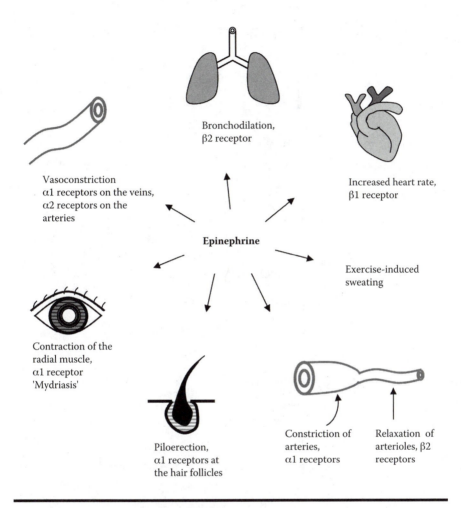

Figure 8.11   The differential effects of epinephrine.

receptor. The best example is the effect produced by *adrenaline* (*epi-nephrine*) in the body once it is released from the adrenals (Figure 8.11). Though norepinephrine is the principal catecholamine neurotransmitter involved in regulating the sympathetic pathway, epinephrine is an equally effective and more stable adrenergic agonist released primarily from the adrenal glands. The steps in the enzymatic biosynthesis of the catecholamines dopamine, norepinephrine (noradrenaline), and epinephrine (adrenaline) are illustrated below (Figure 8.12). The enzyme involved in each catalytic step is indicated in the circles. The first three enzymatic steps occur in *postganglionic sympathetic* nerve terminals, leading to the synthesis of norepinephrine. In the adrenal medulla all the four enzymatic steps occur, resulting in the synthesis of epinephrine. Release of epinephrine

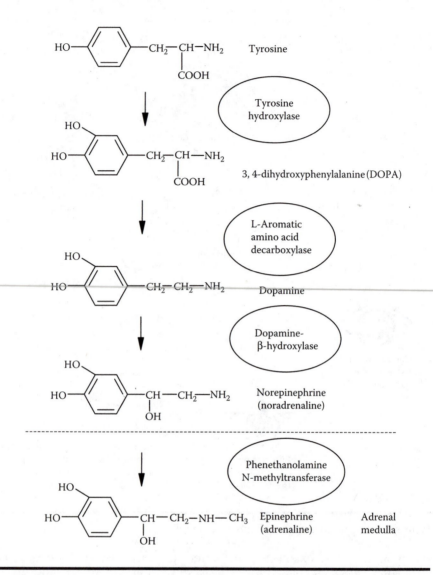

Figure 8.12 The biosynthesis pathway for norepinephrine and epinephrine.

occurs as a result of the activation of the sympathetic nerves innervating the adrenal glands leading to the manifestation of a range of different physiological effects. The ability to produce differential effects by single ligand is a very important phenomenon and being familiar with this important phenomenon is necessary to understand the side effects of drugs.

Epinephrine, an endogenous full agonist released from the adrenal glands, is able to activate all subtypes of adrenergic receptors in the body,

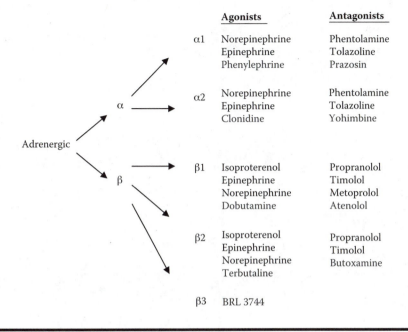

	Agonists	Antagonists
α1	Norepinephrine	Phentolamine
	Epinephrine	Tolazoline
	Phenylephrine	Prazosin
α2	Norepinephrine	Phentolamine
	Epinephrine	Tolazoline
	Clonidine	Yohimbine
β1	Isoproterenol	Propranolol
	Epinephrine	Timolol
	Norepinephrine	Metoprolol
	Dobutamine	Atenolol
β2	Isoproterenol	Propranolol
	Epinephrine	Timolol
	Norepinephrine	Butoxamine
	Terbutaline	
β3	BRL 3744	

Figure 8.13   Adrenergic agonists and antagonists.

producing different effects in different tissues and organs. Similarly, when a drug is injected into the body, it can produce side effects by binding to receptors that are located on a nontargeted tissue and cause side effects. For example, when isoproterenol is used to treat asthma, it could produce an increase in the heart rate by binding to the β1 adrenergic receptors on the heart.

Selective Actions of Adrenergic Agonists and Antagonists

The adrenergic receptors are broadly classified into α and β adrenergic receptors. The α adrenergic receptors are further subdivided into α1 and α2; the β adrenergic receptors are subdivided into β1, β2, and β3. There are agonists and antagonists available that are more specific for each of the types and subtypes of receptors as given in Figure 8.13.

Agonists or antagonists can be very selective and bind to only to a particular subtype of receptors. While binding to a specific subtype of receptors on the tissues or organs, the drugs can produce physiological effects through a single subtype of receptors, while possible side effects resulting from activation of another subtype of receptors will be absent. This concept can be better understood by studying how adrenergic agonists and antagonists change the blood pressure, vascular resistance, and heart rate in an anesthetized dog.

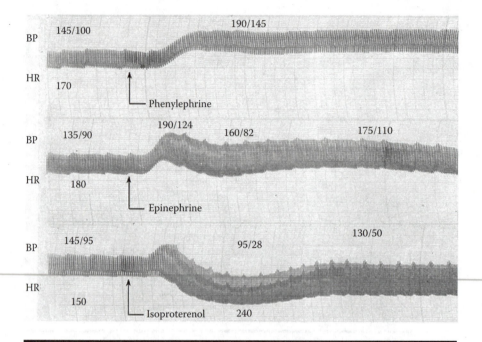

Figure 8.14 **Blood pressure (BP) and heart rate (HR) changes following an intravenous bolus injection of adrenergic α-receptor selective (phenylephrine), β-receptor selective (isoproterenol), and nonselective (epinephrine) agonists to an anesthetized dog. The effects are blunted but not abolished in the anesthetized animal.**

The changes in blood pressure and heart rate after intravenous bolus injections of phenylephrine, epinephrine, and isoproterenol are shown in the tracings given in Figure 8.14. The numbers indicated prior to the injection of agonists, such as 145/100, are initial systolic and diastolic blood pressure, and 170 is the heart rate. When phenylephrine is injected into an experimental animal, both systolic and diastolic blood pressure are increased; this effect is primarily due to relatively selective binding of phenylephrine to the arterial $\alpha1$ receptors, increasing the peripheral vascular resistance and decreasing the venous capacitance. Due to the presence of cardiovascular reflex mechanisms, the rise in vascular pressure leads to a baroreceptor-mediated increase in vagal tone, and slowing of the heart rate (referred to as bradycardia). When a pure $\alpha1$ receptor agonist is used in hypotensive patients, reflex bradycardia is usually not noticed because the blood pressure returns to normal rather than exceeding normal. In the second example, when epinephrine is injected separately as bolus injection, it simultaneously increases the peripheral vascular resistance by binding to the $\alpha1$ receptors and increases the heart rate by binding to the $\beta1$ receptors on the heart. After an initial spike in the blood pressure, both diastolic and systolic pressures are reduced, reaching 160/82. This reduction in pressure occurs because of the activation of the β2 receptors on the arterioles, causing relaxation that reduces the arterial pressure. When isoproterenol is injected, due to its selectivity for binding only to β1 and β2 adrenergic receptors, the heart rate is increased significantly. After a small spike in blood pressure caused by isoproterenol due to increased cardiac output, the vascular resistance is reduced significantly. The reduction in vascular resistance is primarily due to activation of the β2 receptors on the arterioles and relaxing them to increase the blood flow in the skeletal muscle.

When antagonists are used to block receptors, an important consideration for predicting the extent of physiological effect is a possible competition between endogenous or exogenous agonist and the antagonist. Generally, three factors will determine whether an agonist or antagonist is going to control the receptors:

1. Affinity of the agonist or antagonist
2. Concentration of agonist or antagonist
3. Sequence of introduction

The effects of antagonists on blood pressure (BP) and heart rate (HR) are depicted in Figures 8.15 and 8.16. For example, when phentolamine, an α adrenergic blocker, is introduced into the body in sufficient concentrations, it can block the α1 adrenergic receptors on the arteries and reduce the vascular resistance that was originally sustained by endogenous agonists. The drop in the vascular resistance below normal could lead to reflex tachycardia through activation of sensory receptors and cause an increase in the heart rate. On the other hand, if injection of phentolamine is preceded by epinephrine, a master agonist, then the agonist takes control of all α and β adrenergic receptors. Therefore, the α1 adrenergic blocking effect of phentolamine cannot be seen; only the effect of the agonist is perceived. On the contrary, when phentolamine is injected prior to epinephrine, it readily occupies the α1 receptor and blocks the binding of epinephrine to these receptors, and thereby also blocks any increase in the vascular resistance. The greater reduction in the vascular pressure caused by phentolamine in the presence of epinephrine is typically due to the combination of both reduction in vascular resistance by α1 blockade and relaxation of arterioles due to β2 receptor stimulation by epinephrine.

Another example for selective inhibition of the adrenergic receptor is blocking of the β adrenergic receptors by propranolol. Similar to phentolamine, propranolol would be able to block both β1 and β2 adrenergic receptors when injected prior to epinephrine but would not block the α1 adrenergic receptor effect. As a result of the β1 receptor blockade, epinephrine no longer augments the force of contraction nor increases the

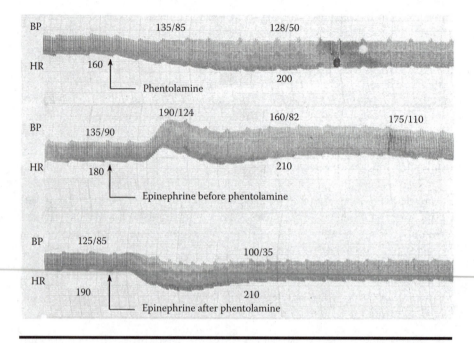

Figure 8.15 *Top*: **Blood pressure (BP) and heart rate (HR) changes following an intravenous bolus injection of an adrenergic α-receptor blocking drug (phentolamine) to an anesthetized dog. The reversal of the effect by epinephrine is demonstrated by response to epinephrine injection before (*middle*) and after (*bottom*) phentolamine injection.**

cardiac rate. However, the vascular resistance is much higher when both propranolol and epinephrine are injected together, as compared to when epinephrine is injected alone. The augmentation in vascular resistance in spite of reduction in the heart rate and cardiac output is due to contraction of arteries by epinephrine through α1 receptors and also simultaneous contraction of the arterioles due to blockade of β2 receptors. The clinical uses of adrenergic agonists and antagonists are listed in Table 8.2.

Atypical Receptors

There are some receptors present in the body that are not very typical in their function or in the way in which they are activated. Many of these receptors are neither activated by a ligand nor initiate a signaling cascade in a typical manner. Some of the atypical receptors are *autoreceptors, heteroreceptors, baroreceptors, chemoreceptors* and *sensory receptors*. The autoreceptors are usually self-limiting receptors; therefore, they are called biological breaks. Typically the autoreceptors control the flow of neurotransmission by controlling the release of neurotransmitters. In the case

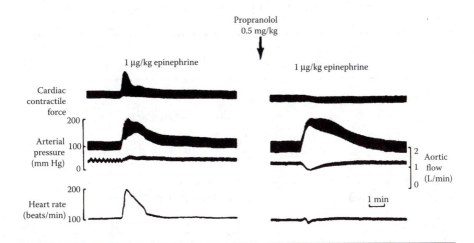

Figure 8.16   Blood pressure (BP) and heart rate (HR) changes following an intra-venous bolus injection of epinephrine before and after the β-adrenergic blocking agent propranolol. In the presence of propranolol, epinephrine is no longer able to increase the force of contraction (measure by a strain gauge attached to the ventricular wall) nor increase the cardiac rate. The blood pressure increase is sustained much longer because of the inhibition of peripheral arteriole dilation by phentolamine.

of heteroreceptors, two different types of receptors that are activated by distinctly dissimilar ligands interact synergistically or antagonistically. The other types of atypical receptors and their specific functions are listed in Table 8.3.

CHOLINERGIC NEUROTRANSMISSION

The central nervous system consists of the brain and the spinal cord. All other nerves in the body comprise the peripheral nervous system. Efferent nerves carry messages from the central nervous system to all parts of the body (the periphery). Afferent nerves carry information from the periphery to the central nervous system. In the peripheral nervous system, there are two types of efferent nerves: the somatic nervous system that goes to skeletal muscles, and the autonomic nervous system that includes the enteric nervous system, which goes to smooth muscles, secretory glands, the heart, the lung, and other organs. The messages, in the form of electrical activity, are conducted along nerve fibers or axons. Between the terminus of two nerves or between the nerve terminal and an effector organ that the nerve controls (innervates), there is a gap called the *synapse* or *synaptic cleft*. When the conducted electrical impulse (action potential) reaches the nerve terminus, it provokes the release of specific chemicals

Table 8.2 Some Examples of Clinical Use of Adrenergic Agonists and Antagonists

Drug	Receptors Involved	Physiological Effect
Agonists		
Phenylephrine	α1	Produce mydriasis; also acts as a nasal decongestant
Clonidine	α2	Acts centrally and decreases norephinephrine release
Isoproterenol	β1	Produces tachycardia
Terbutaline	β2	Used for acute relief of asthma
Antagonists		
Prazosin	α1	Used for treatment of hypertension
Yohimbine	α2	Blocks norepinephrine uptake at the presynaptic site and increases the neurotransmitter level at the synaptic gap
Propranolol	β1	Slows the heart in patients with tachycardia or angina and reduces oxygen requirement that might lead to myocardial infarction

called *neurotransmitters*. These chemicals diffuse across the synaptic cleft and activate the receptors on the postsynaptic membrane. The nerves are then said to be activated or excited, and their activation triggers a series of chemical events resulting ultimately in a biological response such as muscle contraction. The processes involving neurotransmitter release, diffusion, and receptor activation are referred to collectively as *transmission*. There are many types of transmission, and they are named for the specific neurotransmitter involved. Thus, *cholinergic transmission* involves the release of the neurotransmitter, *acetylcholine*, and its activation of the postsynaptic receptor. Acetylcholine is the endogenous agonist for all cholinergic receptors.

Synthesis and Release of Acetylcholine

The neurotransmitter that mediates synaptic transmission between preganglionic and postganglionic nerve fibers in the parasympathetic pathway is *acetylcholine*. The cholinergic neurotransmitter acetylcholine is synthesized in the neurons at neuroeffector and ganglionic junctions from the immediate precursors acetyl CoA and choline by the action of *choline acetyl transferase* (Figure 8.17). The synthesis of acetylcholine takes place in the axoplasm of the neurons with the help of choline that is accumulated

Table 8.3 Different Types of Atypical Receptors and Activating Factors

Receptors	Location	Activating Factors
Autoreceptors	α1 receptors on the presynaptic neurons in the adrenergic pathway	Inhibit the release of NE by feedback mechanism
Heteroreceptors		
Stimulatory (−)	Postsynaptic neurons at the neuroeffector junction	Neuro Peptide Y (NPY) receptor would reduce the effect mediated by NE (norepinephrine) through adrenergic receptors.
Inhibitory (+)	Postsynaptic neurons at the neuroeffector junction	Angiotensin II receptors would augment the effect mediated by NE through adrenergic receptors.
Baroreceptors	In the carotid sinuses and also in the aortic arch	Vascular barometric pressure
Chemoreceptors	Chemoreceptor Trigger Zone (CTZ)	Activated by a variety of anticancer and other drugs
Sensory receptors		
Auditory receptors	Ear	Sound
Visual receptors	Eye	Light
Heat/cold sensing receptors	Skin	Temperature

into the axoplasm from extraneuronal sites by an active uptake process. Once synthesized, this neurotransmitter is packaged in small storage vesicles and stored within the cytoplasm until sufficient action potential at the nerve terminals releases it from the storage vesicles (Figure 8.18). After its release, acetylcholine specifically binds to the cholinergic receptors at the postsynaptic site and initiates a receptor-specific signal. The acetyl choline that is released in to the synaptic gap is finally hydrolyzed by *acetylcholinesterase.*

Differential Effects of Acetylcholine through Cholinergic Receptors

Acetylcholine produces its various effects by binding to (Figure 8.19) specific receptors, called *cholinergic receptors*, present on various organs. These receptors are normally found at the cholinergic synapses and at

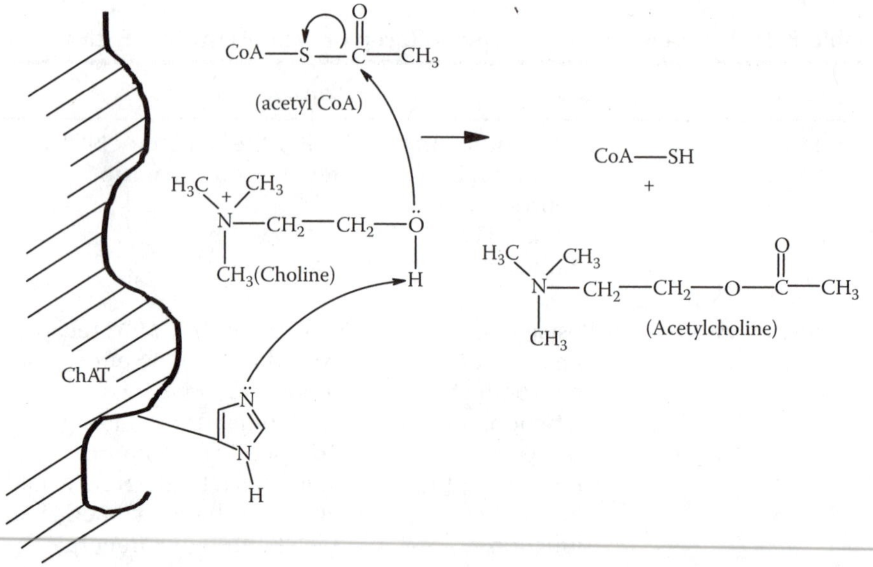

Figure 8.17 Synthesis of acetylcholine in the neurons by choline acetyl transferase.

the neuroeffector junctions in the central and the peripheral nervous systems. The difference in responses elicited by acetylcholine result from actual differences in cholinergic receptors.

Muscarinic and Nicotinic Actions of Acetylcholine

Cholinergic activities are generally designated as muscarinic and nicotinic. Drugs and chemicals that can produce physiological responses by stimulating the parasympathetic nervous system through cholinergic receptors in general are termed *cholinomimetics*. The effects produced are either *nicotinic* or *muscarinic,* depending on the subtype of the receptors activated. A similar distinction is used to classify antagonists at cholinergic receptors as *antimuscarinic* or *antinicotinic.* The muscarinic activities of acetylcholine are those that can be reproduced by the injection of *muscarine,* the active principle of the poisonous mushroom *Amanita muscaria.* The muscarinic effect can be blocked by small doses of atropine. After the muscarinic effects have been blocked by atropine, large doses of acetylcholine produce effects similar to those produced by *nicotine*; this effect is called nicotinic. The muscarinic and nicotinic responses are mediated by a group of specialized receptors; therefore, the receptors that mediate muscarinic and nicotinic effects are subdivided as shown below:

Muscarinic: M_1, M_2, M_3, and M_4
Nicotinic: Ganglionic (N_N) and skeletal muscle (N_M)

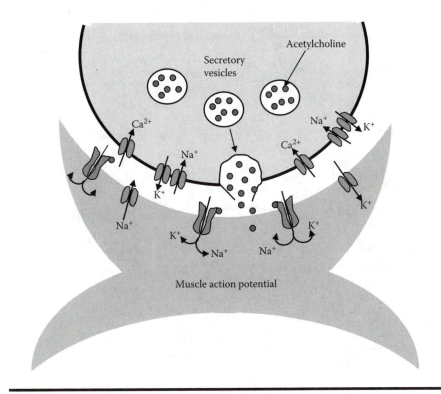

Figure 8.18 The release of acetylcholine from secretory granules and the creation of the membrane potential at the neuroeffector junction.

The Location and Function of Acetylcholine Receptors

Nicotinic receptors fall into two classes, the muscle and neuronal types. Muscle nicotinic receptors (N_M) are normally found at the skeletal neuromuscular junctions (NMJ); neuronal nicotinic receptors (N_N) are found in the autonomic ganglia, and also in the brain where acetylcholine is a neurotransmitter. The molecular structures of these receptors are similar, but they differ pharmacologically. Gene cloning has revealed at least five distinct types of muscarinic receptors, but only four of the receptors have been distinguished functionally and pharmacologically. Three of the muscarinic receptors (M_1, M_2, and M_3) are well characterized. M_1 receptors (neural) are found mainly on the central nervous system (CNS) and peripheral neurons, they mediate slow excitatory response M_2 receptors are found in the heart and also on the presynaptic terminals of peripheral and central neurons. M_2 receptors exhibit an inhibitory effect mainly by increasing K^+ conductance and by inhibiting Ca^{++} channels. M_2 receptor activation is responsible for the vagal inhibition of the heart as well as presynaptic inhibition in the CNS and periphery. M_3 receptors that are found in the glands (e.g., salivary glands,

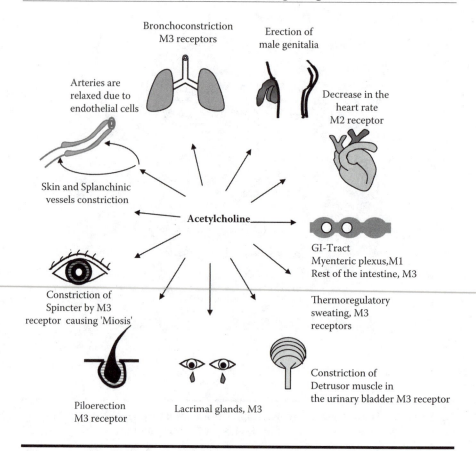

Figure 8.19 The differential effects of acetylcholine.

sweat glands) and smooth muscles produce excitatory effects that result in stimulation of glandular secretions (saliva, sweat, etc.) and contraction of smooth muscles. M_1, M_2, and M_3 receptors are also present in specific locations in the CNS. M_4 receptors are largely confined to the CNS, and their functional role is yet to be defined. In general, all muscarinic receptors belong to the family of G-protein–coupled receptors. The odd-numbered members of the group (M_1 and M_3) act through the inositol triphosphate (IP_3) pathway, and the even-numbered receptors (M_2 and M_4) act by inhibiting adenylate cyclase and thereby reduce intracellular cyclic adenosine monophosphate (cAMP) levels.

Figure 8.20 shows the sites of action of acetylcholine in the autonomic and somatic nervous system.

Cholinomimetics

Cholinomimetics are compounds that can produce pharmacological and physiological effects similar to those of acetylcholine by binding to

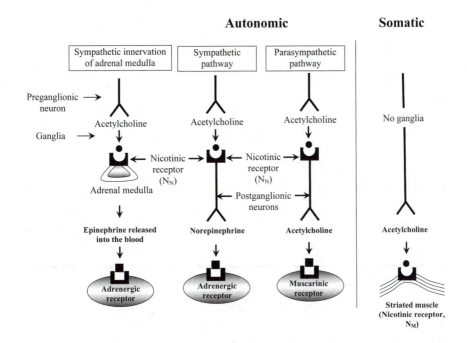

Figure 8.20 Sites of actions of acetylcholine in the autonomic and somatic nervous system.

appropriate receptors. The cholinomimetics are classified into two groups and then further subdivided as shown in Figure 8.21.

Cholinergic Agonists and Antagonists

Cholinergic agonists are direct-acting cholinomimetics. Cholinergic antagonists are receptor-specific blockers with no intrinsic activity. As shown below, in addition to "master" and "submaster" types of agonists and receptor-specific agonists (room key), antagonists also exist with similar specificity. Figure 8.22 lists various cholinergic agonists and antagonists.

Clinical Use of Direct-Acting Cholinomimetics

The direct-acting cholinomimetics can be divided into two main groups: the *choline esters* and the naturally occurring synthetic *alkaloids*. The structures of directly-acting cholinomimetics are shown in Figure 8.23.

Directly-acting cholinomimetics normally produce varying degrees of muscarinic and nicotinic activity. The effects of cholinomimetics that are administered in the usual therapeutic doses are exclusively muscarinic. Some of the organ effects of cholinomimetics are listed in Table 8.4.

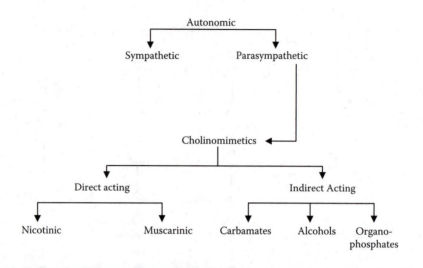

Figure 8.21 Classification of cholinomimetic drugs.

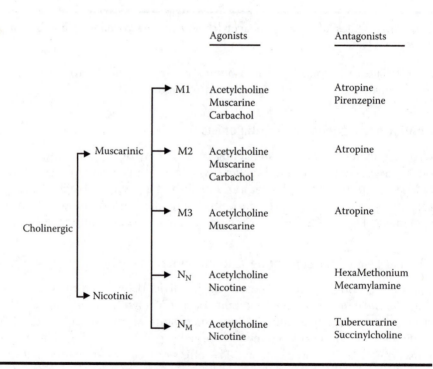

Figure 8.22 Selected cholinergic agonists and antagonists.

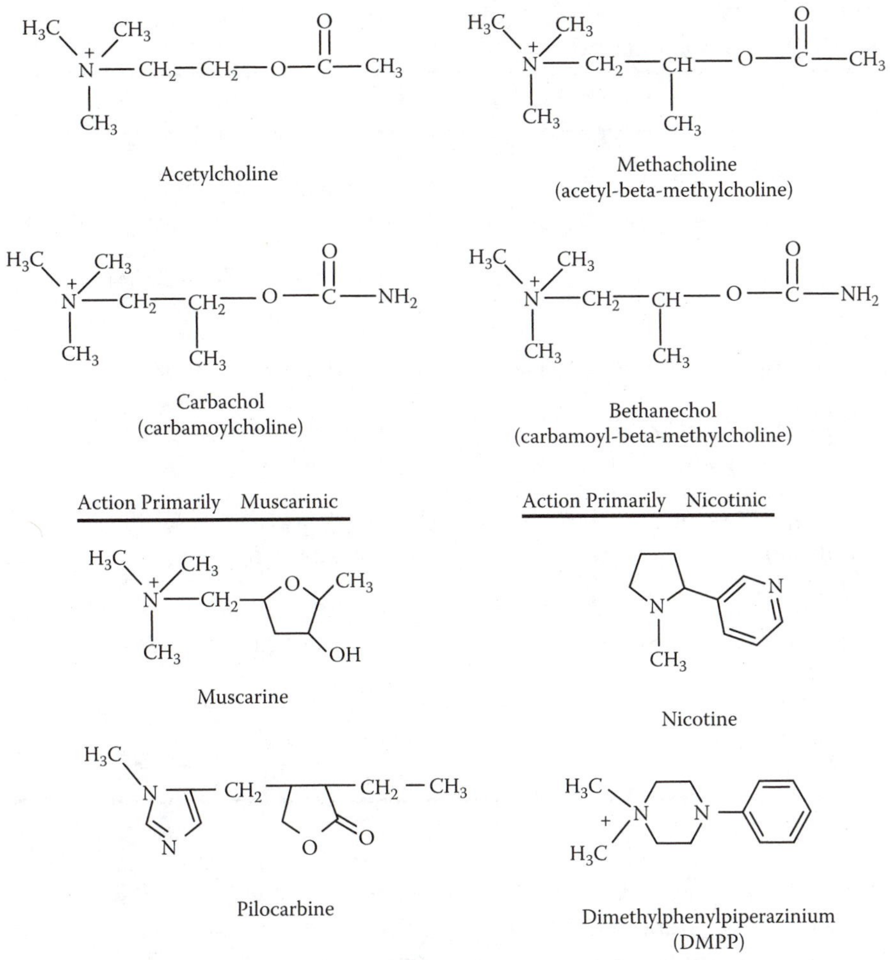

Figure 8.23 Structure of muscarinic and nicotinic (cholinergic) agonists.

Because of its extremely short duration of action, acetylcholine has very limited therapeutic application. In order to obtain any systemic pharmacological effects from exogenously administered acetylcholine, it must be injected intravenously. Even after IV administration, the effects are short lived because of the rapid destruction of acetylcholine by cholinesterases. However, slight modifications of the structure of the acetylcholine molecule have led to three clinically useful choline esters: methacholine (acetyl-β-methylcholine), carbachol (carbamylcholine) and bethanechol (carbaboyl-β-methacholine). These three compounds can bind to the cholinergic receptors in the same manner as acetylcholine does. A primary therapeutic advantage resulting from modifying the acetylcholine

Table 8.4 Specific Types of Muscarinic and Nicotinic Receptors in Different Organs and Tissues

Organ/System	Effect (Receptor Involved)
Eye	
Radial muscle, iris sphincter	Miosis (M_3)
Ciliary muscle contracts	Accommodation for near vision (M_3)
Heart	
Sinoatrial (SA) node	Decelerates, bradycardia (M_2)
Force of contraction	Decreases (M_2)
Blood vessels	
Vascular smooth muscle (EDRF)	Relaxation (M_3)
Lung	
Bronchial muscle	Bronchoconstriction (M_3)
Bronchial glands	Secretion (M_3)
GI tract	
Myenteric plexus	Activates (M_1)
Intestine	Increased motility (M_3)
Urinary bladder	
Detrusor muscle	Contraction (M_3)
Trigone and sphincter	Relaxation (M_3)
Glands	
Lacrimal	Secretion (M_3)
Salivary	Secretion (M_3)
Sweat	Secretion (M_3)

was the resistance of the modified compounds to enzymatic destruction by cholinesterase. This property enables the acetylcholine analogs to have a much longer duration of action than that of the parent compound. The pharmacological actions of choline esters are given in Table 8.5.

Due to its extreme short duration of action, acetylcholine has only one therapeutic application. Acetylcholine chloride (Miochol®) is used during opthalmic surgery to obtain rapid and complete miosis during cataract removal. Methacholine is used for diagnostic purposes to confirm poisoning due to *Atropa belladonna* alkaloids. The diagnosis is confirmed by failure of 10 to 30 mg methacholine, given SC, to elicit characteristic signs of flushing, sweating, salivation, lacrimation, and enhanced gastrointestinal motility. Carbachol produces more prominent actions on the gastrointestinal tract, the urinary bladder, and the iris than acetylcholine does. The cardiovascular effects of carbachol are very minimal in normal doses; however, high doses of carbachol can lead to cardiac arrest. The nicotinic effect of carbachol is greater than that of acetylcholine; therefore, within the therapeutic range, this agent can stimulate autonomic ganglia, the adrenal medulla, and skeletal muscle. Bethanechol is completely resistant

Table 8.5 Pharmacological Actions of Different Choline Esters

Pharmacological Activity	Acetylcholine	Methacholine	Carbachol	Bethanechol
Muscarinic				
Cardiovascular (bradycardia, vasodilation)	++	++	+	+
Gastrointestinal (increased motility)	++	++	+++	+++
Urinary (contraction)	++	++	+++	+++
Nicotinic	++	–	+++	–

Note: + = activity; – = no activity. The number of symbols corresponds to the magnitude of activity.

to breakdown by cholinesterases and is readily absorbed after oral administration. Bethanechol acts more selectively on the gastrointestinal tract and the urinary bladder than does acetylcholine. Therefore, the primary therapeutic application for bethanechol (Urecholine®) is the treatment of urinary retention, both that occurring postoperatively and that of neurogenic origin. Bethanechol is contraindicated in patients with peptic ulcer and in cases in which the strength or integrity of the gastrointestinal wall is weak.

Several naturally occurring alkaloids produce muscarinic activity that is qualitatively similar to that of the choline esters. In addition, many of the naturally occurring alkaloids produce muscarinic effects within the central nervous system. The substance that provided the basis for classification of muscarinic receptors is the alkaloid muscarine. This compound is 100 times more potent than acetylcholine but essentially devoid of nicotinic activity. Muscarine is moderately absorbed from the gastrointestinal tract and is not destroyed enzymatically by cholinesterases. Muscarine can cross the blood–brain barrier and produces cortical arousal. Another alkaloid called pilocarpine is naturally found in the leaves of a species of South American shrub (*Pilocarpus jaborandi*). The effects of pilocarpine on the sweat glands and salivary glands are prominent. Pilocarpine also has marked ability to increase gastric secretions that normally contain pepsin. The cardiovascular effects of pilocarpine are minimal. The sole therapeutic use of pilocarpine (*Pilocar, Carpine,* or *Isopto*) is in lowering the intraocular pressure in the treatment of glaucoma patients by opening the Schlemm's canal and facilitating the drainage of the aqueous humor from the anterior chamber of the eye.

Nicotine is another natural alkaloid; it is found in high concentrations in tobacco leaves, and it stimulates the nicotinic receptors. Nicotine can

Table 8.6   Effects of Atropine on Different Organ Systems

Organ	Effect	When or Use
1. Eye	Mydriasis	Refraction studies, eye examination
2. GI tract	Decreased muscle actions and decreased secretions	Spasm, hypermotility, preoperative medication
3. Bronchiolar smooth muscle	Decreased muscle actions and decreased secretions	Asthma, surgery
4. Brain	Blockade of CNS receptors	Parkinson's disease, motion sickness
5. Urinary bladder	Relaxation of detrusor muscle and constriction of spincter	Urinary incontinence
6. Heart	Tachycardia	*Carotid sinus syncope:* Excessive activity of afferent neurons from the stretch receptors on the carotid sinus provides afferent input to the medulla oblangata and causes pronounced bradycardia
7. Salivary glands	Decreased saliva secretion	Usually a side effect during atropine use. In the past atropine was used before the induction of general anesthesia to block excessive salivary secretion
8. Sweat glands	Decreased thermoregulatory sweating	Usually a side effect

stimulate the parasympathetic ganglia or decrease the heart rate by acting on the parasympathetic ganglia. Nicotine has no therapeutic use. At moderate doses nicotine can produce nausea and vomiting by activating the area postrema. Although this effect may be lifesaving, large doses of nicotine could ultimately depress the central nervous system and cause death. The fatal dose of nicotine is approximately 40 mg, or 1 drop of the pure liquid. This equals the amount of nicotine that can be found in two regular cigarettes. Fortunately, most of the nicotine in the cigarette is destroyed by burning or through the "sidestream" smoke.

Antimuscarinic

Muscarinic blocking drugs are compounds that selectively compete for the muscarinic receptors for binding and thereby block an augmented or unwanted cholinergic response. The muscarinic blocking agents are also called *muscarinic antagonists, antimuscarinic drugs,* and *anticholinergics.* The naturally occurring alkaloid *atropine* and its related compounds are classified as antimuscarinic or muscarinic blocking drugs because they competitively block the action of acetylcholine and its analogs at both central and peripheral muscarinic receptors. Atropine can compete with acetylcholine for both M_1 and M_2 muscarinic receptors. Muscarinic blocking agents are used primarily in ophthalmology and gasteroenterology. In cases of gastrointestinal hypermotility and excessive gastric secretion, atropine is effective in diminishing these activities by blocking parasympathetic stimulation. Atropine is applied topically for preoperative mydriasis (pupil dilation), frequently in combination with phenylephrine. Some of the common uses of antimuscarinics are listed in Table 8.6.

9

DRUG-INDUCED ENZYME INHIBITION

DRUG EFFECTS MEDIATED THROUGH ENZYME INHIBITION

Drugs can produce pharmacological effects by interacting with active proteins such as enzymes. Enzymes, in fact, constitute the primary site of action for many drugs. When drugs and enzymes interact, the pharmacological or toxicological effects of the drugs are exerted through inhibition or activation of specific enzymes. Different types of enzyme inhibitions and a few examples of enzymes that mediate pharmacological as well as toxicological effects of drugs are discussed in this chapter.

Similar to receptor inhibition, enzyme inhibition may also be *reversible* or *irreversible*. An irreversible inhibitor dissociates very slowly from its target (enzyme or receptor) because it becomes very tightly bound to the active site of the target either *covalently* or *noncovalently* (Figure 9.1). Therefore, irreversible inhibition could permanently destroy the enzyme activity. The action of nerve gases on acetylcholinesterase, an enzyme that plays an important role in the transmission of nerve impulses, exemplifies irreversible inhibition. Diisopropyl-phosphofluoridate (DIPF), which is also a nerve poison, can react with a critical serine residues at the active site of enzymes such as acetylcholinesterase to form an inactive diisopropylphosphoryl–enzyme complex that leads to strong inhibition of the enzyme activity. DIPF can inhibit any enzyme with an essential serine residue at its active site. Similarly, alkylating reagents such as iodoacetamide can irreversibly inhibit the catalytic activity of enzymes by modifying cysteine and other side-chain amino acids at the active sites. Some examples of irreversible inhibition of enzymes are shown in Figure 9.2 and Figure 9.3.

Pharmacologically, irreversible inhibition of enzymes is beneficial when the abnormal activity of a particular enzyme is unnecessary for normal biochemical or physiological functions in the body. On the other hand,

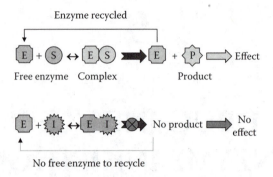

Figure 9.1 Diagram depicts the Enzyme-Substrate interaction and Enzyme-Inhibitor interaction. Both the substrate and inhibitor are able to form complex by binding to free enzyme. When the substrate is converted to product the free enzyme is released for further reaction while the inhibitor keeps the enzyme in an inactive complex.

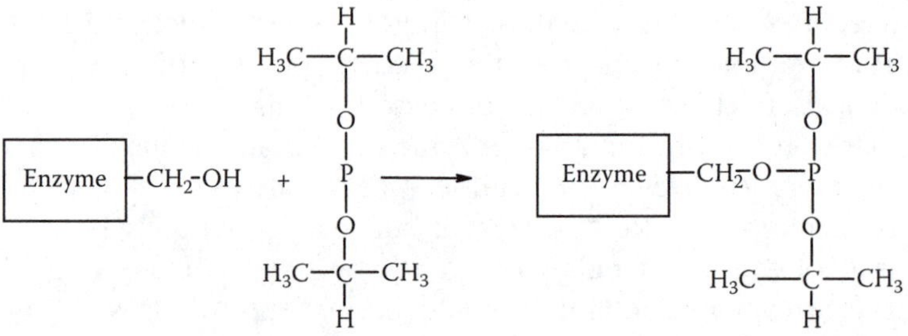

Figure 9.2 Inactivation of enzymes such as *chymotrypsin* and *acetylcholinesterase* by diisopropylphosphofluoridate (DIPF).

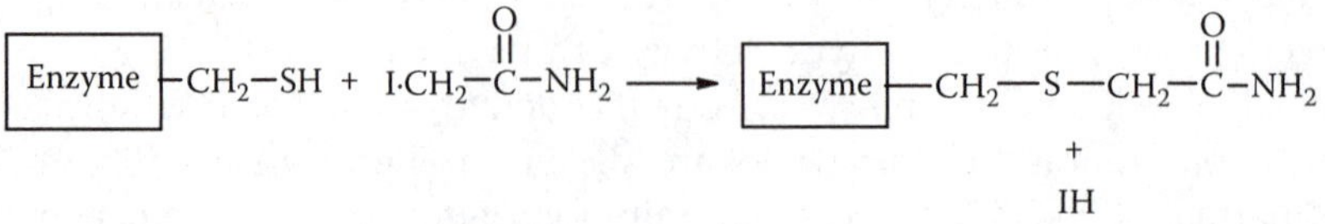

Figure 9.3 Irreversible inhibition of enzymes with critical cysteine residues by iodoacetamide.

irreversible inhibition of enzymes that are essential for normal functioning of cells would lead to toxic and often very serious effects. Irreversible inhibition of enzymes can often produce long-lasting effects. In contrast, reversible inhibition is characterized by the ability of an enzyme–inhibitor complex to dissociate rapidly. Hence, reversible inhibitors usually decrease enzyme activity only temporarily, and full activity returns when the inhibitor is replaced by the substrate in sufficient concentrations. Three major subtypes of reversible inhibition exist: *competitive, uncompetitive,* and *noncompetitive* inhibition.

COMPETITIVE, UNCOMPETITIVE, AND NONCOMPETITIVE INHIBITION

Competitive Inhibition

The hallmark of competitive inhibition is that the inhibitor can combine with the free enzyme in such a way that it competes with the normal substrate for binding at the same active site. Therefore, a competitive inhibitor also reacts reversibly with an enzyme to form an enzyme–inhibitor complex (EI) analogous to the *enzyme–substrate* (ES) complex. However, in an enzyme–inhibitor complex, the inhibitor molecule cannot be changed chemically to a product by the enzyme. Figure 9.4 illustrates competitive inhibition.

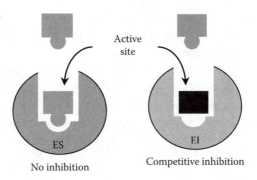

Competitive inhibition

Active site

ES

EI

No inhibition

Competitive inhibition

Figure 9.4   During competitive inhibition both the substrate and the inhibitor bind to the same active site. The competitive inhibitors typically have structural similarities to the substrate.

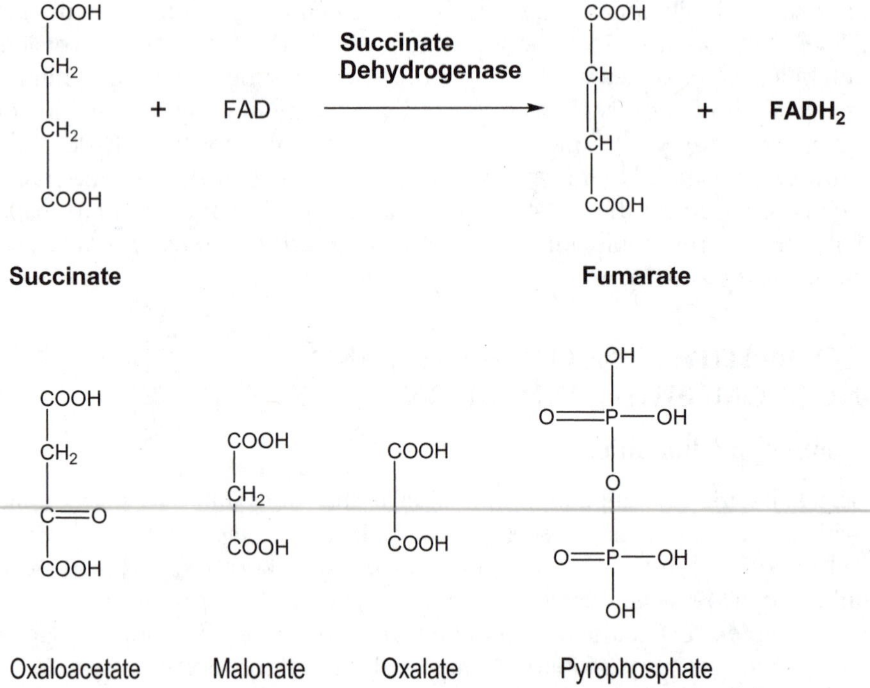

COOH
|
CH₂
| +   FAD   —— Succinate Dehydrogenase ——→
CH₂
|
COOH

Succinate

COOH
|
CH
‖   +   FADH₂
CH
|
COOH

Fumarate

Oxaloacetate   Malonate   Oxalate   Pyrophosphate

Figure 9.5 Competitive inhibition of succinate dehydrogenase by structurally similar inhibitors. All inhibitors contain two anionic groups similar to the substrate.

The classic example of competitive inhibition is the inhibition of succinate dehydrogenase by dicarboxylate anions other than succinate. The enzyme succinate dehydrogenase apparently recognizes its natural substrate succinate by the dicarboxylate moiety and converts it to fumarate, as shown in Figure 9.5. Interestingly, other substances such as malonate, oxalate, and oxaloacetate could also inhibit succinate dehydrogenase because of the presence of dicarboxylate anionic group. Even though pyrophosphate does not have a dicarboxylate moiety, apparently the diphosphate is recognized because of its close resemblance to dicarboxylate; therefore, pyrophosphate is able to bind and inhibit the enzyme. In competitive inhibition, increasing the substrate concentration will reduce the inhibition by the competitive inhibitor.

Uncompetitive Inhibition

In uncompetitive inhibition the inhibitor does not combine with the free enzyme or affect its binding with its normal substrate; however, it does

Uncompetitive inhibition

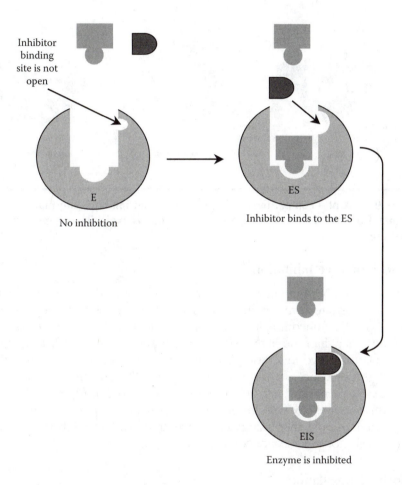

Inhibitor binding site is not open

E

No inhibition

ES

Inhibitor binds to the ES

EIS

Enzyme is inhibited

Figure 9.6 A non-competitive inhibitor binds to a site that is not occupied by the substrate therefore the substrate binding is typically not inhibited by a non-competitive inhibitor. However, a non-competitive inhibitor can prevent the enzyme-substrate complex from dissociating.

combine with the enzyme–substrate complex to create an inactive *enzyme–substrate–inhibitor* complex, which can not undergo further reaction to convert the bound substrate to a normal product. Figure 9.6 illustrates this concept.

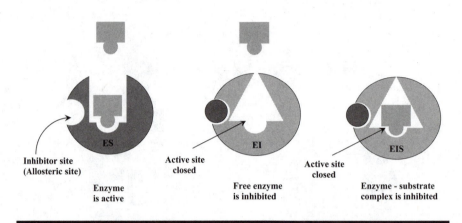

Non-Competitive Inhibition

Inhibitor site (Allosteric site)

ES

Active site closed

EI

Active site closed

EIS

Enzyme is active

Free enzyme is inhibited

Enzyme - substrate complex is inhibited

Figure 9.7 A non-competitive inhibitor binds to an inhibitor site that is totally distinct from the active site of an enzyme that is typically occupied by the substrate.

Noncompetitive Inhibition

A noncompetitive inhibitor can combine with either free enzyme or the enzyme–substrate complex and consequently interfere with the action of both. Usually, noncompetitive inhibitors bind to a separate site on the enzyme other than the active site, as illustrated in Figure 9.7. Binding of the noncompetitive inhibitor often changes the three-dimensional confirmation the enzyme, so that it does not form the enzyme-substrate (ES) complex at its normal rate. If the ES complex has already been formed, the complex does not decompose at the normal rate to yield the products. In general, simply increasing the concentration of the substrate in the system will not reverse noncompetitive inhibition.

Allosteric Regulation

Enzyme regulation is described as *allosteric* when the activity of the enzyme is regulated by reversible binding of an *effector* (inhibitor or stimulator) molecule to a site on the enzyme other than the active site; the site where the effector binds is known as the allosteric site. Most allosteric enzymes are multisubunit enzyme complexes. In a multisubunit enzyme, allosteric sites are commonly located on separate subunits from the active site. Allosteric effectors can be either positive or negative. Negative effectors decrease the reaction rate, whereas positive effectors increase it. A single enzyme may have several different allosteric effectors, both positive and negative.

Allosteric inhibition

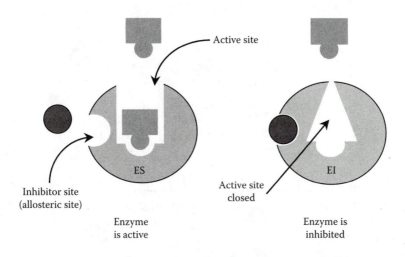

Figure 9.8   An allosteric inhibitor binds to the allosteric site that is distinct from an active site.

Cooperativity

Cooperativity, illustrated in Figure 9.9, is a type of allosteric regulation where the allosteric site may or may not be located on the same subunit as the active site and may or may not affect the binding of substrate to the active site. In simple terms, cooperativity can be defined as the regulation of substrate binding on one subunit by binding of an effector molecule to a site on a different subunit. Cooperativity may also be positive or negative depending on the type of effector molecule binding. If the effector molecule is identical to the substrate, then the cooperativity is called *homotrophic*; if the effector and substrate are different in their molecular structure then the cooperativity is called *heterotropic.* Interestingly, not all allosteric enzymes display cooperativity.

Feedback Inhibition

If an enzyme that catalyzes the very first reaction of a biosynthetic pathway is inhibited by the final product of that same pathway, the inhibition is referred as *feedback inhibition*. The biosynthesis of isoleucine in bacteria illustrates this type of enzyme regulation. Threonine is converted into isoleucine in five steps, the first of which is catalyzed by threonine

Cooperativity:

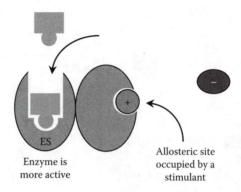

Enzyme is
more active

Allosteric site
occupied by a
stimulant

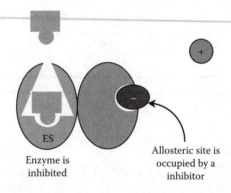

Enzyme is
inhibited

Allosteric site is
occupied by a
inhibitor

Figure 9.9 An active site and the allosteric site that are located on two different subunits of an enzyme could show either positive cooperativity or negative cooperativity.

deaminase. This enzyme is inhibited when the concentration of isoleucine reaches a sufficiently high level. Isoleucine inhibits threonine deaminase by binding to an allosteric site that is distinct from the catalytic site. When the level of isoleucine drops below sufficient levels, threonine deaminase becomes active again and consequently, isoleucine is synthesized once more. (See Figure 9.10.)

EXAMPLES OF DRUG–ENZYME INTERACTIONS

Acetylcholinesterase

Acetylcholinesterases (*AChE; true ChE*) are broadly classified into true (or specific) cholinesterases and pseudo (or nonspecific) cholinesterases.

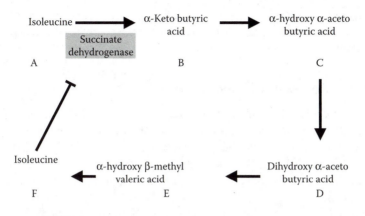

Figure 9.10 Feedback inhibition of the first enzyme (*succinate dehydrogensae*) in a pathway by reversible binding of the final product (isoleucine).

True acetylcholinesterase is responsible for the destruction of the neurotransmitter acetylcholine (ACh) in the neuromuscular junction. Pseudocholinesterase is present in the intestine, plasma, skin, and many other tissues. In the intestine, pseudocholinesterase is believed to act as a local hormone to maintain the tone. Acetylcholinesterase, on the other hand, is primarily found in neurons, at the neuromuscular junction. It is responsible for the hydrolysis of ACh released from the cholinergic nerve terminals within the immediate vicinity of nerve endings. Hydrolysis of acetylcholine is an important means of inactivating the neurotransmitter at the cholinergic junctions. AChE is relatively rich in neurons that give rise to three categories of peripheral cholinergic fibers (postganglionic parasympathetic, preganglionic autonomic, and somatic motor neurons). The concentrations in noncholinergic peripheral neurons are considerably lower. In the neurons, AChE is synthesized in the cell body and then passed along the entire structure of the nerve cell (dendrites, perikarya, and axons) by axoplasmic flow. In ganglion cells acetylcholinesterase formation is induced as a consequence of the release of acetylcholine from the nerve endings.

Butyrylcholinesterase (BuChE)

Butyrylcholinesterase, also known as cholinesterase (ChE) or pseudo cholinesterase (pseudo ChE), is present in the intestine, plasma, and skin and also in various types of glial cells but only to a limited extent in neuronal cells of the central and peripheral nervous system.

Both types of cholinesterases, AChE and BuChE, can hydrolyze ACh and certain other aliphatic and aromatic esters. AChE hydrolyzes ACh at a greater velocity than choline esters with acyl groups larger than acetate.

AChE can effectively hydrolyze methacholine; on the other hand, BuChE hydrolyzes butyrylcholine with maximum velocity and cannot hydrolyze methacholine.

The Active Center of Cholinesterase

There are two binding sites at the active site of AChE, the *anionic site* and the *esteractic site*. The anionic site is an ionized carboxyl group that forms an ionic bond with the positively charged (cationic) head of acetylcholine (Figure 9.11). The esteractic site combines with the ester group. The four amino acids that are normally present in the active site are glu-ser-ala and his.

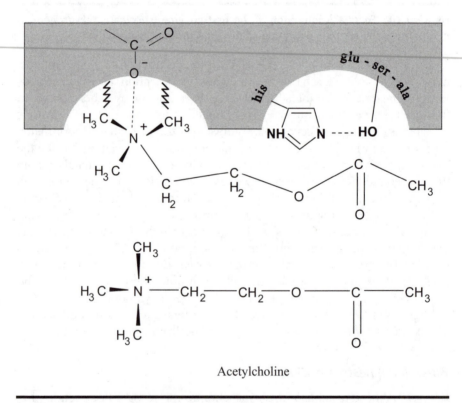

Acetylcholine

Figure 9.11 The two binding sites of the active site of *acetylcholinesterase* are illustrated. The anionic site contains an ionized carboxylic group. The esteractic site contains amino acid sequence *glutamic acid-serine-alanine* and *histidine* residue. The initial binding is by ionic bond between the anionic site and the positively charged nitrogen of the quaternary amine group. The binding is also facilitated by the van der Waals bonds (represented by the zig-zag lines) between the methyl groups and the enzyme.

During hydrolysis the substrate (acetylcholine) binds reversibly to the active site of the enzyme, and the hydrolysis takes place in two stages. The hydrogen atom of the serine hydroxyl group donates electrons to the electrophilic carbon of the carboxylic group of acetylcholine. The hydrogen atom of the serine hydroxyl group is temporarily accepted by a histidine imidazole group in the enzyme. This leads to the breakdown of acetyl choline, after which the hydrolyzed choline is released from the active site of the enzyme, leaving the enzyme acetylated. In the second stage, the acetylated enzyme reacts with water to yield acetic acid, and consequently the enzyme is regenerated. (See Figure 9.12.)

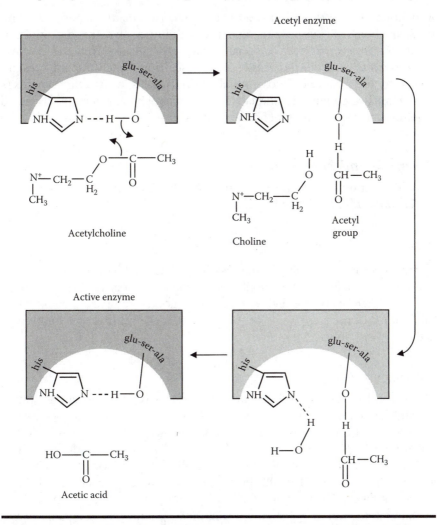

Figure 9.12   Hydrolysis of acetylcholine at the esteractic site of *acetylcholinesterase*. The enzyme is reactivated when acetic acid is removed from the esteractic site by hydrolysis.

Anticholinesterase Drugs

Many drugs inhibit the enzymatic hydrolysis of acetylcholine when added to the enzyme–substrate complex. Most of them cause 50% enzyme inhibition *in vitro* in the concentration range of 1 µmole/liter or less. In whole animals or in isolated tissues, they can readily augment the cholinergic nerve stimulation or potentiate the action of injected acetylcholine by inhibiting the breakdown.

Types of Cholinesterase Inhibitors

Anticholinesterase drugs can be divided into two main classes according to their chemical composition and the stability of the enzyme–inhibitor complex. Those that can dissociate relatively quickly from the enzyme are *reversible anticholinesterases*, and these bear some structural resemblance to acetylcholine. Those which form long-lasting, stable complexes with AChE are chemically unrelated to acetylcholine and may be classified together as *irreversible* anticholinesterases.

Reversible Anticholinesterases

Reversible anticholinesterases are broadly classified into (1) *alcohols* and (2) *carbamates* and related agents.

Alcohols

Edrophonium: This inhibitor possess a quaternary alcohol (Figure 9.13) and binds reversibly to the anionic site. It combines very rapidly with AChE and dissociates very rapidly on dilution (a good example of competitive inhibition). Consequently, its onset of effect is abrupt and the duration of action is very short.

Carbamates

The second group consists of carbamate esters (e.g., neostigmine, physostigmine). These agents undergo a two-step hydrolysis sequence analogous to that described for acetylcholine. A hypothetical depiction of the initial interaction of neostigmine with AChE is shown in Figure 9.13. The strong *onium* charge of neostigmine facilitates its association with the anionic site. At the pH of the body, physostigmine is positively charged and combines with the anionic site in a similar way to neostigmine.

The interaction of neostigmine (Figure 9.14) and physostigmine at the active site of the enzyme resembles the interaction with acetylcholine (Figure 9.12) except that the hydrolysis occurs much more slowly. As a

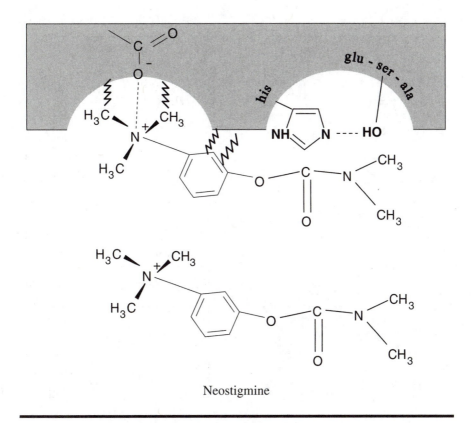

Neostigmine

Figure 9.13   The interaction between neostigmine and *acetylcholinesterase*. The zig-zag lines represent van der Waals' bond.

result, the enzyme remains bound to the carbamates for a longer time. During this time the enzyme cannot combine with acetylcholine, and thus the hydrolysis of acetylcholine is inhibited.

Irreversible Anticholinesterases

Organophosphates

The organophosphorous anticholinesterases are often described as irreversible inhibitors. These agents also undergo initial binding and hydrolysis by the enzyme resulting in a *phosphorylated active site*. The covalent phosphorous–enzyme bond is extremely stable and hydrolyzes in water at a very slow rate (Figure 9.15). This long lasting enzyme–inhibitor complex prevents binding and hydrolysis of acetylcholine.

All of the cholinesterase inhibitors exert their effects by inhibiting acetylcholinesterase and thereby increasing the concentration of endogenous acetylcholine primarily at the neuronal junctions. Most of the anticholinesterases used in medicine are of the reversible type. The main

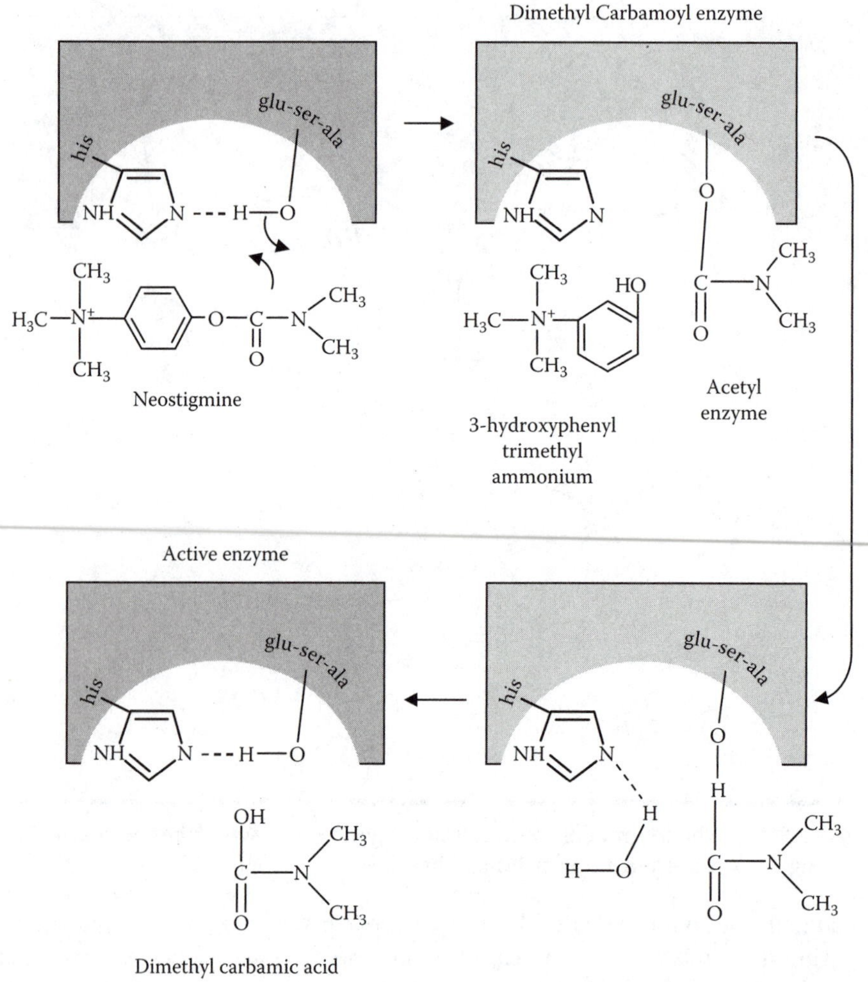

Figure 9.14 Hydrolysis of neostigmine by *acethylcholinesterase*. The reactions at the active site is similar to that of acetylchoiline however, the hydrolysis of dimethylcarbamic acid from esteractic site is slower than the hydrolytic release of acetic acid.

medicinal uses of anticholinesterase drugs are to facilitate cholinergic transmission at the neuromuscular junction.

Effects of Anticholinesterase Drugs

Anticholinesterase drugs produce various pharmacological effects, the most prominent of which involve the cardiovascular and gastrointestinal systems, the eye, and the skeletal muscle neuromuscular junction. Since

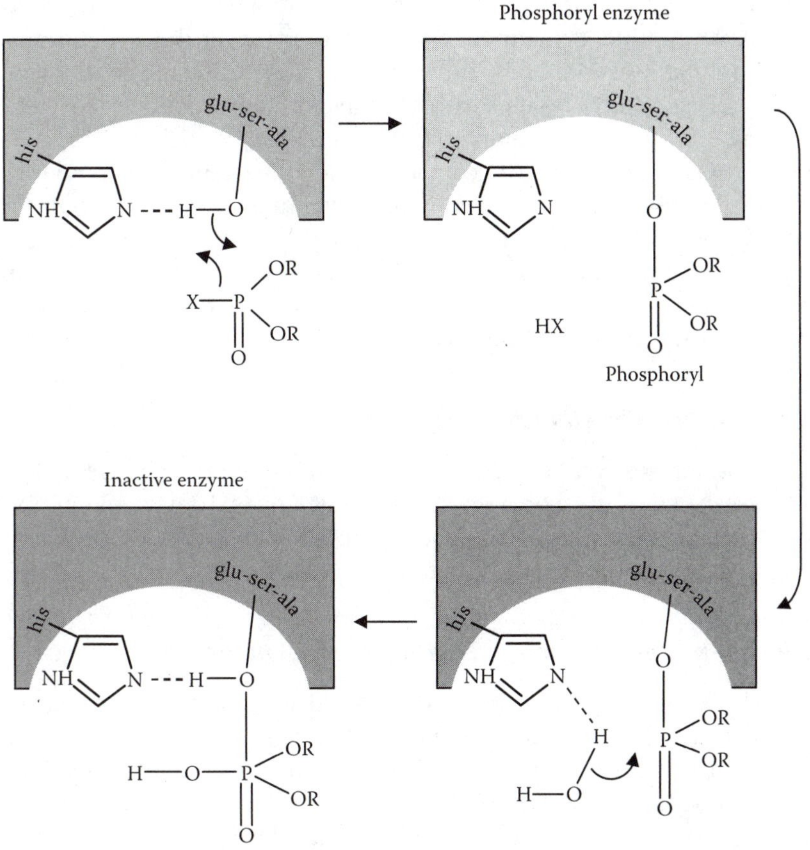

Figure 9.15 **Reaction of organophosphate compound with the esteractic site of** *acetylcholinesterase.* **The hydrolytic removal of phosphoryl group from the ester-actic site is an extremely slow process which might even take several months with some organophosphate inhibitors.**

anticholinesterases amplify the action of endogenous acetylcholine, their effects are similar to those of the direct-acting cholinomimetics. In low concentrations lipid-soluble anticholinesterases produce central nervous system (CNS) effects also. At lower concentrations, CNS effects may start as diffuse activation of the electroencephalogram (EEG) and a subjective alerting response. In high concentrations, anticholinesterases cause generalized convulsions that may be followed by coma and respiratory arrest. In the heart, anticholinesterases produce effects similar to those of vagal nerve activation. Heart rate decreases, atrial contractility decreases, and cardiac output falls as a result of bradycardia. The effects of anticholinesterases on the vascular smooth muscle and on blood pressure are less marked than those of the direct-acting cholinomimetics. The anticholinest-erases have important therapeutic and toxic effects at the skeletal muscle neuromuscular junction. Low concentrations normally intensify the actions of endogenous acetylcholine. At high concentrations antiocholinesterases may cause fibrillation of muscle fibers and fasciculation of the muscle bundles; with marked inhibition of acetylcholinesterase, the membrane depolarization becomes sustained, which eventually causes neuromuscular blockade. Some quaternary carbamate cholinesterase inhibitors, e.g., neo-stigmine, have an additional direct nicotinic agonist effect at the neuro-muscular junction. This may contribute to the effectiveness of these agents in the therapy of myasthenia gravis.

Uses of Anticholinesterase Drugs

Anicholinesterases can be used clinically for the diagnosis or the treatment of diseases such as glaucoma and myasthenia gravis. Irreversible inhibitors such as organophosphates are used as pesticides, and others could be used as weapons of mass destruction (nerve gases).

Antiocholinesterases for the Treatment of Glaucoma

Glaucoma is a group of diseases that can damage the eye's optic nerve and result in vision loss and blindness. Glaucoma can be caused by other diseases that affect the eye, severe trauma to the eye, inflammation, or surgical procedures performed in the eyes. The two major types of glaucoma are open-angle glaucoma and closed-angle glaucoma. In both types the intraocular pressure in the anterior chamber of the eye increases due to the accumulation of aqueous humor that is released from the cilliary epithelium (Figure 9.16). If the condition remains untreated, optic nerve damage and loss of vision could occur. Direct-acting cholino-mimemetics and anticholinesterases can be used to reduce intraocular pressure by facilitating the drainage of the aqueous humor. The primary therapy for open-angle glaucoma is pharmacological. Miotics are useful in treating open angle glaucoma; the most probable mechanism involved in improving aqueous humor outflow is an increased opening of the lamina of the trebecular meshwork due to stretching produced by con-traction of the ciliary muscle. Pilocarpine, methacholine, and carbachol are some of the direct-acting agonists used for the treatment of glaucoma; among these, pilocarpine is the most commonly used. Other cholinesterase inhibitors such as physostigmine, demecarium, echothiophate, and isof-lurophate have also been used. The reduction in the intraocular pressure produced by a single application of organophosphates may last up to 2 to 3 weeks. Timolol, a nonselective β-adrenergic blocker, is supposed to

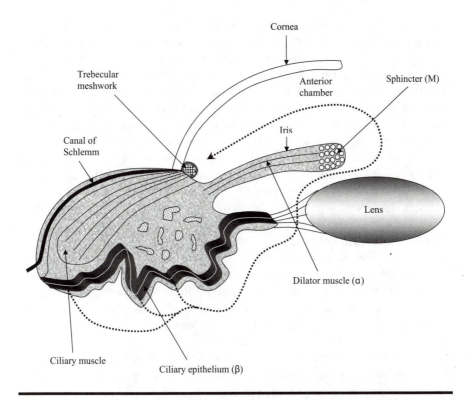

Figure 9.16   Structure of the anterior chamber of the eye. Tissues with significant autonomic function and the associated receptors are shown in this schematic diagram. Activation of the adrenergic receptors associated with the cilliary epithelium is responsible for the release of aqueous humor that flows into the anterior chamber (arrow). Activation of muscarinic receptors associated with the cilliary muscle is responsible for the opening of trabecular meshwork that facilitates drainage of the aqueous humor.

act by primarily decreasing the secretion of aqueous humor. Long-acting anticholinesterase drugs such as echothiophate, demecarium, and isoflu- orophate are reserved for use when the control of intraocular pressure cannot be achieved with other drugs. If a single drug fails to control intraocular pressure, it may be necessary to combine two or more drugs from different classes.

Anticholinesterase for the Treatment of Myasthenia Gravis

Myasthenia gravis is an autoimmune disease in which the cholinergic receptors on the skeletal muscles are decreased due to attack by autoan- tibodies. Down regulation (reduction) in the number of cholinergic recep- tors results in a decreased sensitivity of the muscle to acetylcholine. This disease may affect many skeletal muscles but most often affects the small muscles of the head, neck, and extremities. Severe disease may affect all the muscles, including those necessary for respiration. The characteristic symptoms are weakness, fatigability, ptosis, diplopia, difficulty in speaking and swallowing, and weakness in the extremities. In these patients, fatigability and weakness remit with rest and worsen with exercise. This disease often resembles the neuromuscular paralysis produced by tubocurarine, succinylcholine, and similar neuromuscular blockers. Anticholinesterases play a key role in the diagnosis and therapy of myasthenia gravis because they increase muscle strength by elevating the concentration of acetylcholine in the synaptic cleft, by inhibiting its hydrolysis by acetylcholine esterase. During diagnosis, the patient's muscle strength is examined before and immediately after the intravenous injection of edrophonium chloride. An increase in muscle strength for few minutes immediately after injection would be a confirmation of myasthenia gravis. Pyridostigmine and neostigmine are the major anticholinesterase agents used in the therapy of myasthenia gravis. Pyridostigmine has a slightly longer duration of action than neostigmine and causes fewer muscarinic effects. The pronounced weakness that may result from inadequate therapy of myasthenia gravis can be distinguished from that due to anticholinesterase overdose (cholinergic crisis) by the use of edrophonium. In cholinergic crisis, edrophonium will briefly cause a further weakening of muscles, whereas improvement in muscle strength is seen in patients whose anticholinesterase therapy is inadequate.

Table 9.1 lists cholinomimetic drugs and their uses.

Table 9.1 Therapeutic Uses and Duration of Action of *Acetylcholinesterase* **Inhibitors**

Cholinomimetics (Indirect)	Uses	Approximate Duration of Action
Alcohols		
Edrophonium	Myasthenia gravis (diagnosis/confirmation)	5 to 15 min
Carbamates		
Neostigmine	Myasthenia gravis	1/2 to 2 hr
Physostigmine	Glaucoma	1/2 to 2 hr
Organophosphate		
Echothiophate	Glaucoma	100 hr

Poisonous Effects of Irreversible Anticholinesterases

Irreversible anticholinesterases are *pentavalent* phosphorous compounds containing fluoride as in dyflos (isoflurophate) or an organic group (*p*-nitrophenyl) as in parathion or malathion. When these groups are released either spontaneously at physiological pH or by metabolism, the active portion of the molecule is attached covalently to the acetylcholinesterase through the phosphorous atom. Many organophosphate compounds have been developed as war gases and pesticides as well as for clinical use. Organophosphates interact mostly with the esteractic site and have no cationic group. Echothiophate is an exception, having a quaternary nitrogen group that enables this compound to bind to the anionic site also. Organophosphates are highly lipid soluble and therefore can penetrate the blood–brain barrier and exert their poisonous effects in the central nervous system. War gases are highly volatile, nonpolar substances that are rapidly absorbed through the mucous membranes in the lungs, even through unbroken skin and intact cuticles.

The inhibition caused by organophosphates is very stable; with drugs such as dyflos, no appreciable hydrolysis of phosphate occurs, and recovery of enzymic activity depends on the synthesis of new enzyme molecules, a process that may take weeks. With drugs like echothiophate, slow hydrolysis occurs over the course of a few days; therefore, they are not strictly irreversible inhibitors.

Cholinesterase-Regenerating Compounds

A group of compounds that are capable of regenerating active enzyme from the organophosphorous–cholinesterase complex is also available for treating organophosphorous poisoning. These compounds include pralidoxime (PAM), diacetylmonoxime (DAM), and the prototype compound hydroxylamine (HAM). The structures of PAM and DAM are shown in Figure 9.17. The oxime (=NOH) group has a very high affinity for the phosphorous atom; therefore, these compounds are able to hydrolyze the phosphorylated enzyme if the complex has not "aged" and reactivate the enzyme. When inhibition of acetylcholinesterase enzyme is allowed to persist, one of the hydroxyl groups from the phosphate is replaced by an alkyloxy group (Figure 9.18), which makes the enzymes more resistant to reactivation. Pralidoxime is the most extensively studied in humans of the three agents mentioned above and the only one available for clinical use. Pralidoxime is administered by intravenous infusion, 1 to 2 g given over a period of 15 to 30 min. Administration of pralidoxime over several days may be useful in severe poisoning. Another approach to protection against excessive AChE inhibition lies in pretreatment with reversible inhibitors of the enzyme to prevent irreversible organophosphate inhibitors

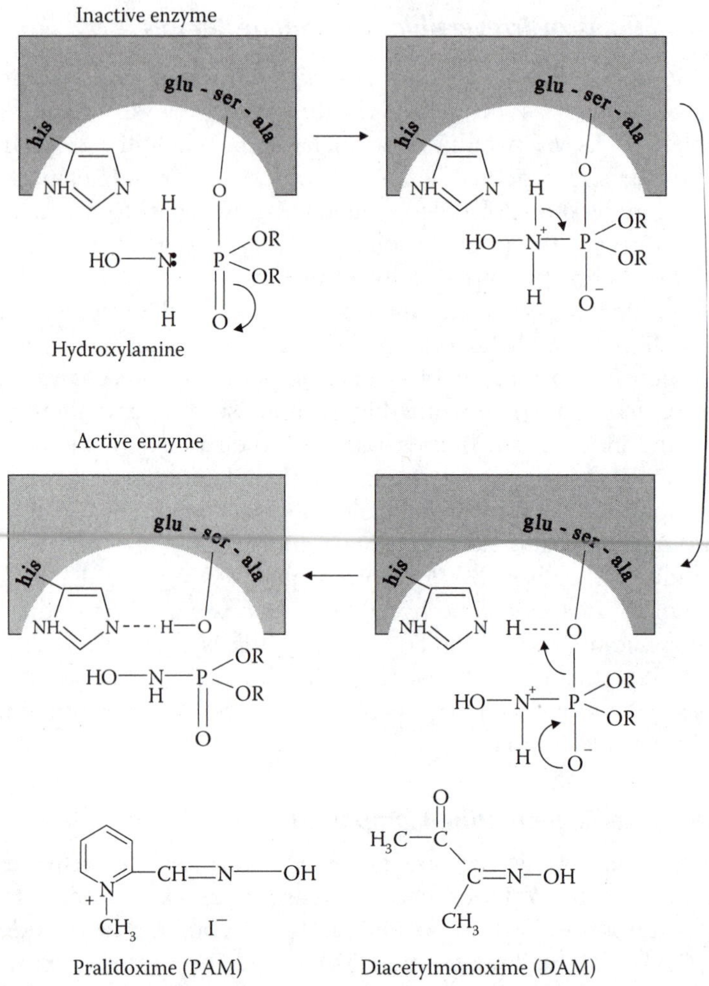

Figure 9.17 **Reactivation of the acetylcholinesterase by nucleophilic agents such as hydroxylamine or an oxine (pralidoxime or diacetylmonoxime) can facilitate the hydrolytic removal of phosphate from phosphoryl-enzyme.**

from inhibiting the enzyme. This prophylaxis can be achieved with physostigmine or pyridostigmine in conditions when lethal poisoning is feared. The toxic symptoms consist of effects associated with overactivity of the parasympathetic nervous system coupled with powerful fasciculation of skeletal muscles. If poisoning is not treated immediately, death is usually caused by pulmonary edema or by depression of the respiratory center. Therefore, simultaneous use of atropine is required in all attempts to treat organophosphate poisoning. Atropine blocks the muscarinic receptors and prevents excessive stimulation of the nerves.

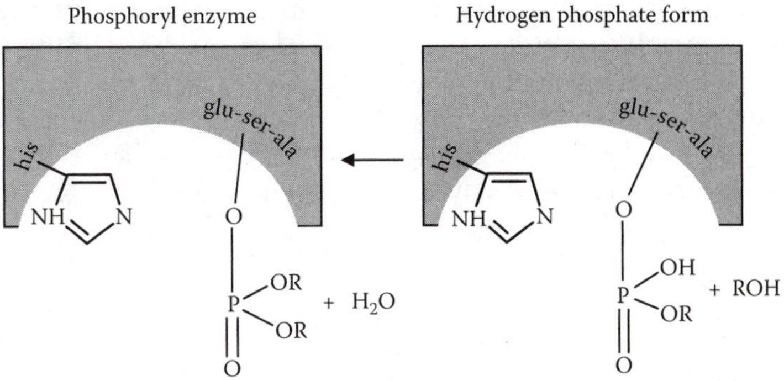

Phosphoryl enzyme   Hydrogen phosphate form

Figure 9.18 When an alkyloxy (e.g., isopropoxy from isofluorophate)) group is removed by hydrolysis from the phosphoryl-enzyme the organophosphate is converted to a hydrogen phosphate form. This process is termed as *aging* which results in the strengthening of the bond between phosphate and the *ser* residue of the esteractic site. Once *aging has* occurred reactivation of the acetylcholine esterase enzyme by removing the hydrogen phosphate becomes very difficult.

TRANSPEPTIDASE-PENICILLINASE INHIBITION PRODUCING PHARMACOLOGICAL EFFECTS

Transpeptidase

Inhibition of transpeptidase is a good example for understanding how *penicillins* produce an antibacterial effect by inhibiting an essential bacterial enzyme. The normal functions of *transpeptidase* as well as the consequences of enzyme inhibition are discussed in this section.

Bacterial Cell Wall Synthesis

In contrast to animal cells, most bacteria have an outer cell wall around the cytoplasmic membrane that helps them to live even in a hypotonic environment. The cell wall confers mechanical support and prevents bacteria from bursting due to their high internal osmotic pressure. The cell wall also confers upon these bacteria their characteristic morphology and *Gram stain* retaining property. Christian Gram discovered that bacteria could be divided into *Gram-positive* (those retaining violet-iodine dye after washing with alcohol) and *Gram-negative* (those did not retain violet-iodine dye). The difference in staining correlates with a fundamental difference in cell wall structure. Generally, the Gram-positive bacterial cell is surrounded by an inner cytoplasmic membrane and a thick cell wall on the outside, consisting of 20 to 30 layers of a sugar–amino acid heteropolymer (*peptidoglycan*). Gram-negative bacteria have the inner cytoplasmic membrane and a much thinner cell wall consisting of only three to five layers of peptidoglycan; this cell wall is surrounded by a second outer membrane comprised of lipids, lipopolysaccharide, and proteins (phospholipid bilayer). Figure 9.19 shows the structures of the outer cell layers in Gram-positive and Gram-negative bacteria.

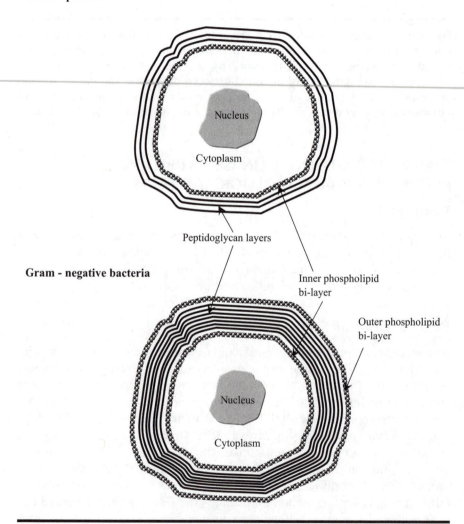

Figure 9.19 Cell wall structures of Gram-positive and Gram-negative bacteria.

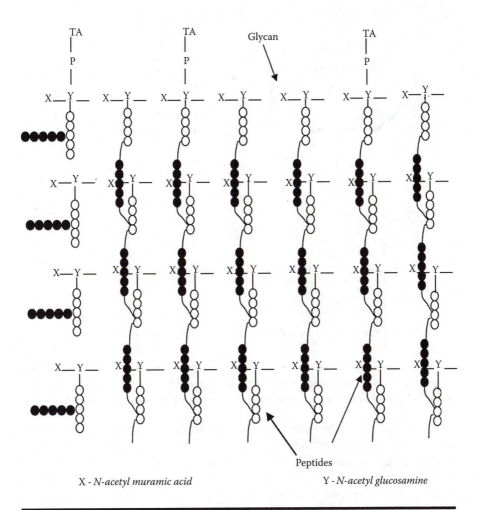

X - N-acetyl muramic acid   Y - N-acetyl glucosamine

Figure 9.20 Structure of the peptidoglycan cell wall in *Staphylococcus aureus*. Acetylglucosamine (X) and acetylmuramic acid (Y) are the two sugars in the peptidoglycan. Open circles represent the four amino acids of the tetrapeptide *L*-alanyl-*D*-γ-glutamyl-*L*-lysyl-*D*-alanine. Closed circles are pentaglycine bridges that interconnect peptidoglycan strands. The nascent peptidoglycan units containing open pentaglycine chains are shown at the left side of each strand. TA-P is the teichoic acid antigen of the organism, which is attached to the polysaccharide through a phosphodiester linkage.

Peptidoglycans

The cell wall macromolecule peptidoglycan consists of linear polysaccharide chains that are cross-linked by short peptides (Figure 9.20). The peptidoglycans have a polymeric structure composed of a chain of amino

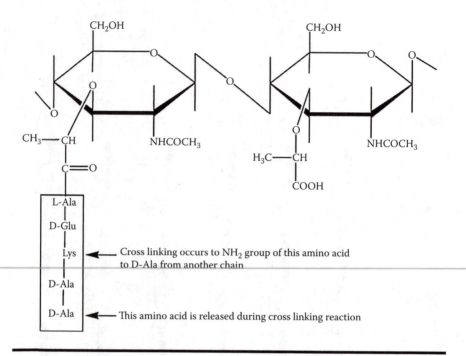

Figure 9.21 The peptidoglycan with pentapeptide showing the *lysine* and *D-alanine* amino acids that are involved in cross-linking of the peptidoglycan strands.

sugars (*glycans*) in one dimension cross-linked to a branch of polypeptides in the other dimension (Figure 9.21).

The amino sugars in the glycan strands are *N*-acetylglucosamine and *N*-acetylmuramic acid. These amino sugars are strictly alternated while forming the polymeric aminoglycan strand. To the *N*-acetylmuramic acid in the polymeric aminoglycan a short peptide chain (pentapeptide) is attached, and the whole assembly including aminoglycans and the peptide is called a peptidoglycan.

Transpeptidase

During bacterial cell wall synthesis, the final step is cross-linking of the peptidoglycans through *pentaglycines* by means of an interpeptide bridge. This final cross-linking is catalyzed by the enzyme *transpeptidase* (Figure 9.22). Bacterial cell walls are unique in containing D-amino acids, which form cross-links by a mechanism entirely different from that used to synthesize proteins. The transpeptidase normally forms an *acyl intermediate* with the penultimate D-alanine residue of the D-Ala-D-Ala-peptide. This acyl–enzyme intermediate then reacts with the amino group of the

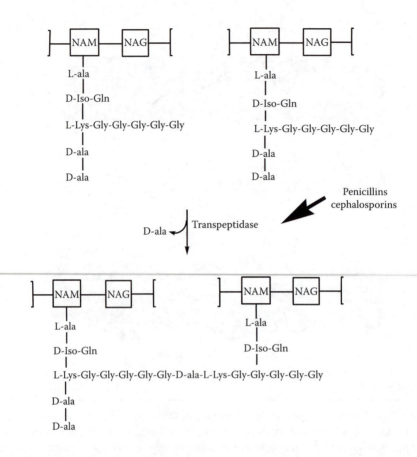

Figure 9.22   The transpeptidase reaction in *Staphylococcus aureus* that is inhibited by beta-lactam antibiotics.

terminal glycine of the pentaglycine that has already been attached to another peptidoglycan chain (Figure 9.22). The location of transpeptidase in the bacterial structure is shown in the Figure 9.23.

The susceptibility of bacteria to beta-lactam antibiotics depends on various structural and functional characteristics. In order to reach the enzymes, the drug must permeate the outer layers of the cell envelope. In Gram-negative bacteria, there is an outer phospholipid membrane that may hinder passage of these drugs. Sometimes, hydrophilic molecules (e.g., ampicillin, amoxicillin) may penetrate more readily through pore molecules (porins) in the membrane than penicillin G does. In Gram-positive bacteria the phospholipid membrane is lacking, and its barrier function is absent.

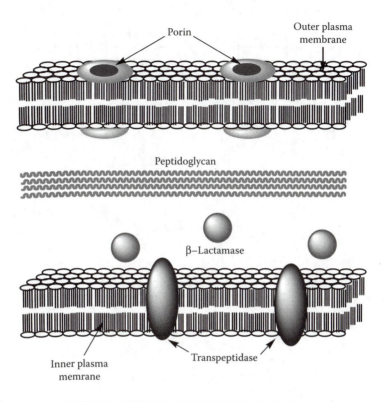

Figure 9.23 A simplified cell wall structure of the Gram-negative bacteria show-ing the outer lipid bi-layer. The cell wall is penetrated by *porins*, special proteins that provide hydrophilic access to cytoplasmic membrane. The peptidoglycan layer is unique to bacteria and provides additional strength to the bacterial cell wall. The penicillin binding proteins (PBPs) are the *transpeptidases*, which exist as the transmembrane or peripheral proteins on the cytoplasmic membrane. In Gram-negative bacteria *beta-lactamase*, when produced, may reside in the periplasmic space or on the outer surface of the cytoplasmic membrane. In resistant bacteria *beta-lactamase* destroys the beta-lactam antibiotics that penetrate the outer mem-brane.

Transpeptidase Inhibitors

Pencillins and cephalosporins are known inhibitors of bacterial cell wall synthesis. Penicillin blocks the last step in cell wall synthesis by blocking the cross-linking enzyme transpeptidase. Molecular models show that penicillin closely resembles one of the possible conformations of acyl-D-Ala-D-Ala; hence, it binds to the active site of the *transpeptidase* and acylates the active site. The mechanism of action of cephalosporin is similar to that of the penicillins. Figure 9.24 illustrates the structures of

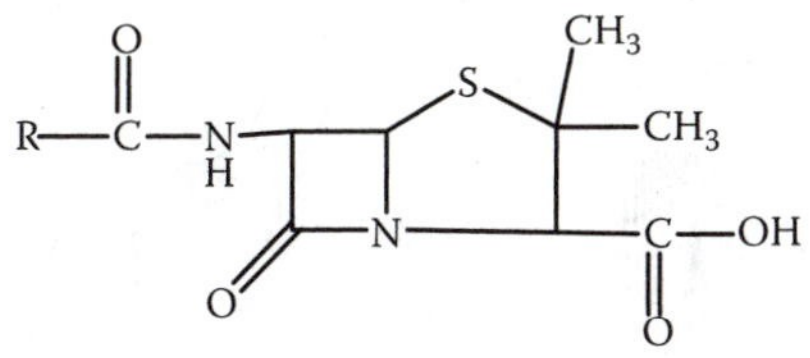

Penicillin 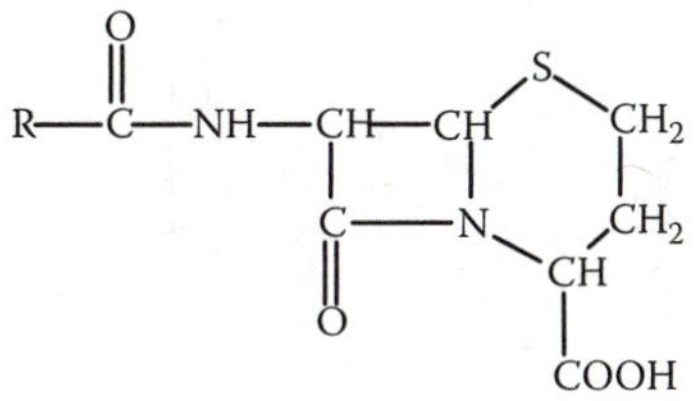   Cephalosporin

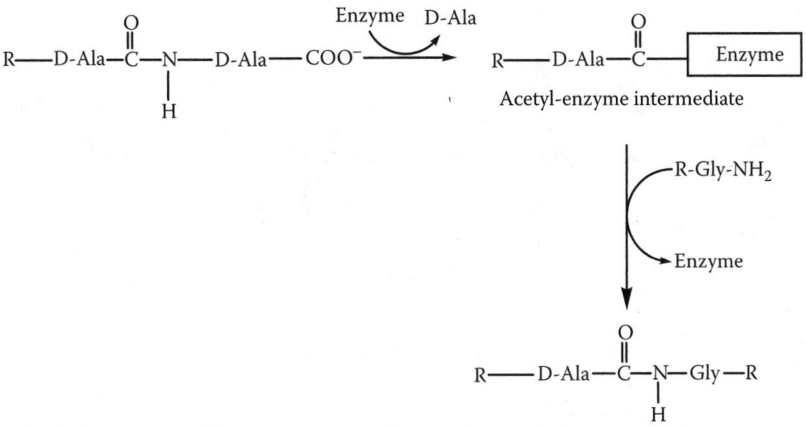

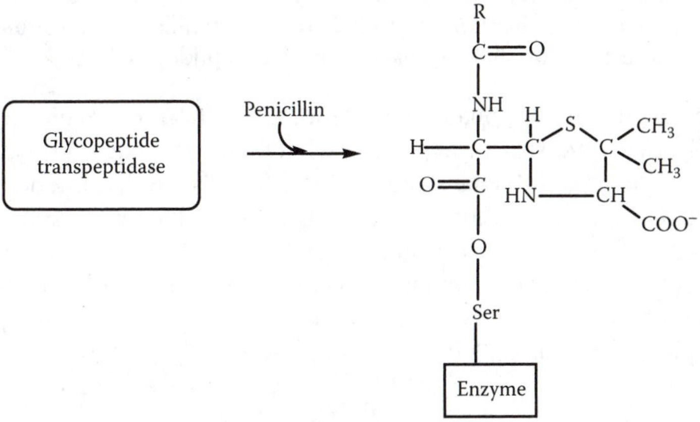

Acetyl-enzyme intermediate

Figure 9.24   Formation of penicilloyl-enzyme complex results in the irreversible inhibition of the *transpeptidase* enzyme. Irreversible inhibition of the *transpeptidase* enzyme causes a disruption to the cross-linking of peptidoglycan layers.

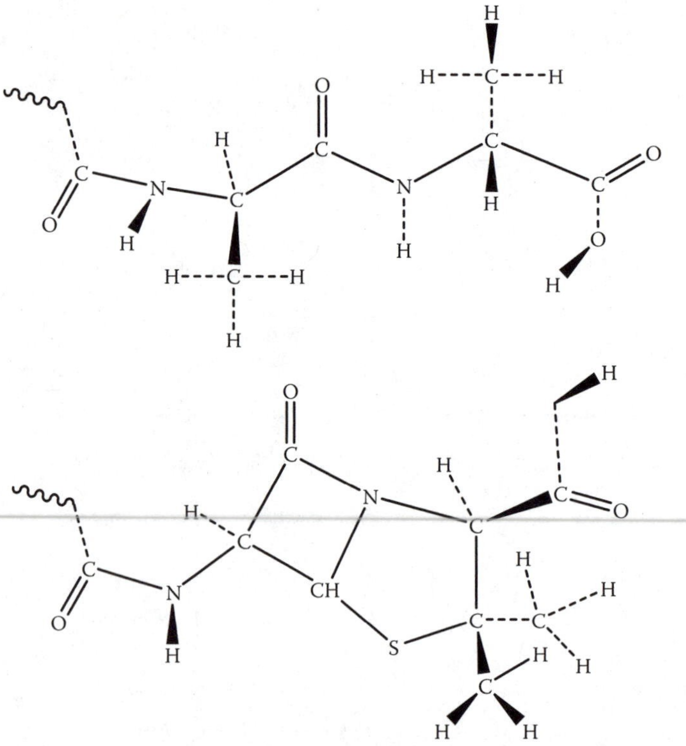

Figure 9.25 Comparison of the structures of D-ala-D-ala (A) and beta-lactam (B) portion of the penicillin by molecular modeling. Both A and B have similar shape, and structures, therefore can bind to the pencillin-binding proteins (PBPs) that catalyze the cross-linking reaction during peptidoglycan cell wall synthesis.

penicillin and cephalosporin and the action of penicillin. Figure 9.25 illustrates the structural similarity between penicillin and acyl-D-Ala-D-Ala.

The remarkable lack of toxicity of beta-lactam antibiotics to mammalian cells must be attributed to the absence of bacterial type cell walls with peptidoglycan layers in animal cells. The differences in susceptibility of bacteria to various penicillins or cephalosporins probably depends on the structural differences in their cell walls (e.g., amount of peptidoglycan, lipids, the nature of cross-linking, etc.)

Penicillins

Penicillins represent a large group of compounds with the same basic chemical nucleus. The essential constituents of the penicillin nucleus are a beta-lactam ring and a thiazolidine nucleus. The antimicrobial activity of penicillin resides in the β-lactam ring of the penicillins. The penicillins can be divided into three groups: *naturally occuring penicillins* (penicillin G and penicillin V); *penicillinase-resistant penicillins* (methicillin, naficillin, oxacillin, cloxacillin, and dicloxacillin) and *broad-spectrum penicillins* (ampicillin and amoxicillin). Penicillins differ greatly in their oral absorption, binding to proteins, metabolism, and excretion. Structures of some of the penicillins are shown in Figure 9.26.

Penicillinases

Almost all bacterial resistance to the penicillins comes from the effects of enzymes that catalyze the hydrolysis of the beta-lactam ring of penicillins. This enzyme is often referred as *penicillinase* but is more appropriately called *beta-lactamase*. Penicillinases (β-lactamases) catalyze the hydrolysis of penicillin to inactive penicilloic acid, as shown in Figure 9.27.

The function of the beta-lactamase is to destroy, by hydrolysis, the bond between the amino and the carbonyl groups in the beta-lactam ring of the penicillin. When this bond is destroyed, the beta-lactam ring is no longer active as an acylating agent, and the penicillin molecule is not able to participate in its usual beta-lactam–mediated actions. In Gram-positive bacteria such as *staphylococci* and *bacilli*, the enzyme is present extracellularly. In these microbes the enzyme is produced at higher levels when the organism comes in contact with the antibiotic. In Gram-negative bacteria the enzyme is cell bound. The beta-lactamses have been broadly classified, on the basis of amino acid sequence, into three classes: A, B, and C. The key amino acid residue in class A beta-lactamase is serine. The class B enzymes are *metalloenzymes* that require Zn^{++} for activity. Several of the penicillins are not affected by the beta-lactamase of staphylococci; they are referred to as the *beta-lactamase–resistant* penicillins. These include methicillin, oxacillin, cloxacillin, dicloxacillin, and naficillin. Actions of gastric acid also could result in the formation of penicilloic acid. On the other hand, the actions of bacterial *amidases* result in formation of 6-aminopenicillanic acid, which may have residual transpeptidase inhibiting ability. The penicilloyl derivatives may combine with protein carriers to become major determinants of penicillin allergy.

Beta-Lactamase Inhibitors

Alkoxy penicillins (methicillin), oxazolyl penicillns (oxacillin, cloxacillin, and dicloxacillin) and isoxazolylpenicillins (ticarcillin) can inhibit beta-lactamase by themselves. These agents act as competitive inhibitors but are also hydrolyzed at a very slow rate. Thus, the oxazolyl penicillins are considered competitive substrates for beta-lactamases. Izumenolide, a sulfated

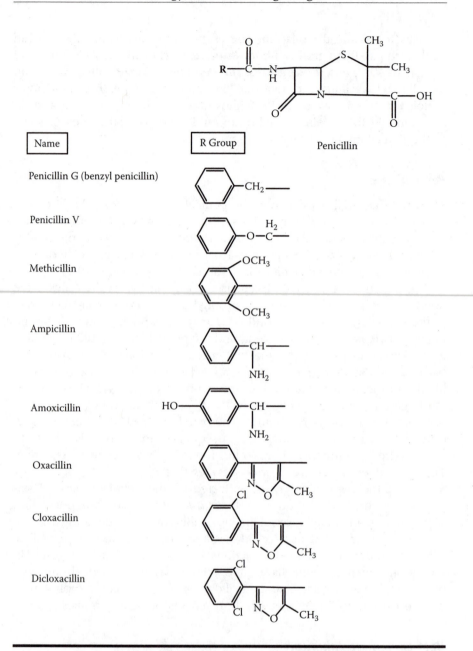

Figure 9.26 Core structure of beta-lactam antibiotics and different substitutions that can be made in place of R to produce various penicillins.

macrolide (erythromycin), is a noncompetitive inhibitor that binds to a site other than the active site of the enzyme and acts as an irreversible inhibitor. A subset of beta-lactamase–specific, irreversible inhibitors are

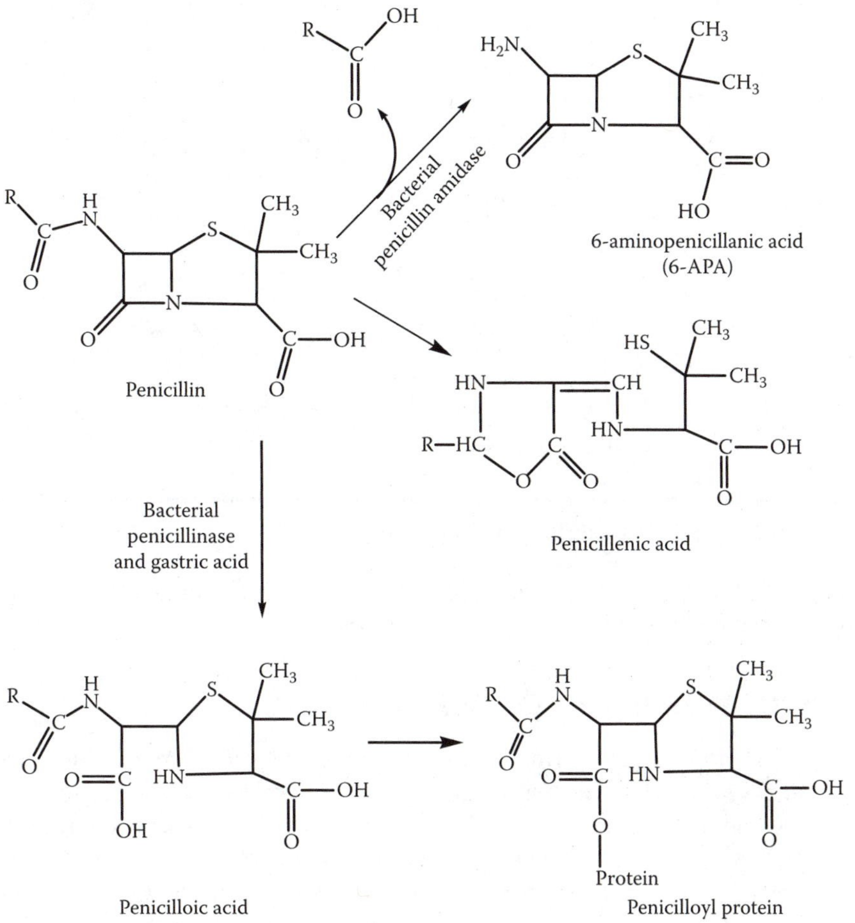

Figure 9.27   Enzymes and pathways leading to the inactivation of penicillins in resistant bacteria.

called *suicide inactivators*. These inhibitors initially bind to the active site of the beta-lactamase very poorly, but as a result of the enzyme action they produce highly reactive intermediary compounds. These reactive compounds eventually form covalent bonds at the active site of the enzyme leading to irreversible inhibition of the beta-lactamase. Clavulanic acid, shown in Figure 9.28, is an example of a suicide inhibitor. Clavulanic acid appears to bind to the serine amino acid at the active site of the beta-lactamase and inhibit its enzyme activity. Other suicide beta-lactamase inhibitors are the penicillanic acid sulfones such as sulbactam, which act very similar to clavulanic acid. Inhibition of beta-lacatamase would normally reverse the resistance to penicillins, and there are some penicillins that are

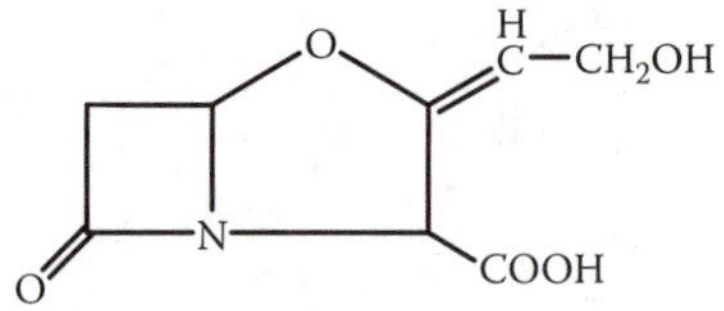

Clavulanic acid

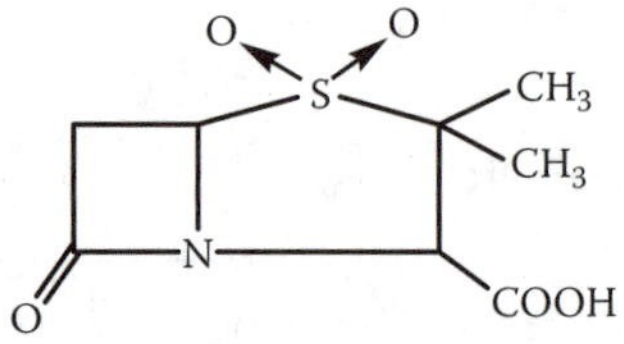

Sulbactam

Figure 9.28 Suicide inhibitors of *beta-lactamase*.

inherently resistant to beta-lactamase. The beta-lactamase–resistant penicillins include methicillin, oxacillin, nafacillin, cloxacillin, and dicloxacillin.

SUICIDE INHIBITION OF ENZYMES

Structural analogs of normal substrates (*pseudo substrates*), which are chemically unreactive in their original state, generate highly reactive intermediates in the active site of the target enzymes. If these chemically reactive intermediates covalently link to some amino acid residue or cofactor molecule in the active site, the target enzyme may lose catalytic activity irreversibly. This mechanism-based enzyme inactivation is called *suicide inhibition* of enzymes. The substrate analogs have also been widely termed *suicide substrates* in a loose concept that they induce target enzymes to commit suicide at some stage in the catalytic cycle.

Suicide Inhibition of Thymidylate Synthetase (TS)

Fluorouracil (or fluorodeoxyuridine), a clinically useful anticancer drug, is converted *in vivo* into *fluorodeoxyuridylate* (F-dUMP). This analog of dUMP irreversibly inhibits thymidylate synthetase after acting as a normal substrate through part of the catalytic cycle, as shown in Figure 9.29. First, the enzyme thymidylate synthetase is attached to the C-6 of the F-dUMP through a SH group. Second, N^5, N^{10}-methylenetetrahydrofolate adds a CH_2 to the enzyme–nucleotide intermediate. If the nucleotide is dUMP, a hydride ion of the folate is subsequently shifted to the methylene group, and a proton is taken away from C-5 of the bound nucleotide. In case

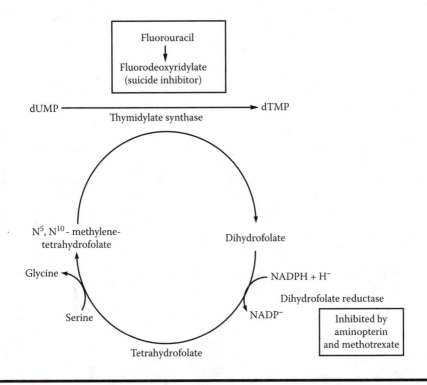

Figure 9.29   The enzyme target for suicide inhibitor 5-fluorouracil is *thymidylate synthetase*. The active metabolite fluorodeoxyuridylate inhibits the methylation of dUMP to dTMP.

of F-dUMP the nucleotide has a fluorine substitution at the C-5 position. Since F$^+$ cannot be abstracted from F-dUMP by the enzyme, the catalysis is blocked at the stage of the covalent complex formed by F-dUMP, methylene tetrahydrofolate, and the sulfhydryl group of the enzyme (Figure 9.30).

Suicide Inhibition of Xanthine Oxidase (XO)

Allopurinol is an analog of hypoxanthine in which the N and C atoms at positions 7 and 8 are interchanged (Figure 9.31). This compound is used to treat gout, where there is excessive accumulation of uric acid produced by the action of xanthine oxidase on hypoxanthine and xanthine, the purine metabolites. Allopurinol first acts as a substrate; once alloxanthine is formed, it acts as an inhibitor of xanthine oxidase (Figure 9.32). When this enzyme hydroxylates allopurinol to alloxanthine, the alloxanthine remains tightly bound to the active site of the enzyme. The molybdenum atom of xanthine oxidase is kept in the +4 oxidation state by the binding of alloxanthine instead of returning to the +6 oxidation state as it does in a normal catalytic cycle. This is another example of suicide inhibition.

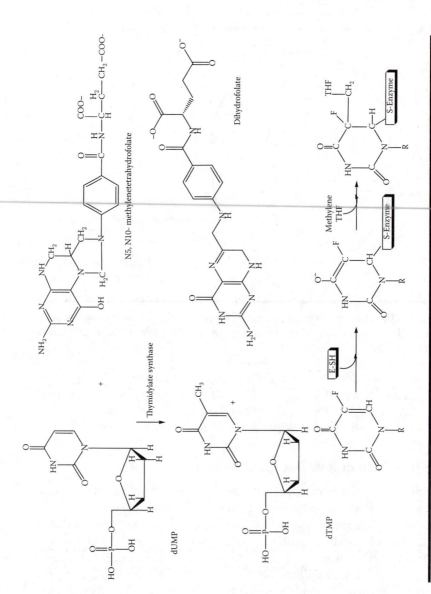

Figure 9.30 *Thymidylate synthetase* is irreversibly inhibited by fluorodeoxyuridylate (F-dUMP). This analog forms a covalent complex with both a sulfhydryl residue of the enzyme and methylenetetrahydrofolate.

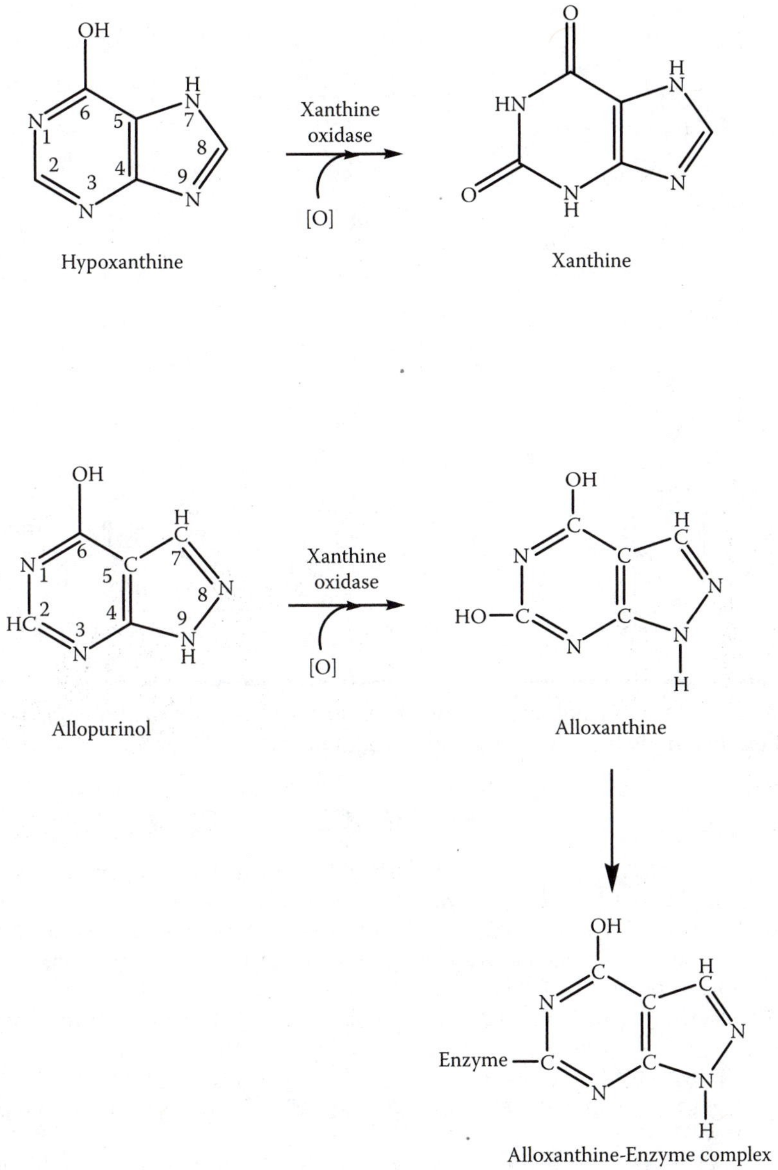

Figure 9.31   Suicide inhibition of *xanthine oxidase* by alloxanthine.

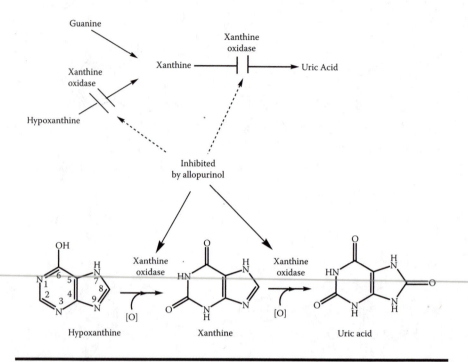

Figure 9.32 Allopurinol can inhibit *Xanithine oxidase* as suicide inhibitor in multiple locations to reduce uric acid production.

REFERENCES

1. Lehninger Principles of Biochemistry by David L. Nelson and Michael M. Cox, 3rd Edition, Chapters-8 (Enzymes), 2000, Worth Publishers Inc., New York.
2. Textbook of Pharmacology by W.C. Bowman and M. J. Rand; chapter-10 (Peripheral Autonomic Cholinergic mechanisms: Inactivation of acetylcholine), 1980, Blackwell Scientific Publications, Edinburgh, London, Melbourne, and Oxford.
3. Biochemistry by William M. Sutherland, Chapter-2 (Enzymes), 1990, Churchill Livingstone, New York, Edinburgh, London, and Melbourne.
4. Biochemistry by Lubert Stryer, 4th edition, Chapter-8 (Basic concepts and kinetics) & chapter-9 (Catalytic strategies), 1995, W. H. Freeman and Company, New York.
5. Biochemistry by Geoffrey L. Zubay, Chapter 8 (Enzyme kinetics) and Chapter 10 (Regulation of enzyme activities), 1998 Wm. C. Brown Publishers, Boston, Buenos Aires, Chicago, London, Mexico City, Sydney, and Toronto.
6. Modern Pharmacology with Clinical applications by Charles R. Craig and Robert E. Stitzel, 5th edition, 1994, Chapters 11-16, Little Brown and Company, Boston, New York, Toronto, and London.
7. Basic & Clinical Pharmacology by Bertram G. Katzung, 8th edition, Chapter 7 (Cholinoceptor-Activating & Cholinesterase-inhibiting Drugs), 2001, Lang Medical Books/McGraw-Hill, New York, St. Louis, San Francisco, Lisbon, London, Madrid, Montreal, New Delhi, Singapore, Tokyo, and Toronto.

10

DRUG–RECEPTOR DYNAMICS AND THEORIES

Numerous mathematical, thermodynamic, and biochemical models have been put forth to describe the interaction of drugs with drug receptors. Currently, several theories are in existence that propose various mathematical correlations for quantifying drug–receptor interaction and the consequent effects produced. Though many theories are in existence, all theories are basically categorized into two major types:

1. *Occupation theory*, which states that the response is a function of the occupation of receptor molecules by an agonist. The receptors produce responses only when they are occupied by appropriate drug molecules (agonists).
2. *Rate theory*, which states that the response is a function of the rate of occupation of receptors by agonist molecules.

OCCUPATION THEORY (CLARK)

According to occupation theory, a linear relationship exists between occupation (binding) of a receptor molecule and the cellular response produced as a result of that receptor occupation. Furthermore, as shown in Figure 10.1, this theory also proposes that the effect produced in a cell is proportional to the fraction of the receptors occupied and therefore, the maximal response occurs when all the available receptors are occupied or saturated by agonist molecules. While considering the occupation theory, it is necessary to make the following assumptions:

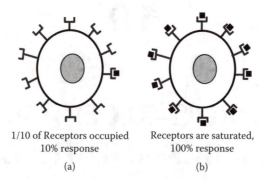

1/10 of Receptors occupied   Receptors are saturated,
10% response   100% response

(a)   (b)

Figure 10.1   Ten percent and 100% saturation of a receptor by drug molecules.

1. The stimulus is elicited when a receptor molecule is occupied by an agonist.
2. The drug–receptor complex is formed by readily and rapidly reversible chemical bonds.
3. Maximal stimulus occurs when all available receptor sites are occupied by an agonist.
4. The occupation of one receptor does not affect the tendency of other receptor molecules to be occupied.

The simplest assumption about the formation of a drug–receptor complex is that it may be expressed as a chemical reaction, thus:

$$\text{Drug} + \text{Receptor} \Leftrightarrow \text{Drug–Receptor Complex}$$

(or)

$$D + R \underset{k_2}{\overset{k_1}{\Leftrightarrow}} DR \qquad\qquad (10.1)$$

where k_1 and k_2 are rate constants for association and dissociation respectively for the drug–receptor complex. According to the law of mass action the rate of forward reaction is given by k_1 [D] [R] and the rate of reverse reaction is given by k_2 [DR]; the square brackets signify the concentration of the entity they have enclosed. The concentrations of receptors and the drug–receptor complex are formal concepts rather than the actual concentrations in the strict chemical sense. At equilibrium the rate of association and dissociation of the complex are equal, that is:

$$k_1 [D] [R] = k_2 [DR] \qquad (10.2)$$

therefore,

$$\frac{k_2}{k_1} = K_D = \frac{[D][R]}{[DR]} \qquad (10.3)$$

where K_D is the dissociation constant

In this situation, the total number of receptors $[R_T]$ is the sum of the receptors in the complex $[DR]$ plus the free receptors $[R]$ or

$$[R] = [R_T] - [DR]$$

Substituting for $[R]$ in Equation (10.3):

$$K_D = \frac{[D]\big[[R_T]-[DR]\big]}{[DR]}$$

$$K_D = \frac{[D][R_T]}{[DR]} - \frac{[D][DR]}{[DR]}$$

By rearranging the equation:

$$\frac{K_D + D}{[D]} = \frac{[R_T]}{[DR]}$$

$$\frac{[DR]}{[R_T]} = r = \frac{[D]}{[D]+K_D} \qquad (10.4)$$

where $[DR]/[R_T]$ is the proportion of the receptors occupied by the drug by forming the complex; this can also be referred to as the fraction of the receptors occupied and is represented by the letter *r*. According to Clark's occupation theory, the effect observed in cells is directly proportional to the receptor occupancy

$$r = \frac{[DR]}{[R_t]} = \frac{B}{B_{max}} \frac{E}{E_{max}} \qquad (10.5)$$

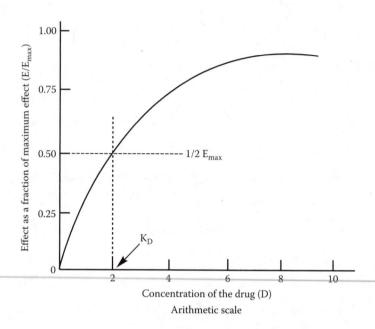

Figure 10.2   A concentration–response curve showing the relationship between drug concentration and the fractional response produced.

where B and B_{max} are measures of *binding* and *maximum binding* respectively. E and E_{max} are the *effect* and *maximum effect* that can be produced by drug binding to receptors in the system. By substituting E/E_{max} for r in Equation (10.4), the equation can be rewritten as below:

$$\frac{B}{B_{max}} = \frac{E}{E_{max}} = \frac{[D]}{[D] + K_D} \qquad (10.6)$$

Thus Clark's equation correlated the fraction of binding to the fraction of the effect produced. Clark's equation can also predict that the plot of binding as a fraction of the maximal binding (B/B_{max}) against the concentration of the drug [D] can produce a hyperbolic (Figure 10.2) curve starting from the origin and approaching B_{max} asymptotically. The plot of fractional response (B/B_{max}) against the logarithm of the drug concentration is predicted to be a symmetrical sigmoid curve, as shown in Figure 10.3.

As indicated in Figure 10.2, the K_D value can be determined from the plots; it equals the concentration of the drug that produces half-maximal binding (50% binding). When the concentration of agonist is such that the binding obtained would be half the maximal binding, then [D] is equal to K_D as shown below:

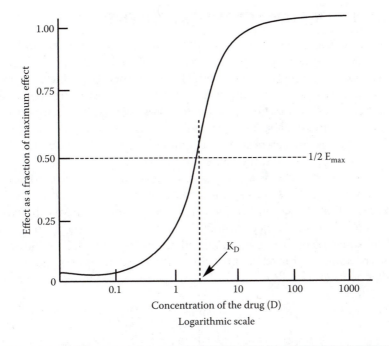

Figure 10.3   A concentration–response curve showing the relationship between drug concentration and the fractional response produced. The drug concentration is plotted on a logarithmic scale.

$$\frac{B}{B_{max}} = \frac{[D]}{[D] + K_D}$$

$$\frac{1}{2} = \frac{[D]}{[D] + K_D}$$

$$[D] + K_D = 2[D]$$

$$K_D = 2[D] - D$$

$$K_D = D$$

Another way of expressing the affinity of a ligand for a receptor is by giving the PD_2 value. The PD_2 value is generally calculated as shown below:

$$PD_2 = \text{negative log of } K_D \text{ value}$$

MODIFIED OCCUPANCY THEORY (ARIËNS)

The most obvious weakness in Clark's occupation theory is an underlying assumption that the response produced in cells is linearly proportional to the fraction of the receptor occupied. However, the observations of Ariëns in several cases were unsupportive of Clark's assumption because in certain cases, even though the receptor sites were fully occupied (saturated) by drug molecules, the drugs were not able to produce the maximal response. Ariëns further noticed that, though certain drugs were able to bind to the receptors with the same affinity as many others in their group, they were not able to produce maximal response even after saturating the receptors. Thus, Ariëns's observation was not fully coherent with Clark's equation, Equation (10.5), where the assumption was that whenever maximal receptor occupation (saturation) is achieved, that would yield maximal response. To accommodate his findings Ariëns introduced a proportionality factor termed *intrinsic activity* (denoted α) and modified Clark's equation as follows:

$$\frac{E}{E_{max}} = \frac{\alpha[DR]}{[R_T]} = \frac{\alpha[D]}{[D] + K_D} \tag{10.7}$$

Thus, the intrinsic activity was defined as the property of the agonist that produces the effect per unit of drug–receptor complex. The limits of α are zero to one. For example, $\alpha = 1$ for full agonists, $\alpha = 0$ for antagonists and $0 < \alpha < 1$ for agonists that are incapable of producing the maximal response even at full receptor occupation. Drugs in this latter class are called *dualists* because they possess the dual properties of producing below-maximal responses and at the same time having the ability to antagonize response from full agonists. Thus, Ariëns's theory still employs Clark's original assumption that the tissue response is linearly related to receptor occupancy; however, Ariëns modified the theory by suggesting that intrinsic activity determined the strength of pharmacological stimuli that can be exerted by agonists. Ariëns reiterated that maximal receptor occupancy for full agonists is still required for maximal tissue response.

RATE THEORY (PATON)

An alternative model available to determine the effects produced by drug molecules by binding to the receptors are based on the rates of *association* and *dissociation* of drugs to and from the receptors. This model was introduced as an alternate to occupation theory by Paton and is widely referred to as *rate theory*. Paton's model accounts for a general observation that antagonists act much more slowly than agonists do and hence, the

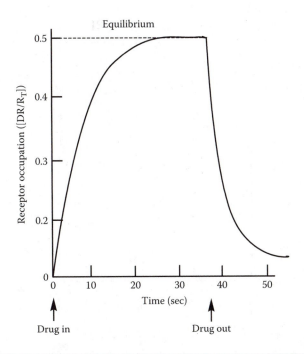

Figure 10.4 A graph showing a time-stimulus relationship predicted by occupation theory. The receptor occupancy decreases gradually when the drug is removed from the system.

rate of dissociation is inversely proportional to the potencies of antagonists while it is directly proportional to the potencies of agonists. In contrast to rate theory, the occupation theory predicts that the stimulus increases gradually once the agonist (drug) is introduced into the system and decreases gradually after the removal of the drug (Figure 10.4). Also, Clark's occupation theory cannot account for a unique phenomenon called *fade*, which is observed when an agonist produces a very transient *peak effect* (E_{peak}) initially, followed by a steady-state response (equilibrium effect) of a lower magnitude that is equal to E_{max} in this case. The difference between E_{peak} and E_{max} was the fade that occurred when an equilibrium was being reached during drug-receptor binding. This is illustrated in Figure 10.5.

Using the rate of association and dissociation of drug molecules, Paton was able to explain the reason for the peak effect that is produced by certain full agonists and also provide a logical explanation for fading of response while reaching an equilibrium effect. Thus, the whole rate theory is based on the premise that it is not just the occupation of the receptor by an agonist, but rather the rate of drug–receptor association that is responsible for the response produced. Initially, when all receptor sites

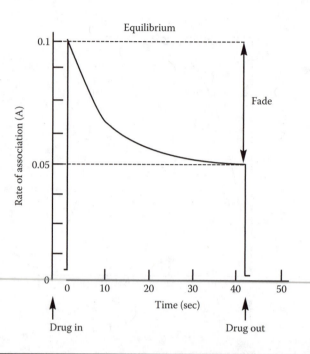

Figure 10.5 A graph showing a time–stimulus relationship based on rate theory. The graph illustrates the peak and equilibrium effects and also the "fade." The receptor occupancy comes to zero when the drug is removed from the system.

are available for binding, the drug molecules can associate with a maximum rate that leads to a transient peak effect in the beginning. Thus, the agonist activity depends on the rate of association A of [D] to [R] given by the equation:

$$A = \frac{k_1 [D][R]}{[R_T]} \tag{10.8}$$

In the above equation k_1 is the rate of onset and R_T is the total concentration of receptors. At equilibrium the rate of dissociation is equal to the rate of association, i.e.,

$$k_1 [D][R] = k_2 [DR],$$

therefore

$$A_{eq} = \frac{k_2 [DR]}{[R_T]} \tag{10.9}$$

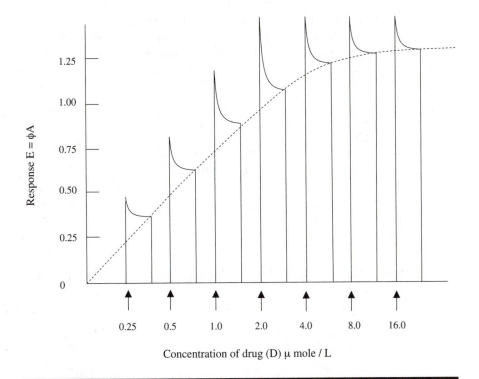

Figure 10.6 **Individual responses to increasing concentrations of an agonist drug molecule with the same duration of effect. As predicted from rate theory, each dose is producing a peak effect that is transiently larger than the equilibrium effect. At all doses, the response becomes zero when the drug is removed from the system.**

according to Equation (10.4).

$$\frac{[DR]}{[R_T]} = r = \frac{[D]}{[D] + K_D} \tag{10.4}$$

Then substituting for $[DR]/[R_T]$ between Equations (10.4) and Equation (10.9),

$$A_{eq} = \frac{k_2[D]}{[D] + K_D} = \frac{k_2}{1 + K_D/[D]} \tag{10.10}$$

Paton proposed the response

$$E_{peak} = \phi A \tag{10.11}$$

where ϕ is a factor relating the intensity of stimulation to the effect produced in the system. From Equation (10.10), as the concentration of the drug [D] is increased, $A \rightarrow k_2$. The maximal response is therefore given by

$$E_{peak} = \phi k_2 \qquad (10.12)$$

Since the maximal response is proportional to the rate constant for dissociation, drugs that dissociate rapidly will tend to be potent agonists, whereas drugs that dissociate slowly from their receptor complex will produce a small or negligible effect. In this situation, the half-maximal equilibrium response will be given by:

$$\frac{E_{eq}}{E_{peak}} = \frac{1}{2} = \frac{\phi k2 / (1 + KD/[D])}{\phi k2} = \frac{1}{1 + KD/[D]}$$

$$\frac{E_{eq}}{E_{peak}} = \frac{1}{2} \qquad = \frac{[D]}{D + KD}$$

Hence, the concentration of drug producing half the maximal response is equal to the dissociation constant K_D, which is the same conclusion as that reached by simple occupation theory.

On removal of the drug, rate theory predicts that the response should immediately fall to zero since, from Equation (10.8)

$$A = \frac{k_1 [D][R]}{[R_T]}$$

$$A = 0 \text{ when } [D] = 0.$$

That is, the response should terminate abruptly when the concentration of the free drug binding to the receptor is zero.

The changes predicted from rate theory in peak and plateau (E_{max}) responses with increasing concentrations of drug is shown in Figure 10.6. The changes in plateau responses, according to rate theory, are the same as those predicted from the occupation theory. However, in rate theory, the peak (E_{peak}) responses may greatly exceed the maximal response (E_{max}) achievable according to occupation theory.

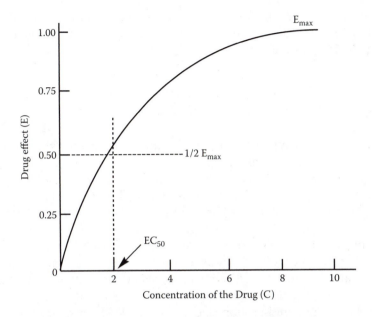

Figure 10.7 A graph showing the concentration of the drug [C] versus the response (E) relationship that can be used to determine EC_{50}.

RELATIONSHIP BETWEEN CONCENTRATION AND RESPONSE

The relation between dose of a drug and the clinically observed response may be quite complex. In carefully controlled *in vitro* systems, however, the relation between concentration of a drug and its effect is often as simple as the correlation proposed by Clark.

CONCENTRATION–EFFECT CURVES

In intact animals or in humans, the responses to low doses of a drug usually increase in direct proportion to dose. As doses increase, however, the incremental response diminishes; finally, doses may be reached at which no further increase in response can be achieved. In idealized or *in vitro* systems, the relation between drug concentration and effect is described by a hyperbolic curve (Figure 10.7), according to the following equation:

$$E = \frac{E_{max} \times C}{C + EC_{50}} \qquad C = [D]$$

where E is the effect observed at concentration C, E_{max} is the maximal response that can be produced by the drug, and EC_{50} is the concentration of drug that produces 50% of maximal effect.

In these systems, the relation between drug bound to receptors (B) and the concentration of free (unbound) drug (C) depicted in Figure 10.8 is described by an analogous equation:

$$B \quad \frac{B_{max} \times C}{C + K_D}$$

in which B_{max} indicates the total concentration of receptor sites (i.e., sites bound to the drug at infinitely high concentrations of free drug). K_D (the equilibrium dissociation constant) indicates the concentration of free drug at which half-maximal binding is observed. This constant characterizes the receptor's affinity for binding the drug in a reciprocal fashion: If the K_D is low, binding affinity is high, and vice versa.

Graphic representation of dose–response data is frequently improved by plotting the drug effect (ordinate) against the *logarithm* of the dose or concentration (abscissa). The effect of this purely mathematical maneuver is to transform the hyperbolic curve on Figure 10.9 into a sigmoid curve with a linear mid-portion (Figure 10.10). This transformation makes it easier to graphically compare different dose–response curves because it expands the scale of the concentration axis at low concentrations (where the effect is changing rapidly) and compresses it at high concentrations (where the effect is changing slowly). This transformation has no special biologic or pharmacologic significance.

DRUG ANTAGONISM

The Clark, Arien, and Paton theories discussed earlier describe the relationship between concentration and occupancy when a single drug is present. The situation commonly arises in pharmacology where the effect of one drug is diminished or completely abolished in the presence of another drug; that phenomenon is called *antagonism*. The classification of antagonism is very similar to that of enzyme inhibition and includes the following major categories:

1. Competitive antagonism
2. Noncompetitive antagonism

The consequences of receptor antagonism are as follows:

1. Receptor antagonists bind to the receptor but do not activate it.
2. The effects of antagonists result from preventing agonists (other drugs or endogenous regulatory molecules) from binding to and activating receptors.

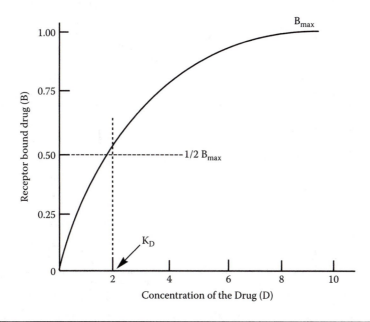

Figure 10.8 A graph showing the concentration of the drug [C] versus the receptor binding (B) relationship that can be used to determine K_D.

3. Such antagonists are divided into two classes depending on whether or not they reversibly compete with agonists for binding to receptors. The two classes of receptor antagonists produce quite different concentration–effect and concentration–binding curves *in vitro* and exhibit important practical differences in therapy of disease.

Competitive Antagonism

Competing means that two drugs (D and A) compete for the same binding site. The competitive antagonism can be further classified into:

- Reversible competitive antagonism
- Irreversible, or nonequilibrium, competitive antagonism

A reversible competitive antagonist may be regarded as a drug that interacts reversibly with receptors to form a complex. When the agonist molecules alone are present in the system, as shown in Figure 10.10, they fully occupy the receptors and produce maximum response. However, when an antagonist is introduced into the system, the antagonist molecules compete and occupy the same binding sites but produce no response (Figure 10.12). Even though an antagonist could have the same affinity

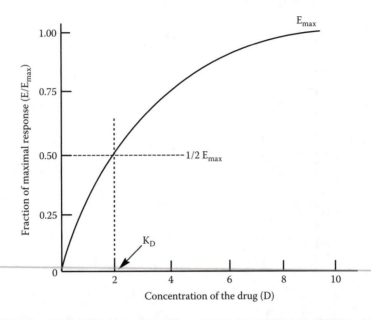

Figure 10.9 A theoretical concentration–response curve, where the drug concentration is plotted on an arithmetic scale showing K_D value.

as an agonist toward a particular type of receptors, the intrinsic activity of the antagonist is zero. The original equation to predict the quantitative effects of such an antagonist on the agonist dose–response curves was derived by Gaddum. The equilibrium interaction of the free receptor [R] with an agonist [D] and competitive antagonist [A] can be described by the reactions

$$[D]+[R] \underset{K_{2D}}{\overset{K_{1D}}{\Leftrightarrow}} [DR] \qquad [A]+[R] \underset{K_{2A}}{\overset{K_{1A}}{\Leftrightarrow}} [AR]$$

where K_1 and K_2 are the respective rates of onset and offset of either D or A for the receptor, and [DR] and [AR] are the complexes formed between the receptor and the drug and the antagonist. The total receptor population $[R_T]$ is given by

$$[R_T] = [R] + [DR] + [AR]$$

The equation for the association of drug–receptor formation at equilibrium according to the law of mass action is

$$K_{1D} [D] \{[R_T] - [DR] - [AR]\} = K_{2D} [DR]$$

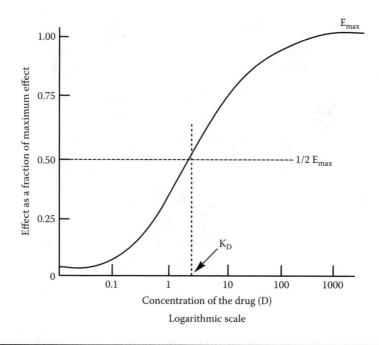

Figure 10.10 A theoretical concentration–response curve, where the drug concentration is plotted on a logarithmic scale showing K_D value.

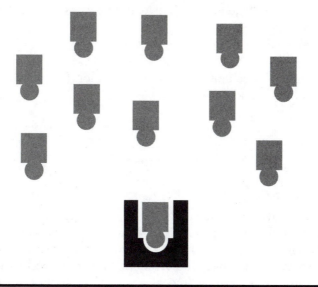

Figure 10.11 Agonist molecules with complementary structure binding to receptors.

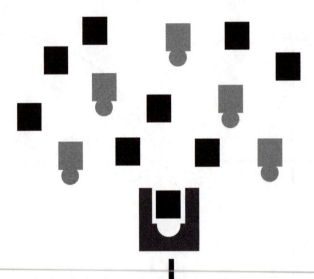

No response

Figure 10.12 Antagonist molecules present in higher concentration competing with agonist molecules and binding to the receptors.

The equation for equilibrium between antagonist – receptor is

$$K_{1A} [A] \{[R_T] - [DR] - [AR]\} = K_{2A} [AR]$$

From these two equations, the classic equation for competitive antagonism derived by Gaddum is

$$\frac{[DR]}{[R_T]} = \frac{[D]}{[D] + K_D \left(1 + [A]/K_A\right)}$$

where $K_A = K_{2A}/K_{1A}$ and $K_D = K_{2D}/K_{1D}$

This equation gives the fractional receptor occupancy by an agonist [DR]/[R_T] for any given concentration of antagonist that is present simultaneously (Figure 10.13). This equation also predicts that in the presence of a competitive antagonist, the fractional receptor occupancy by the agonist will be lower than in the absence of antagonist since the two drugs compete for the same receptors.

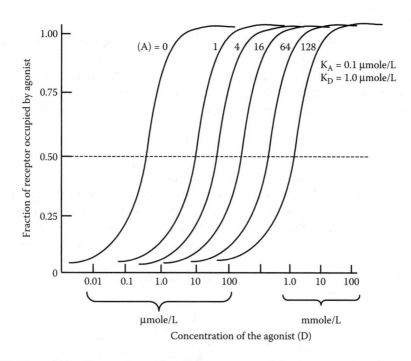

Figure 10.13 Dose–response curves in the presence and absence of antagonists, plotted on a logarithmic scale. The graph illustrates the requirement for a higher concentration of agonist to produce the same effect in the presence of a competitive antagonist. As the concentration of the antagonist is increased, the fractional occupancy by the agonist is decreased, imposing the necessity for a higher concentration of the antagonist to produce the same maximal effect.

SCHILD'S EQUATION

To describe the effects of a competitive antagonist on the response produced by a range of agonist concentrations, it was assumed by Schild that, when a given concentration of an agonist [D] occupies a fraction of the receptors pA in the absence of the antagonist, then in the presence of concentration [A] of the antagonist (which also competes and occupies a fraction of receptors), the fractional occupancy by [D] will be reduced. In order to attain the same fractional occupancy pA, the concentration of the drug [D] must be increased. From the graph given below it can be seen that the curve is shifted to the right, which indicates that to produce the same exact effect in the presence of an antagonist you would need to use a higher concentration of the agonist drug. Therefore, the multiple increase in agonist concentration that is required to achieve the same original response in the presence of an antagonist is termed the dose ratio.

Since the dose ratio can be determined experimentally, this parameter functions as a scale for comparing competitive antagonist potencies. An empirical scale developed for comparing antagonist potencies based on the dose ratio, termed as the pA scale, was introduced by Schild. The term pA_x is defined as the negative logarithm of the molar concentration of antagonist that reduces x times the potency of the agonist.

$$pA_x = -\log [A]_x = \log (1/[A]_x)$$

Following Schild's lead, it has become common practice to determine the pA_2 or pA_{10} or both values for competitive antgonists in comparing their relative antagonistic potency. A high specificity of antagonism is indicated by a high pA_2 value (i.e., a low concentration of the antagonist is effective). The pA_{10} values are less than the pA_2 value for a given agonist–antagonist interaction.

Shild's equation is based on the drug, receptor, and antagonist reaction shown below:

$$[D]+[A]+[R] \Leftrightarrow [AR]+[DR] \rightarrow E \downarrow$$

$$\frac{[D]_A}{[D]_o} = \frac{[A]}{K_A}+1 \quad \text{Schild's equation}$$

It may be written as

$$\frac{C'}{C} = 1+\frac{[I]}{K_D}$$

In the equation above C' is the agonist required to produce a given effect in the presence of a fixed concentration [I] of a competitive antagonist, which is greater than the agonist concentration (C) required to produce the same effect in the absence of the antagonist. The ratio of these two agonist concentrations (the *dose ratio*) is related to the dissociation constant ($K_D = K_I$) of the antagonist using a different format.

When Shild's equation is rearranged, then it becomes:

$$\frac{[D]_A}{[D]_o} - 1 = \frac{[A]}{K_A} \quad \text{and if,} \quad \frac{[D]_A}{[D]_o} = x$$

Then

$$x - 1 = \frac{[A]_x}{K_A}$$

Taking logarithms,

Log $(x - 1)$ = Log $[A]_x$ – Log K_A ← Let us call this *Schild's correlation*

In this equation x is the dose ratio and $[A]_x$ is the concentration of the antagonist producing the dose ratio x. Also, in the above equation $[D]_o$ and $[D]_A$ are the concentrations of the agonist in the absence ([D]$_o$) and presence ([D]$_A$) of an antagonist 'A'.

If the concentration of the antagonist is such that, if it produces a dose ratio of 2, then

$$[D]_A = 2[D]_0$$

Therefore:

$$\frac{[D]_A}{[D]_o} = \frac{2}{1} \quad \text{and} \quad x = 2$$

Therefore

$$2 - 1 = \frac{[A]_x}{K_A}$$

$$K_A = [A]_x$$

$$\text{Log } K_A = \text{Log } [A]_x$$

$$-\text{Log } K_A = -\text{Log } [A]_x$$

Since

$$-\text{Log } [A]_x = pA_x$$

$$-\text{Log } K_A = pA_x$$

In the above condition the value for x = 2, therefore

$$-\text{Log } K_A = pA_2$$

Since

$$-\text{Log } [A]_x = pA_x$$

$$\text{Log } [A]_x = -pA_x$$

$$\text{Log } (x - 1) = \text{Log } [A]_x - \text{Log } K_A \leftarrow \textit{Schild correlation}$$

By substituting pA_2 for $-\text{Log } K_A$ and $-pA_x$ for $\text{Log } [A]_x$ in Schild's correlation, the equation becomes:

$$\text{Log } (x - 1) = -pA_x + pA_2$$

when rearranged:

$$\text{Log } (x - 1) = pA_2 - pA_x$$

This is the equation that is used to test the competitive antagonism. In this equation, if pA_{10} is substituted for pA_x then,

$$\text{Log } (10 - 1) = pA_2 - pA_{10}$$

$$\text{Log } 9 = 0.95 = pA_2 - pA_{10}$$

Therefore, for a good competitive antagonist the difference between pA_2 and pA_{10} should be around 0.95. On the other hand, a gross departure from the value of 0.95 for pA_2 minus pA_{10} would indicate that the interaction is not competitive. Table 10.1 and Table 10.2 list some of the pA2 and pA10 values of antagonists.

WHAT IS THE IMPORTANCE OF THIS MATHEMATICAL RELATIONSHIP?

For clinicians this mathematical relationship has two important therapeutic implications:

1. The degree of inhibition produced by a competitive antagonist depends upon the affinity towards the receptor and the concentration of antagonist in the system. Thus, the extent and duration of action of such a drug will depend upon its concentration in plasma

Table 10.1   The pA_2 and pA_{10} Values for Some Antagonists against Acetylcholine and Histamine Agonists

| Antagonist | Comparison of pA_2 and pA_{10} Values | | | | Tissue |
| | Acetylcholine | | Histamine | | |
	pA_2	pA_{10}	pA_2	pA_{10}	
Atropine	9.0	8.1	5.6	4.6	Guinea pig
Diphenhydramine	6.6	5.4	8.0	7.0	ileum
Pethidine	5.9	4.8	6.1	5.0	

Table 10.2   A Comparison of pA_2 and pA_{10} Values for Some Antagonists against Acetylcholine, Histamine, and Adrenaline Agonists

| Antagonist | Comparison of pA_2 Values of Different Antagonists | | | Tissue |
	Acetylcholine pA_2	Histamine pA_2	Adrenaline pA_2	
Promethazine	7.7	9.2	—	Guinea pig ileum
Desipramine	6.1	6.7	—	
Imipramine	3.4	7.8	—	
Diphenhydramine	6.6	7.5	—	Rat intestine
Propranolol	5.0	5.5	—	
Oxprenolol	4.8	6.2	7.5	Rabbit atria
Sotalol	5.1	3.6	6.1	

and also will be critically influenced by the rate of its metabolic clearance or excretion. (Different patients receiving a fixed dose of propranolol, for example, exhibit a wide range of plasma concentrations, owing to differences in clearance of the drug.)

2. The Gaddum and Schild's equations also define variability in clinical response to a competitive antagonist depending on the concentration and affinity of the antagonist that might be already present in the system. When the competitive beta-adrenoceptor antagonist, propranolol, is administered in doses sufficient to block the effect of basal levels of the neurotransmitter norepinephrine, the resting heart rate is decreased. However, the increase in release of norepinephrine and epinephrine that occurs with exercise, postural changes, or emotional stress may overcome competitive antagonism and increase heart rate.

IRREVERSIBLE ANTAGONISM

When an antagonist forms a strong bond with receptors, the antagonism becomes irreversible. This type of antagonism cannot be reversed by washing the tissues or perfusing the organs with a drug-free solution since the antagonists form a stable bonding with the receptors (e.g., acetylcholinesterase inhibitors: organophosphates). When an antagonist forms a strong bond with receptors, the rate of dissociation of the antagonist–receptor complex is so slow as to be virtually zero. This type of antagonism has the following characteristics:

    a. The receptors available for interaction with the drug molecules are reduced; hence, the maximal response (E_{max}) is reduced. Therefore, the types of antagonists capable of producing irreversible inhibition are widely known as *chemical scalpels*.

    b. The irreversible antagonism cannot be reversed simply by increasing the concentration of an agonist; however, the occupation of the receptors by antagonists can be reduced by simultaneous presence of high concentrations of the agonist.

    c. Irreversible antagonism is time dependent; i.e., the longer the antagonist is in contact with the receptors, the greater the magnitude of the observed antagonism.

Graphs of the dose–response relationship in the presence of various degrees of inactivation of receptors by an irreversible antagonist are shown in Figure 10.14 and Figure 10.15. Even in the presence of an irreversible antagonist the curves approach asymptotically to responses that are proportional to the number of receptors remaining. However, as can be seen in the graphs, the dissociation constant K_D for the agonist is not altered in the presence of an irreversible antagonist because the half-maximal responses before and after receptor inactivation could be produced by the same concentration of agonist.

If the proportion of receptors inactivated by an irreversible agonist is designated r_i, the equation for the response and agonist concentration is:

$$\frac{E}{E_{max}} = \frac{\left[D\right]\left(1 - r_i\right)}{\left[D\right] + K_D}$$

where 1 = total receptors and r_i = fraction of the receptors bound by the irreversible antagonist.

Phenoxybenzamine, an irreversible alpha-adrenoreceptor antagonist, is used to control the hypertension caused by an excessive release of

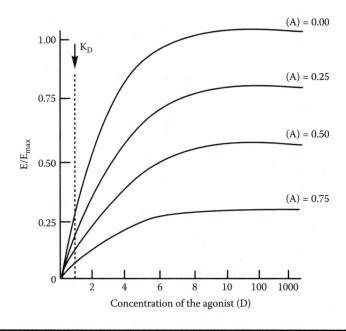

Figure 10.14   The effect of an irreversible antagonist on the response produced by different concentrations of an agonist. [A] = antagonist concentrations that are producing inactivation of the receptor fraction indicated.

catecholamines coming from pheochromocytoma, a tumor of the adrenal medulla. If administration of phenoxybenzamine lowers blood pressure by inhibiting the adrenergic receptors, that blockade will be maintained even when the tumor episodically releases very large amounts of catecholamines. In this case, the ability to prevent responses to varying and high concentrations of agonist is a therapeutic advantage.

NONCOMPETITIVE ANTAGONISM

Another type of blockade of agonist response is by interaction of an antagonist with a binding site that is intimately associated with the receptors but distinct from the site for agonist binding. In this case it is assumed that the binding of antagonist to this site precludes the activation of the receptor by the agonist. Experimental studies with competitive antagonist drugs often provide graphs as shown in Figure 10.16.

From the graph it appears that the noncompetitive antagonist acts competitively in low concentrations and similarly to irreversible inhibitors in higher concentrations. This behavior is sometimes explained by using the concepts of efficacy and spare receptors. If the agonist has a high efficacy, there may be spare receptors when the maximal response is

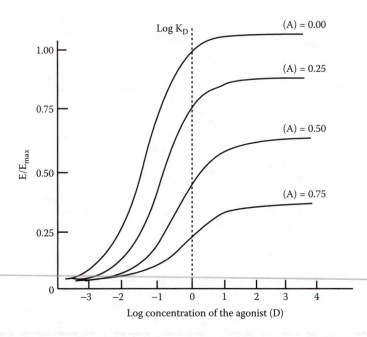

Figure 10.15   The effect of an irreversible antagonist on the response produced by different concentrations of an agonist, plotted on a logarithmic scale. [A] = the concentration of the antagonist that is producing inactivation of the receptor fraction indicated. The graph clearly indicates that the concentration of the drug that is required to produce an achievable 1/2 E_{max} may remain the same; however, the E_{max} is gradually reduced.

produced. Therefore, inactivation of receptors by a purely noncompetitive antagonist will not reduce the maximal response until the entire reserve of spare receptors is inactivated. When a noncompetitive antagonist inhibits all the spare receptors present in a cell, the maximal response will start to decrease, similar to the decrease seen with irreversible antagonist.

PARTIAL AGONISTS

Agonists with full intrinsic activity will generally previously produce full response when all the receptors are saturated. However, as previously discussed by Ariën, not all drugs would be able to produce maximal response even when 100% of the receptors are saturated. Therefore, based on the maximal pharmacologic response that is produced when all receptors are occupied, agonists can be divided into two classes: *full agonists* and *partial agonists*. The full agonist changes receptor conformation in a way that initiates subsequent pharmacological effects of receptor occupancy.

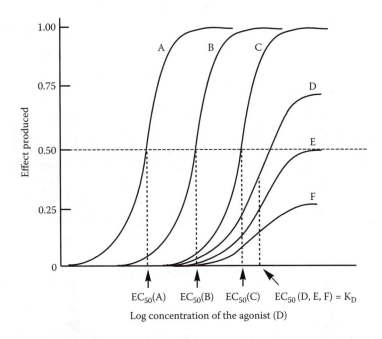

Figure 10.16 Theoretical dose–response curves of an agonist in the presence of increasing concentrations of a noncompetitive antagonist. At lower concentrations the noncompetitive antagonists behave like competitive antagonists and do not affect the E_{max}. However, at higher concentrations noncompetitive antagonists, similar to irreversible antagonists, reduce the E_{max}.

When compared to full agonists, the partial agonists produce concentration–effect curves that resemble curves observed with full agonists in the presence of a noncompetitive antagonist that blocks the receptor response. Partial agonists may occupy all receptors but fail to produce a maximal response due to lack of full intrinsic activity (Figure 10.17).

Even though combining a partial and a full agonist is not a common occurrence in a therapeutic situation, the graphs in Figure 10.18 and Figure 10.19 indicate how two drugs can compete for the same receptors and as a result tissue responses can change when they are introduced individually or in combination with each other. When two drugs having same affinity (K_D) are introduced individually into the system, full agonists can produce maximum response at the saturating concentrations, while partial agonists can only produce partial response even at 100% saturation of the receptors because of lower intrinsic activity. However, when a partial agonist is added to displace the full agonist in the system, as the concentration of the partial agonist is increased to saturating concentrations, the effect of the full agonist will decrease gradually. The final effect produced

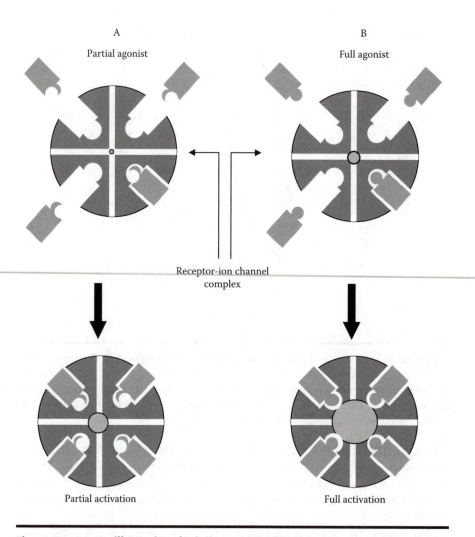

Figure 10.17 An illustration depicting an ion channel–receptor complex that is activated by full and partial agonists. This complex requires cooperativity of all four receptor sites for producing 100%. Partial agonists are not able to produce maximum effect even after saturating the ion channel–receptor complex.

in this system, after the full agonists are completely displaced from the receptors by the partial agonist, would equal the effect of the partial agonist alone as shown in Figure 10.20. In this situation, the factor that determines whether agonist or antagonist is going to occupy the receptor molecules would be the *concentration,* provided the affinity of both agonist and antagonist toward that receptor are similar.

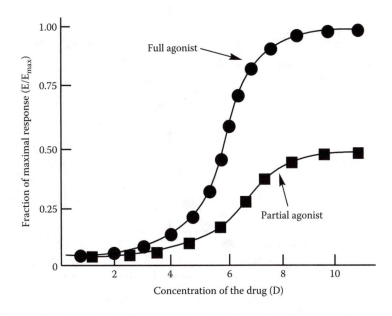

Figure 10.18   The dose–response relationship for full and partial agonists.

VARIOUS FACTORS THAT CAN REGULATE A DRUG'S EFFECT

A drug can produce a pharmacological effect when the concentration or quantity of the drug at the site of a responsive tissue attains a certain critical minimum level. The magnitude of this *effective* level is determined by four general factors:

1. Affinity between the drug and the tissue receptors
2. Intrinsic ability of the drug to cause confirmation changes
3. Responsiveness of the target tissue to the changes that occur at the cellular level
4. Effectiveness of cellular and systemic reflexes in resisting or modifying the changes induced by the drug

Due to the four major factors outlined above, drug actions are subject to considerable variation from individual to individual. Therefore, the pharmacologic variability in general can be ascribed to three causes:

1. Variation in the purity or composition of the drug
2. The constantly changing physiologic and biochemical state of the body
3. The differences in physiological and biochemical state of individuals.

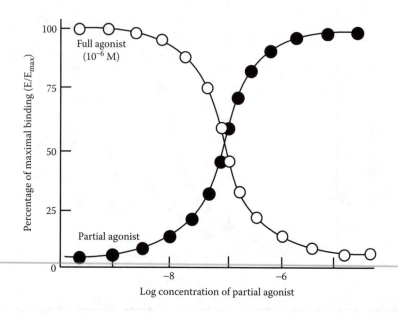

Figure 10.19   A graphic illustration of the receptor binding displacement that would take place as the concentration of the partial agonist is increased. At approximately 10 times higher concentration of a partial agonist, all the agonist molecules are displaced from the receptors.

The vast majority of drugs used in medicine are chemically pure and reasonably stable; therefore, variations in their purity or composition make only a minor contribution to pharmacologic variability. Most of the variation in therapeutics lies in the wide ranges of physiologic, biochemical, and pathologic conditions that confront the drug when it is administered to a living organism.

Factors That Can Determine the Dose–Response Relationship

Potency and Efficacy

To choose among drugs and to determine an appropriate drug, pharmacologists must know the relative *pharmacologic potency* and *maximal efficacy* of the drug in relation to the desired therapeutic effect.

Potency

The concentration–response curves for a series of agonists that can bind to the same type of receptors and produce the same maximum effect are

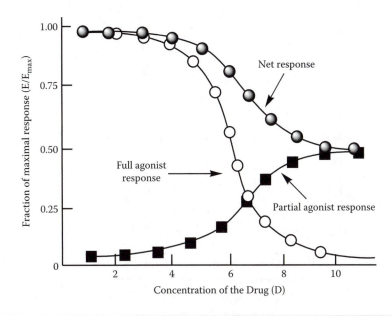

Figure 10.20 A theoretical dose–response relationship, illustrating a decrease in the agonist response that was originally produced by a single concentration of that agonist. As the concentration of the partial agonist is increased, the receptor occupancy by the agonist is gradually decreased and reaches zero. However, the net response detected in the system is only partially reduced and stabilizes at the level that is equal to the response produced by the partial agonist alone.

shown schematically in Figure 10.21. Among the five drugs shown, drug A is the most potent of the five because it can produce 50% of the maximum effect with the smallest concentration. Drug E is the least potent because this drug requires a much higher concentration to achieve the 1/2 maximal effect. The most potent drug has the smallest apparent K_D and the least potent has the largest K_D.

Efficacy

This term applies to a series of agonists that can bind to the same receptor subtype with almost similar potency but a different degree of ability to produce maximal effects (Figure 10.22). The agonist with the maximal efficacy is defined as the one with the ability to produce the greatest maximum effects (Drug A). Drug D is an example of an agonist with same affinity for the receptor as a full agonist (A) but with lower intrinsic activity. When a drug is selected, it is desirable to have the maximum of both efficacy and potency, as seen for Drug A (Figure 10.23).

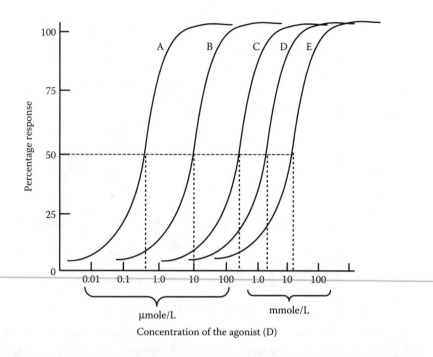

Figure 10.21   Log concentration–response curves for a series of agonists (A, B, C, D, and E). All drugs are exhibiting the ability to produce E_{max}. However, each of the five drugs has a different potency. The most potent drug is the one that produces 1/2 maximal effect with the lowest concentration.

Dose–Response Curves

There are two basic types of dose-response relationships:

1. *Graded* curves that relate the dose of a drug to any size of response that can be detected in a single biologic unit.
2. *Quantal* or all-or-none type curves in which the relationship is between the dose of the drug and the total number of biological objects that are displaying a predetermined level of pharmacological response. The biological material that is used to establish this type of data may be an intact organism, an isolated tissue, or even a single cell.

Graded Dose–Response Curves

An example of a graded curve is given in Figure 10.24. As the dose administered to a single subject or to a discrete organ or tissue is increased,

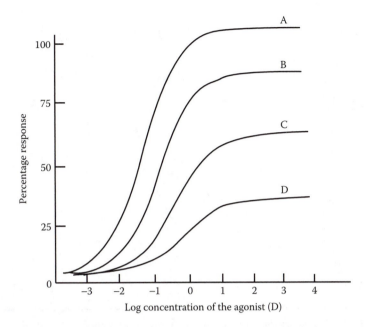

Figure 10.22   Log concentration–response curves for a series of agonists (A, B, C, and D). These drugs seem to have essentially the same potency; however, the ability to produce E_{max} by these drugs is different. The most efficacious drug is the one that produces maximal effect (A), and the least efficacious is the one that produces the least effect.

the pharmacological response will increase in a gradual, smooth fashion, provided the dose has exceeded a critical level called the *threshold dose.*

The degree of effect produced by increasing doses of a drug will eventually reach a steady-state level, the so-called *ceiling effect*. The drug dose that can produce the ceiling effect can be referred to as the *ceiling dose*. In general, drug doses beyond the ceiling dose do not elicit any further increase in therapeutic effect. In fact, doses exceeding the ceiling dose may actually provoke undesirable effects such as toxicity. However, the ceiling dose has a considerable importance in therapeutics, where the aim often is the achievement of a maximum pharmacologic effect. The ceiling dose also serves as the basis for a systematic comparison of the therapeutic efficacy of drugs. In the graded response curve, the main body of the curve lies between threshold dose and the ceiling dose. The graded curve may be a symmetric sigmoid curve, or an asymmetric sigmoid curve where either end may be distorted, or even one-half of a sigmoid curve (the upper half), which would then make it a hyperbolic function. Knowledge of the general shape of the graded curve for a given drug has

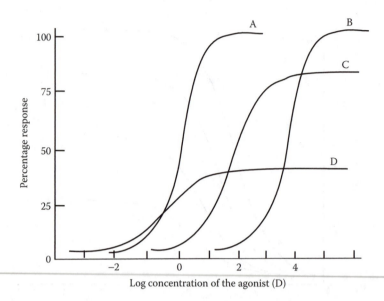

Figure 10.23 Dose–response curves for a series of agonists (A, B, C, and D). These drugs seem to have different efficacies and potencies. Drug A is a good example of an agonist that combines good potency and efficacy.

practical use in medicine when a patient has to be virtually titrated with the drug in order to obtain the optimum result. It is usual that the central part of the graded curve is linear for a range so that the rate of change of response is directly related to the rate of change of dose.

Quantal Dose–Response Curves

The quantal, also known as all-or-none, curve relates the frequency with which any dose of a drug evokes a predefined pharmacologic response. It is, therefore, essentially a curve describing the distribution of minimum doses that produce a given effect in a population of experimental (biological) objects. For a large group of subjects, one can organize the results by noting the minimum concentration of a drug that is needed to obtain a defined response in the experimental subjects. By plotting the number of subjects that respond versus the minimum concentration of dose required for that response, the distribution curve can be obtained with most of the subjects clustered around the *median dose*. In its most basic form, the quantal dose-response curve takes the shape of a Gaussian or normal distribution (Figure 10.25). The Gaussian distribution suggests that the observed variation in doses needed to produce the response is due to simple random variation.

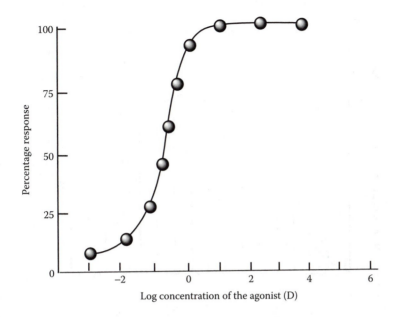

Figure 10.24 A graphic representation of graded response that can be detected in an isolated aortic strip in response to increasing concentration of norepinephrine treatment.

It is usual to obtain dose distributions that are imperfect normal distributions, because either one or the other end of the distribution is not available (truncation). In a symmetric normal or bell-shaped curve, the value that has the greatest frequency is called the *mode*; it is equal to the mean (average value) and median (the value that bisects the population of values into equal halves).

The histogram or normal distribution function is not a practical form in which to use dose–response data for various important purposes. Therefore, a more linearized presentation of the quantal response data is preferred for several reasons. The linearization is accomplished by replotting the data as the *cumulative percentage responding* versus the dose as shown in Figure 10.26. This converts the bell-shaped curve into an S-shaped plot, with the region between approximately 20 and 80% forming a straight line.

Statistics That Can Be Derived from the Quantal Dose–Response Curve

Arithmetic Mean Dose

The arithmetic mean (average) dose of a drug is the dose computed as the sum of all the doses required to produce a stated response, divided by the number of such doses in the summation $x = \Sigma x/N$.

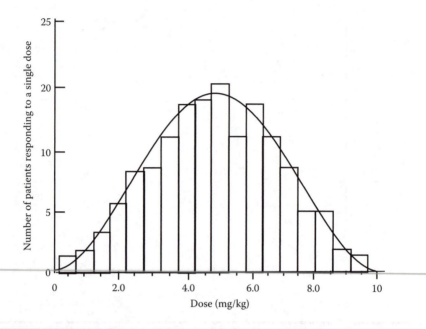

Figure 10.25 A quantal response curve. The data used are collected after administration of increasing doses of drug to a group of subjects and observed for the number of individuals who were showing a predefined level of effect. Each bar represents the total number of people who responded fully to a given dose.

Median Dose

The median dose is the smallest dose that is effective in 50% of individuals. The median effective dose is expressed symbolically as ED_{50} for *effective dose in 50% of the population.*

Confidence Limits

Every statistic derived from experimental data is only an estimate of the "true" value of the statistic in a population of infinite size, and each estimate is associated with an error, which is expressed generally as the standard error for the statistic. Another more meaningful way of indicating the precision of a statistic is the use of *confidence limits.* These are the boundaries that are expected to contain the "true" value of a statistic. When the 95% confidence limits are calculated for an ED_{50} value, the assertion is made that the true ED_{50} for the drug in an infinite population of experimental subjects will be found with a probability of 95%.

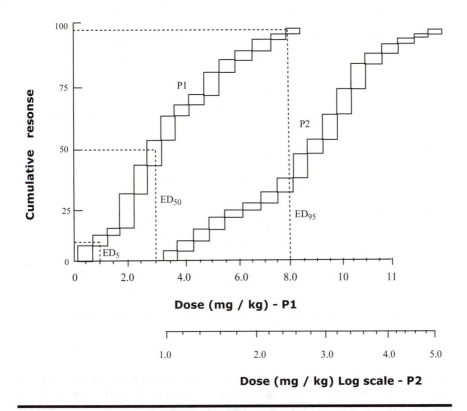

Figure 10.26 Plots with cumulative number (percentage) of individuals who would be responding to each dose of drug versus the doses administered. The plot produces a hyperbolic curve when plotted on an arithmetic scale (P1) and a sigmoidal curve when plotted on a log scale (P2).

THERAPEUTIC INDEX

The therapeutic index of a drug is an approximate statement of the relative safety of the drug expressed as the ratio of the lethal or *toxic dose* (LD) to the therapeutic or *effective dose* (ED). The larger the ratio, the greater the relative safety of the drug. A ratio of one, for example would indicate that, the dose that is effective in producing pharmacological response in 50% of the population would also be lethal to the same percentage of individuals in that population. It is not sufficient to merely state the therapeutic index in terms of *lethal dose* and *therapeutic dose* without specifically defining where on the quantal dose–response curves these doses occur. Most often the therapeutic index is based on the estimates of the ED_{50} and the median lethal dose (LD_{50}) of a drug as shown in Figure 10.26.

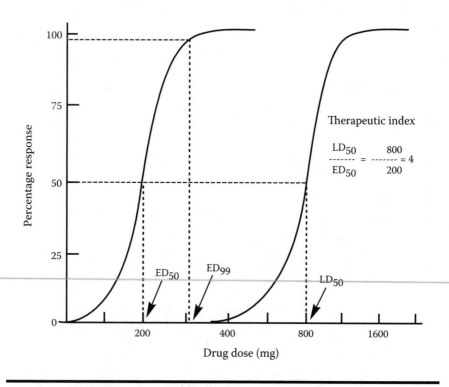

Figure 10.27 Cumulative quantal response curve for a drug that can produce pharmacological effect at lower doses and cumulative quantal response curve for lethal effects at higher doses.

The dose of a drug required to produce a specified intensity of an effect in 50% of individuals (population) is known as *median effective* dose and is abbreviated as ED_{50}. If death is the end point, the median effective dose producing death in 50% of the population is called *median lethal* dose and is abbreviated as LD_{50}.

$$\frac{LD_{50}}{ED_{50}} = \text{Therapeutic Index}$$

The use of the median effective (ED_{50}) and median lethal (LD_{50}) doses for safety assessment has some disadvantages. The median doses tell nothing about how close they are to the toxic effects or to the related dose. One method suggested to overcome this deficiency uses the ED_{99} or $ED_{99.9}$ for the desired drug effect and the LD_1 or even the $LD_{0.1}$ for the undesired effect. Using these levels of response, the therapeutic index is denoted by:

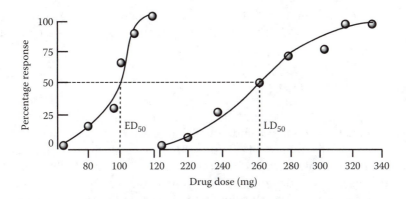

Figure 10.28 Cumulative quantal response curve for phenobarbitol that produces therapeutic lethal effects.

Table 10.3 Therapeutic Index (TI) and Standard Safety Margins (SSM) Calculated by Different Methods for the Drug Data Shown in Figure 10.28

Therapeutic Index and Standard Safety Margin for Phenobarbitol	Value of Index
Therapeutic index LD_{50}/ED_{50}	2.62 (262%)
Standard safety margin $[(LD_1/ED_{99}) - 1] \times 100$	34%
Standard safety margin $[(LD_{0.1}/ED_{99.9}) - 1] \times 100$	8%

Sometimes, instead of therapeutic index, a better notation called the *safety margin* or *standard safety margin* is used. The standard safety margin is defined as the percentage increase of a dose above the therapeutic dose that is lethal to a given proportion of the subjects. The dose–response curve and the safety margins calculated by different methods for phenobarbitol are shown in Figure 10.28 and Table 10.3.

$$\left(\frac{LD_1}{ED_{99}} - 1 \right) \times 100 = \text{Standard Safety Margin}$$

For example, item no. 2 in the table states that the dose of phenobarbitol that is effective in producing sleep in 99% of the subjects needs to be increased 34% before 1% of the experimental subjects die. Similarly item no. 3 shows that the dose that is effective in 999 out of 1000 experimental subjects has to be increased by only 8% in order to be lethal for 1 out of 1000 animals. Thus, this index of safety is more precise and conservative in terms of assessing the safety of a drug and its therapeutic doses.

TIME–ACTION CURVES

When drugs are introduced into the body, the drug effects do not develop instantaneously or continue indefinitely; instead, they change with time. Therefore, the magnitude of a drug effect at any given moment is a function of not only of the dose but also the amount of time elapsed since the drug has made contact with the reactive tissues. The time–action properties of drugs have considerable importance in applied pharmacology, where they form the basis for the selection of the best drug and *optimum dosage schedule*, either for sustained therapeutic effect or for transient effect. The basic ideas of time action are summarized in Figure 10.29. There are three distinct phases in all time–action curves; a fourth phase is present and pronounced with some drugs and absent with others:

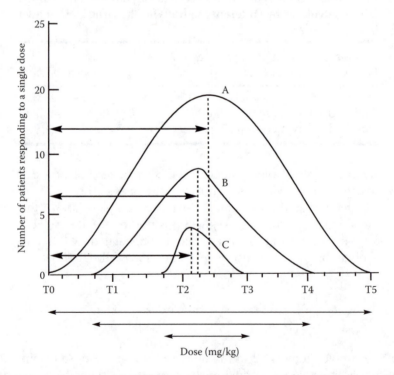

Figure 10.29 Time action curve for three doses of a drug that shows different *duration of effect* for the three doses and the *time(s) to peak effect*.

Phase I: Time to Onset of Action

Following the administration of a drug to an organism or to isolated tissues, there is a delay in time before the first signs of the drug's effect are manifested.

Phase II: Time to Peak Effect

The maximum response will occur when the most resistant cell has been affected to its maximum or when the drug has reached the most inaccessible cells of the responsive tissue.

Phase III: Duration of Action

The duration of action of a drug extends from the moment of onset of perceptible effects to the time when an action can no longer be measured.

Phase IV: Residual Effects

When a drug is administered, even after its primary actions are terminated, it is possible for the drug to exert a residual action. This residual action may be unmasked only when another dose of the same drug is administered and exaggerated response is evoked. Residual effects can be observed when an entirely different drug is given and the phenomenon of synergism or antagonism is manifested. Residual effects are also referred to as *carryover.*

Thus, various factors determine the amount and duration of the pharmacological effects produced in a system. Among different factors discussed in this chapter, affinity, intrinsic activity, concentration, presence of antagonists, and presence of partial agonists are some of the most important factors that could significantly influence the amount of response produced in an intact or isolated system. Time and time-related events can also be included as additional important factors for accurate determination of the total pharmacological effect that can be quantified in a biological system.

SAMPLE PROBLEMS

Problem 1

If 8 μmol/L concentration of a drug produces 32% effect by binding to the specific receptors on the cell, what is the K_D value?

$$[D] = 8 \ \mu \ moles/L$$

$$[E] = 32\%$$

$$[E_{max}] = 100\%$$

$$K_D = ?$$

$$\frac{E}{E_{max}} = \frac{[D]}{[D] + K_D}$$

$$\frac{32}{100} = \frac{8 \ \mu \ moles}{8 \ \mu \ moles + K_D}$$

$$K_D = 17 \ \mu \ moles/L$$

Problem 2

A 10^{-6} M concentration of a full agonist initially produced 100% effect by binding to the receptors on a target tissue. Subsequently, when 2×10^{-7} M concentration of a partial agonist with the same binding affinity as the full agonist for that particular receptor is added to that system, what would be net effect produced?

$$[D] = 1 \ \mu mol \ / \ L \ (10^{-6} \ M)$$

The concentration of the partial agonist to produce 75% binding:

$$[A] = 0.2 \ \mu mol/L \ (2 \times 10^{-7} \ M)$$

$$K_D = KA$$

Therefore, if

$$K_D = 0.01 \ \mu mol/L$$

$$K_A = 0.01 \ \mu mol/L$$

Method I:

$$\frac{E}{E_{max}} = \frac{[D]}{[D] + K_D \left(1 + [A]/K_A \right)}$$

$$\frac{E}{100} = \frac{1}{1+0.01\left(1+0.2/0.01\right)}$$

$$E = \frac{1}{1+0.01\left(201\right)}$$

$$= \frac{1}{1+0.201} = 0.8326$$

$$\frac{E}{100} = 0.8326$$

therefore,

$$E = 83.26\%$$

Method II

$$\frac{E}{100} = \frac{[D]K_A}{K_D K_A + K_D [A] + K_A [D]}$$

$$= \frac{1 \times 0.01}{\left(0.01 \times 0.01\right)+\left(0.01 \times 0.2\right)+\left(0.01 \times 1\right)}$$

$$= \frac{0.01}{0.0001+0.002+0.01}$$

$$= \frac{0.01}{0.0121}$$

$$\frac{E}{100} = 0.8333$$

$$E = 83.33\%$$

Problem 3

A 10 µmol/ L concentration of a drug produces 40% effect. The K_D value for the drug is 5 µmol/L. Calculate the intrinsic activity and determine whether the drug is a full agonist, partial agonist, or antagonist.

$$[D] = 10 \ \mu mol/L$$

$$[E] = 40\%$$

$$[E_{max}] = 100\%$$

$$K_D = 5 \ \mu mol/L$$

$$\frac{E}{E_{max}} = \frac{\alpha[D]}{[D] + K_D}$$

$$\frac{40}{100} = \frac{\alpha \times 10 \ \mu \ moles}{10 \ \mu \ moles + 5}$$

$$0.4 \times 15 = \alpha \times 10$$

$$\alpha = 0.6$$

Problem 4

If a drug that dissociates at the rate of $5 \times 10^{-7} \ \alpha$ mol/L/sec produces 130% "peak effect" when given at a concentration of $1 \times 10^{-6} \ \mu mol/L$. The K_D value for this drug is 2×10^{-8} mol/L. Calculate the intensity factor ϕ for this drug when it is producing the peak effect.

$$[E] = 130\%$$

$$[D] = 5 \times 10^{-7}$$

$$K_D = 1 \times 10^{-6} \ \mu mol/L$$

$$E = \phi \ A$$

$$A = \left(\frac{K_2[D]}{[D] + K_D} \right)$$

$$E = \phi \left(\frac{K_2[D]}{[D] + K_D} \right)$$

$$130 = \phi \left(\frac{\left(5 \times 10^{-7}\right) \times \left(1 \times 10^{-6}\right)}{1 \times 10^{-6} + 2 \times 10^{-8}} \right)$$

$$130 = \phi \frac{5 \times 10^{-13}}{1.02 \times 10^{-6}}$$

$$130 = \phi \times (4.901 \times 10^{-7})$$

$$\phi = 2.653 \times 10^8$$

Problem 5

If 5 µmol/L concentration of an antagonist increases the concentration of the agonist from 10 µmol/L to 1.0 mmol/L, in order to produce the same effect, determine the dissociation constant for the antagonist.

$$[D]_A = 1 \text{ mmol}$$

$$1 \text{ mmol} = 1000 \text{ µmol}$$

$$\frac{[D]_A}{[D]_0} = \frac{[A]}{K_A} + 1$$

$$\frac{1000}{10} = \frac{5}{K_A} + 1$$

$$100 = \frac{5}{K_A} + 1$$

$$100 - 1 = \frac{5}{K_A}$$

$$99 = \frac{5}{K_A}$$

$$K_A = \frac{5}{99}$$

$$= 0.050 \text{ µ moles/L}$$

302 ■ Basic Pharmacology: Understanding Drug Actions and Reactions

Problem 6

If the dose ratio of a drug [D] is 100 in the presence of 8.5 μmol/L of an antagonist, calculate the pA_{10} value for the antagonist. Also, determine whether it is a competitive antagonist for the drug D.

$$\log (x - 1) = pA_2 - pA_x$$

Value for x = 100

Therefore,

$$\log (100 - 1) = pA_2 - pA_{100}$$

since

$$\pi A_{100} = -\log \text{ of } 8.5 \times 10^{-6} = 5.070$$

$$\log 99 = pA_2 - 5.070$$

$$1.995 = pA_2 - 5.070$$

$$1.995 + 5.070 = pA_2$$

$$7.065 = pA_2$$

Again, use the above formula,

$$\log(x - 1) = pA_2 - pA_x$$

$$\log(10 - 1) = 7.065 - pA_{10}$$

$$\log 9 = 7.065 - pA_{10}$$

$$0.954 = 7.065 - pA_{10}$$

$$pA_{10} = 7.065 - 0.954$$

$$pA_{10} = 6.111$$

Answer to the second part of the problem:

$$pA_2 - pA_{10} = 7.065 - 6.111 = 0.954$$

It is a competitive antagonist.

PRACTICE PROBLEMS

1. If 5×10^{-8} mol/L concentration of an agonist drug produces 80% of the maximum effect, calculate the K_D value for the drug using Clark's equation.

2. If 8 μmol/L concentration of a drug produces 50% effect by binding to the specific receptors on the cell, what is the K_D value?

3. If the concentration of the drug used is 1/3 of the K_D value, what percentage of maximal effect will that antagonist produce in the system according to Clark's occupation theory?

4. If 1×10^{-7} mol/L concentration of a partial agonist produced only 45% effect even when all the receptors were occupied, calculate the intrinsic activity of this partial agonist. The K_D value for this partial agonist is 1×10^{-8} mol/L.

5. If 20 μmol/L concentration of a drug with the K_D value of 3 μmol/L binds to the receptors in a tissue, what percent effect will that drug produce? The α value for this drug is zero.

6. The original effect produced by 5×10^{-9} mol/L concentration of an agonist was reduced from 100 to 60% after the introduction of an irreversible antagonist. The K_D value for that agonist is 8.6×10^{-11}. Determine the fraction of the total receptor that might be occupied by the irreversible antagonist at this concentration in this experimental system.

7. Three hundred eighteen milligrams of atropine inhibited 55% (it did not bring the effect down to 55%) of salivary secretion stimulated by 300 mg of carbachol by forming a drug–receptor complex by binding to 9×10^9 receptor molecules on that gland. Calculate the total number of receptors that might be present on the salivary gland. (In this experimental system, the K_D values for carbachol and atropine respectively are 70 and 75 μmol/L).

8. If the dose ratio for an agonist in the presence of 1×10^{-7} mol/L concentration of an antagonist is 50, calculate the pA_{10} value for this antagonist that imposed the dose ratio and determine whether it is a competitive antagonist.

9. Injection of a 8.5×10^{-6} mol/L concentration of a competitive antagonist A to an experimental animal that was already receiving an agonist imposed a dose ratio of 30 on that agonist to produce the same effect. For the same agonist, injection of 3.8×10^{-5} mol/L concentration of a second competitive antagonist B imposed a dose ratio of 22 in the same experimental system. Calculate the pA_2 and pA_{10} values for the antagonists A and B, and also determine which one is a potent antagonist.

10. Among the four concentrations listed below, two represent the concentrations that had provided the pA_2 values and two represent the concentrations that had provided the pA_{10} values for antagonists A and B.

a. 1.00 x 10-6 moles/liter
b. 2.51 x 10-9 moles/liter
c. 1.12 x 10-7 moles/liter
d. 2.23 x 10-8 moles/liter

Find out the corresponding pA_2 and pA_{10} value providing concentrations for antagonists A and B from the list. Also determine which one could be a competitive antagonist (Hint: the pA_{10} value for drug A is 6.)

11. Solve the problems given for three related situations using appropriate equations and verify Gaddum's theory.

Situation 1. Calculate the percent effect produced by 10 µmol/L concentration of a drug whose K_D value is 0.3 mol/L

Situation 2. If you introduce 9 µmol/L concentration of a competitive antagonist whose K_A value is 3 µmol to the above-mentioned system, what will be the effect (E) produced? After introducing the competitive antagonist, does the effect (E) increase from situation 1 or decrease? By how much?

Situation 3. Now increase the concentration of the antagonist to 900 µmol/L and determine what percentage of maximal effect will be produced by the agonist.

12. The concentrations of antagonists imposing the dose ratio of two on the same agonist are given below. Based on the pA_2 values given below, determine which of the listed drugs is the least potent antagonist.

Drug A: 5.6×10^{-9}
Drug B: 5.0×10^{-10}
Drug C: 1.0×10^{-10}
Drug D: 8.9×10^{-10}
Drug E: 3.5×10^{-8}

13. The K_D values (µmol/L) for five different drugs that can bind to the same receptors are given below. Which one of the drugs listed below has the highest affinity for that particular receptor?

The K_D value for drug A is 8×10^{-3} mol/L.
The K_D value for drug B is 5×10^{-9} mol/L.
The K_D value for drug C is 9×10^{-7} mol/L.
The K_D value for drug D is 2×10^{-8} mol/L.
The K_D value for drug E is 1×10^{-6} mol/L.

14. An agonist concentration of 8 µmol/L initially produced 100% effect. The K_D value for this drug is 0.5 µmol/L. When 2 µmol of a competitive antagonist was introduced into the same system, the effect (E) was reduced to 25% of the maximum. Calculate the dissociation constant (K_A) for that competitive antagonist.
15. The ED99 for four different drugs A, B, C, and D (that can be used for treating the same condition), respectively are 100, 125, 150, and 200. The LD_1 concentrations for these drugs, respectively, are 125, 150, 175, and 275. Calculate the standard safety margin (SSM) and determine which of the drugs would be the safest.

ANSWERS FOR THE PROBLEMS

1. 6.25×10^{-8} mol/L
2. 8 µmol/L
3. 25%
4. 0.495
5. 0 (zero)
6. 0.039
7. 2×10^{10} receptor molecules
8. $pA_{10} = 7.74$; it is a competitive antagonist based on calculated pA_2 and pA_{10} values.
9. The pA_2 and pA_{10} values for antagonist A are 6.53 and 5.58, respectively. The pA_2 and pA_{10} values for antagonist B are 5.74 and 4.79, respectively.
10. The pA_2 imposing concentrations for antagonists A and B are 1.12×10^{-7} and 2.51×10^{-9}; pA_{10} imposing concentrations for A and B are 1×10^{-6} and 2.23×10^{-8}.
11. In situation 1 the value of E = 97%; in situation 2 the value of E = 89%; in situation 3 the value of E = 9.97%.
12. Drug E
13. Drug B
14. $K_A = 0.0425$ µmol/L
15. SSM for drug A = 25%, drug B = 20%, drug C = 16%, drug D = 37.5. Drug D is the safest of the four listed.

REFERENCES

1. Basic & Clinical Pharmacology by Bertram G. Katzung, 8th edition, Chapter 2 (Drug Receptor and Pharmacodynamics), 2001, Lang Medical Books/McGraw-Hill, New York, St. Louis, San Francisco, Lisbon, London, Madrid, Montreal, New Delhi, Singapore, Tokyo, and Toronto.
2. Textbook of Pharmacology by W.C. Bowman and M. J. Rand; Chapter-39 (Principles of Drug Action), chapter 41 (Quantitative Evaluation and Statistical Analysis), 1980, Blackwell Scientific Publications, Edinburgh, London, Melbourne, and Oxford.
3. Pharmacologic analysis of Drug-Receptor Interaction by Terry Kenakin, 2nd Edition, Chapter 1 (Drug-receptor theory)
4. Molecular Biology of The Cell by Bruce Alberts, Dennis Bray, Julian Lewis, Martin Raff, Keith Roberts, James D. Watson, Chapter 13 (Chemical Signaling Between cells), Garland Publishing Inc, New York & London.
5. Human Pharmacology by Theodore M Brody, Joseph Larner, Kenneth P. Minneman and Harold C. Neu, 2nd edition, Chapter 3 (Concentration Response Relationship), 1994, Mosby, St. Louis, Baltimore, Berlin, Boston, Carlsbad, Chicago, London, New York, Sydney, Tokyo & Toronto.

11

RECEPTOR REGULATION AND SIGNALING MECHANISMS

SPARE RECEPTORS

Frequently, the measure of biological response elicited by a drug, by binding to receptors, is proportional to the fraction of the receptors that are occupied by that drug. In some instances, however, the maximal response may be achieved even when a small fraction of the receptors is occupied. This phenomenon occurs due to the presence of *spare* receptors. In the above-mentioned situation the receptors are said to be in spare (in excess) for a given drug; hence, the maximal response is elicited by a dose that does not result in the complete occupancy (100%) of all the receptor sites (saturation). The spare receptors that are present on the cells are usually not different from nonspare (original) receptors, and they are not hidden, either. When the spare receptors are occupied by ligands, they also produce responses similar to those of any other normal receptors.

Experimentally, the presence of spare receptors may be demonstrated by using an irreversible antagonist or noncompetitive antagonist. Even though irreversible antagonists can prevent the binding of agonists to a fraction of available receptors, at high concentrations the agonist can still produce an undiminished maximal response. This is because the irreversible antagonists have blocked only spare receptors, and therefore the receptors necessary to produce the maximal effect are still available for binding by agonists. Thus, a maximal ionotropic response of heart muscle to catecholamines can be elicited even under conditions where up to 90% of the β receptors are occupied by a quasiirreversible antagonist. This is possible because the myocardium is said to contain a large proportion of spare receptors.

The spare receptor concept explains how the sensitivity of a cell or tissue is dependent not only on the affinity of the receptor for binding, but also on the total concentration of the receptors that could be found on a target tissue or cell. Normally, it is the K_D value of an agonist that would determine what fraction (B/B_{max}) of the total receptors will be occupied at a given free concentration (C) of the agonist, regardless of the concentration of the receptors.

$$\frac{B}{B_{max}} = \frac{C}{C + K_D}$$

If a tissue with **100** (100%) total receptors has **90** (90%) spare receptors, this tissue would require only **10** (10%) of the receptors' occupancy to produce maximal (E_{max}) response. In that case, the half-maximal response will be produced by an agonist concentration (EC_{50}) that results in occupancy of only **5** (5%) of the total receptors per cell. If the receptor concentration is doubled to 200 per cell due to activation of protein synthesis, it will still require the occupancy of only **10** receptor molecules per cell to produce maximal response and **5** receptors per cell for half-maximal response. Now, since the number of total receptors has increased to **200**, after the increase, **10** receptors per 200 is equal to 5% and **5** per **200** is equal to 2.5% of total (**200**) receptors. If the affinity (K_D) of the drug does not change, a lower concentration of agonist will be sufficient to occupy 2.5% (a total of **5** receptors) rather than 5% of receptors, and consequently the EC_{50} value will be decreased. Thus, the sensitivity of the cell can change with spare receptors. An important biologic consequence of spare receptors is that they allow an agonist with low affinity to produce full response at lower concentrations.

From these concepts it is clearly evident that the spare receptors can increase the sensitivity of tissues to a drug. For example, if the concentration of a free drug is 1/3 of the K_D value, it will be sufficient to occupy 25% of the receptors (one out of four) on the membrane and produce 25% effect (Figure 11.1). On the other hand, if the number of receptors on the membrane is increased fourfold to a total of 16 receptors, the same concentration of the drug with the same K_D value can now occupy 25% of the receptors (four out of 16). Since it is required to activate only four receptor-coupled effector molecules to produce 100% effect, the same concentration of the drug can produce 100% effect when the concentration of the receptors is increased by a factor of four (Figure 11.2).

OVERSHOOT

The phenomenon of overshoot follows withdrawal of certain drugs. Overshoot may occur with either agonists or antagonists. When an antagonist is used to block an undesirable effect of an endogenously present hormone or neurotransmitter, a complete blockade by the antagonist may increase the total number of receptors during treatment by increasing the synthesis

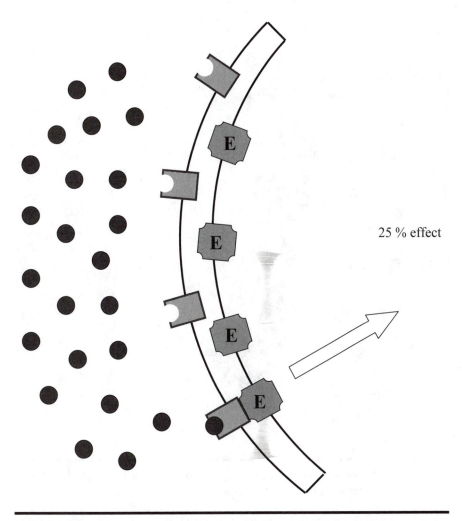

25 % effect

Figure 11.1   When a drug concentration equal to 1/3 of the K_D value was administered, a 25% effect was observed in the cells. The cells produce a 25% effect because of 25% receptor saturation.

or by preventing the down regulation of receptors. When the antagonist is withdrawn, the elevated number of receptors (spare) can produce an exaggerated response to physiologic concentrations of agonist that were originally present in the system. This is referred to as overshoot.

DOWN REGULATION

Down regulation is a process by which the number of total receptors present on the cell membrane is decreased subsequent to continued

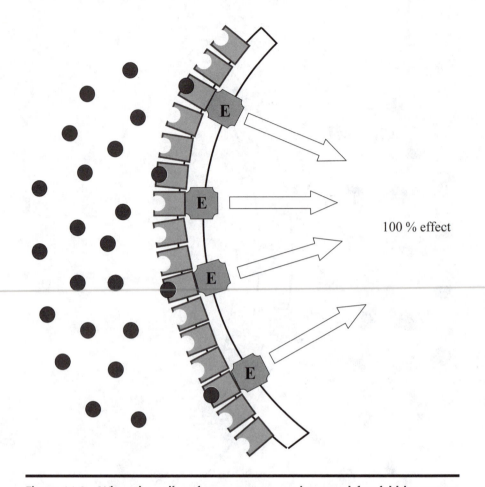

Figure 11.2   When the cell surface receptors are increased fourfold by up regulation, 25% saturation can produce 100% effects.

stimulation of the receptors by an agonist. Down regulation of receptors is primarily mediated by a process called *endocytosis*, which is a receptor internalization process. The receptor internalization process is depicted in Figure 11.3. The internalization process is generally initiated when the receptor proteins on the cell surface form a complex with a specific agonist. Subsequent to agonist binding, the ligand–receptor complexes cluster in small regions of the membrane. This region of the membrane is coated with a protein called *clathrin* on the cytoplasmic side of the plasma membrane. The clathrin-coated areas form pits called *coated pits,* which eventually form vesicles. These vesicles (*endosomes*) take the receptor–agonist complex to the inside of the cell, where they fuse with other vesicles called *sorting endosomes*. The sorting endosomes have an internal pH of ~5.0, which causes the receptors to dissociate from their

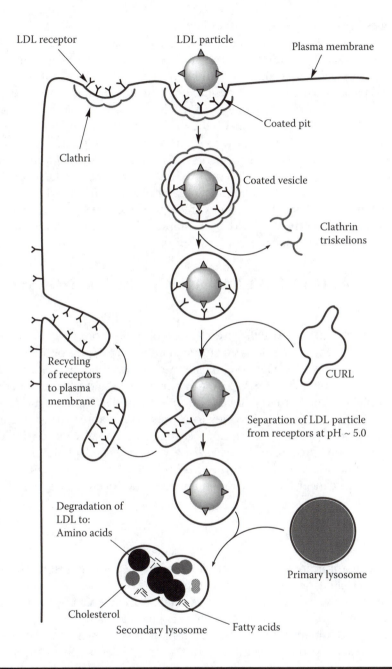

Figure 11.3 The endocytosis of low-density lipoprotein (LDL) and receptor through the endosomes. The same pathway is followed by other receptors that are internalized subsequent to ligand binding. Internalization can lead to down regulation when the recycling mechanism is very slow or absent.

agonists. The free receptors then concentrate in one section of these vesicles, which ultimately buds to form a separate vesicle, which is transported back to the membrane surface. The ligand is segregated into a different vesicle that ultimately fuses with a lysosome, where proteases and other hydrolytic enzymes degrade the ligand. During this process the receptors may also be delivered into the lysosomes, which could eventually result in the degradation of the receptors. The degradation of the receptors in the lysosomes normally leads to a decrease in the total number of cell surface receptors; this process is called *down regulation.* Subsequent to down regulation the normal responses can be achieved only when new receptor molecules are synthesized and transported to the cells' surface. In general, synthesizing new receptors is a slow process; therefore, a long duration of time would be required to bring the total number of receptors and the response back to normal.

OTHER FACTORS THAT CAN AFFECT DRUG RESPONSE

Tolerance

The word *tolerance* is usually used to describe the more gradual decrease in the effectiveness of a drug given repeatedly over a long period of time. This term is usually applied to clinically used drugs when larger and larger doses have to be given to produce the same desired effect (e.g., tolerance to morphine). The term tolerance is frequently used to describe the relative insensitivity of a particular species to a drug (e.g., rabbits are particularly insensitive to atropine). *Individual tolerance* is the relative insensitivity of some members of one species. *Acquired tolerance* is adaptation by secreting enzymes that will degrade the drug (e.g., resistance to penicillin and resistance to cancer chemotherapeutic agents can occur due to degrading enzymes).

Tachyphylaxis

Successive application of the same dose of a powerful agonistic drug such as acetylcholine or histamine usually produces consistently reproducible responses. However, with some drugs such as angiotensin II, the response gets smaller and smaller when the drug is given at high doses or by rapid and repeated administration. This phenomenon is known as *tachyphylaxis* (loss of response on repeated administration), which implies that a fairly rapid diminution in response occurs. The occurrence of tachyphylaxis is sometimes explained based on the rate of agonist dissociation from the receptor. As discussed in Chapter 10, if the dissociation occurs at sufficiently slow rate, then the receptors are still occupied (not free to engage new agonists), and therefore the receptors cannot produce any further effects.

Idiosyncratic Drug Response

Individuals may vary considerably in their responsiveness to a drug. A single individual may respond differently to the same drug at different times during the course of treatment. For example, peripheral neuropathy may occur following insoniazid therapy in some individuals who are genetically slow acetylators of isoniazid. Another example is precipitation of acute hemolysis in some patients who are using sulfonamides. The acute hemolysis occurs frequently among patients who are genetically deficient in the enzyme glucose-6-phosphate dehydrogenase. These variations in general are related to the genetic make-up of an individual.

RECEPTOR SIGNALING AND SECOND MESSENGER SYSTEMS

The amount of response produced by a receptor also depends on the type of second messenger–producing systems that are linked to that receptor. For easy understanding, the different modes of receptor signal transduction mechanisms for the receptors can be classified into four superfamilies:

1. Intracellular receptors (DNA-linked receptors)
2. Receptors linked to enzymes
3. Receptors linked to ion channels
4. Receptors linked to G-proteins

Four Basic Mechanisms of Receptor Signaling

In general, as mentioned earlier, there are four different mechanisms by which ligands can transmit their signals across the plasma membrane (Figure 11.4):

1. Lipid-soluble ligands could cross the plasma membrane and activate intracellular receptors that eventually lead to enzyme activation or gene transcription.
2. Ligands that are soluble in water (hydrophilic) can primarily bind to the transmembrane receptor protein and activate intracellular enzymes by inducing conformation change.
3. The transmembrane ion-channels can be opened or closed by allosteric regulation following ligand binding to an extracellular site.

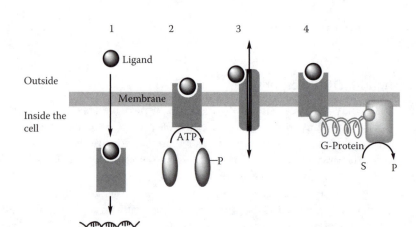

Figure 11.4 Different transmembrane signaling mechanisms. 1. A lipophilic drug (ligand) crosses the plasma membrane and regulates gene transcription. 2. A hydrophilic drug (ligand) binds to the extracellular binding site on the cell surface receptors and initiates phosphorylation by stimulating kinase activity. 3. The drug (ligand) binds to the ion channel or ion channel–receptor complex and opens the ion channel. 4. A hydrophilic drug binds to cell surface receptors and activates the second messenger system through G-proteins.

Table 11.1
Approximate Time Required for Different Signaling Systems to Work

Type of Receptors	Time Required to Produce Effect
Ion channel linked	Milliseconds
Receptors linked to second messenger–producing enzymes	Seconds
Receptors linked to protein kinases that phosphorylate target proteins	Minutes
DNA-linked	Hours

4. By interaction with a transmembrane receptor protein such as GTP-binding protein (G-protein) the signal transduction pathway is activated, which in turn can generate the intracellular second messengers (cAMP [cyclic adenosine monophosphate], cGMP [cyclic guanosine monophophate], diacylglycerol [DAG], inositol 1,4,5-triphosphate [IP_3] and Ca^{2+} ion).

The times required for each system to work are shown in Table 11.1.

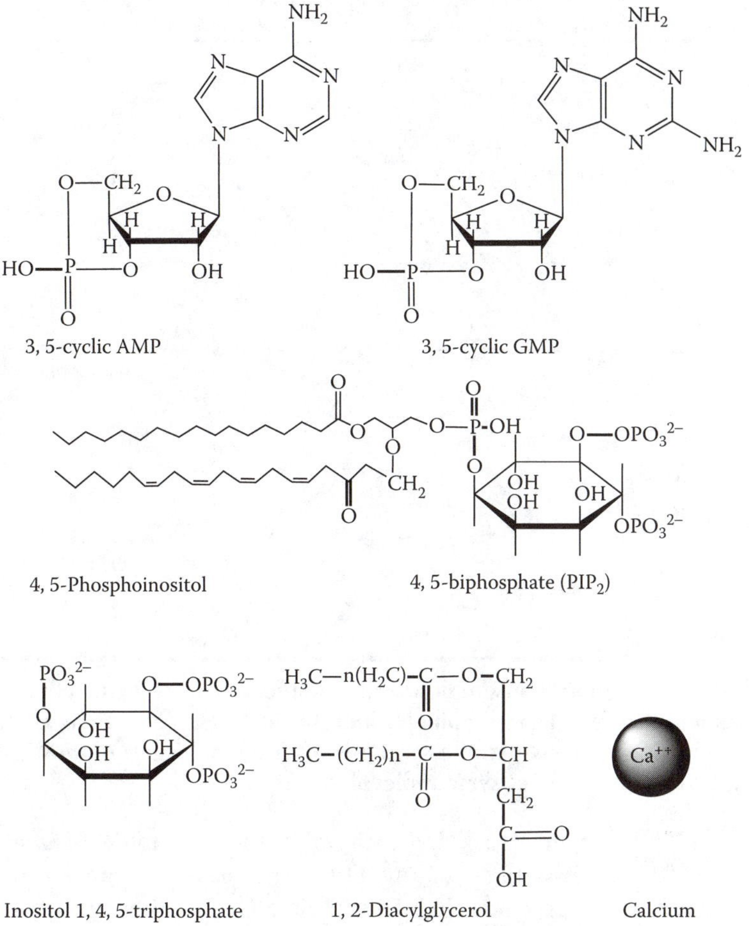

Figure 11.5   Structures of important second messengers.

The Four Major Types of Second Messengers

In general, hormones, neurotransmitters, cytokines, etc. that can bind to receptors are considered *first messengers*. The small molecules that carry signals inside the living cell are called *second messengers*. At least three biochemicals and a divalent cation (Ca^{2+}) are widely known as second messengers (Figure 11.5). These second messengers are produced in response to the activation of the membrane-bound receptors by ligands; they conduct the signals further towards an ultimate target that can produce cellular responses. While conducting the signals from the receptor molecules,

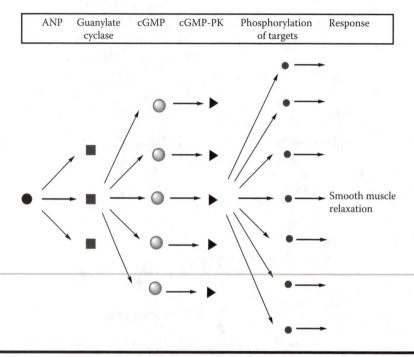

ANP	Guanylate cyclase	cGMP	cGMP-PK	Phosphorylation of targets	Response

Smooth muscle relaxation

Figure 11.6 Initiation, transduction, and amplification of an extracellular signal that was initiated by a ligand (epinephrine). In this example, binding of a single ligand (epinephrine) results in the synthesis of many molecules of cAMP, which, in turn, activate multiple enzyme molecules.

the second messenger also helps to amplify the amounts of signals and produce sufficient responses (Figure 11.6). The messages carried by these second messengers are modulated by their concentration, which in turn is determined by the rate of synthesis and degradation of second messengers by specific enzymes (Figure 11.7). These enzymes switch *on* and *off* rapidly in response to activation and inhibitory responses, allowing them to modulate the concentration of the second messengers in milliseconds. The physical nature of the second messengers and their solubility in water or lipid bilayer has important consequences in terms of what targets they can activate. For example, lipid-derived second messengers such as phosphoinositol 4,5-biphosphate, inositol 1,4,5-triphosphate, diacylglycerol, phosphatidic acid, and arachidonic acid (Figure 11.8) can easily reach targets in the lipid bilayer or hydrophobic targets elsewhere. Calcium acts primarily in the cytoplasm, where a high concentration of binding sites for calcium is present. On the other hand, cyclic nucleotides (cAMP and cGMP) act globally because they diffuse rapidly throughout the cytoplasm.

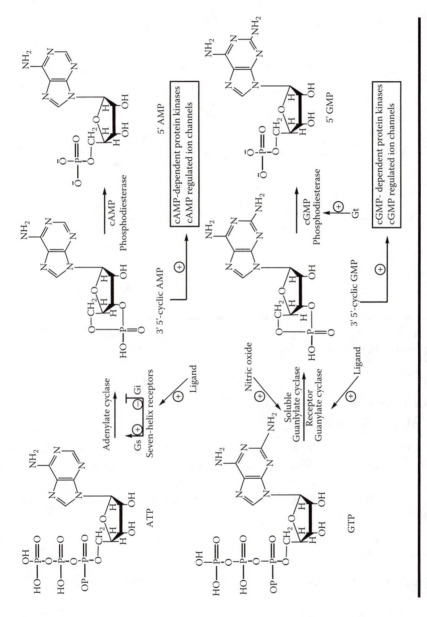

Figure 11.7 Pathways leading to production or degradation of cAMP and cGMP. The pathway also indicates the G proteins, regulatory inputs, and targets.

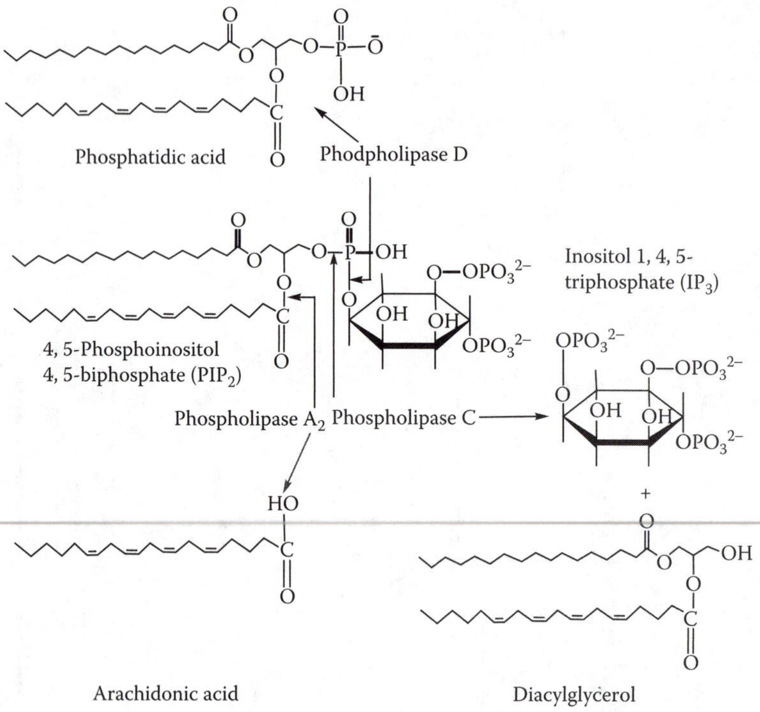

Figure 11.8 Production of lipid second messengers by enzymatic hydrolysis of PIP_2 (phosphatidylinositol 4,5-biphosphate).

HORMONES ACTING THROUGH INTRACELLULAR RECEPTORS

Several steroid hormones bind to intracellular receptors and cause cellular responses. Examples include corticosteroids, mineralocorticoids, sex steroids, and thyroid hormone. The general mechanisms involved in activation of intracellular receptors and the consequent responses are outlined below.

Mechanism of Action

The location of the intracellular receptors are affected as follows:

a. Glucocorticoid receptor reside in the cytoplasm of the cells until it binds with the ligand, and then the receptor–hormone complex moves to the nucleus to activate specific genes (Figure 11.9).

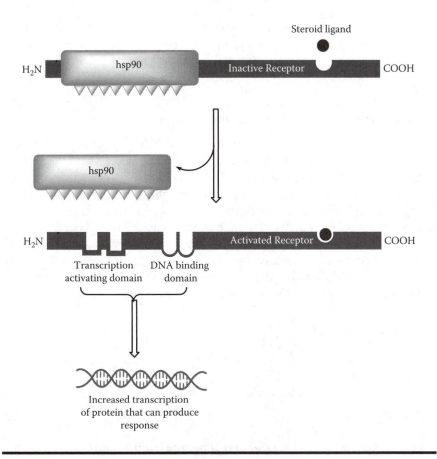

Figure 11.9 Mechanism of steroid (glucocorticoid) action. The steroid receptor is schematically depicted in dark shade, inhibited by the heat-shock protein (*hsp90*) before ligand (steroid) binding. When activated by ligand, the *hsp90* dissociates from the receptor and allows the receptor to obtain an active configuration.

b. In some cases, the receptors seem to be located in the nucleus even in the absence of their respective ligands (examples: estrogen and thyroid hormone receptors).

The mechanism used by hormones that act by regulating gene expression has two therapeutically important consequences:

1. The steroid hormones in general produce their effects after a characteristic lag period of 30 min to several hours. This means that the gene-active hormones cannot be expected to alter a pathologic state within minutes (e.g., steroids can not relieve inflammatory conditions immediately).

2. The effect of steroid hormones can persist for hours or days even after the agonist concentration has been reduced. The toxic effects of a gene-active hormone will usually decrease slowly after the administration of the hormone is stopped.

Ligands Acting through Cell Surface Receptors

Many hormones and drug molecules, especially those that are hydrophilic in nature, bind to membrane-bound cell surface receptors and activate cellular responses. In these cases, subsequent to the occupation of the binding sites, the receptor molecules go through a series of conformational changes that result in the activation of coupled enzymes and further transmission of the signals. The activated enzymes may be part of the cytoplasmic portion of the receptor molecules, or they could be separate entities linked by intermediary components such as *G-proteins*. There are many kinds of receptor-coupled enzymes that belong to different categories; some of them are *protein kinases, guanylate cyclase,* and *adenylate cyclase*.

Protein Kinases

Protein kinases are enzymes that can phosphorylate receptor proteins and enzyme proteins. Many different protein kinases are coupled to various receptor molecules and function in different ways in response to receptor activation.

Phosphorylation and the Effects of Phosphorylation

Transfer of the terminal phosphate group from ATP (adenosine triphosphate) to serine, threonine, or tyrosine amino acids of substrate proteins by protein kinases is called *phosphorylation* (Figure 11.10). Examples of kinases activating biochemical pathways are depicted in Figure 11.11. Phosphorylation can transform inactive enzymes, receptors, and ion channels to active forms or *vice versa*. The activity of phosphorylated proteins, receptors, or ion channels will persist until the particular protein is dephosphorylated by a *protein phosphatase*. Activation of protein kinase is one way of transmitting a signal from the cell surface to the inside of a cell. Insulin, epidermal growth factor (EGF), platelet-derived growth factor (PDGF), and several other tropic hormones mediate their signals through activation of protein kinases.

Two Types of Protein Kinases

The protein kinases are classified into two broad groups based on their target amino acid in the protein molecule that is phosphorylated:

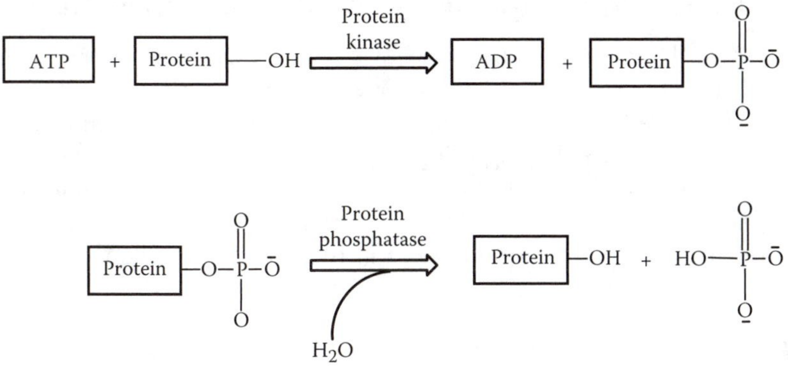

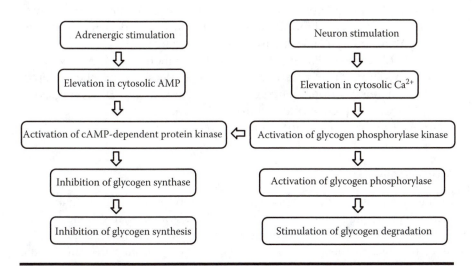

Figure 11.10 Phosphorylation and dephosphorylation of proteins by kinases and phosphatases.

Figure 11.11 Activation of protein kinases such as glycogen phosphorylase kinase and cAMP-dependent protein kinase is involved in conducting a signal along a biochemical pathway.

1. *Tyrosine kinases* phosphorylate tyrosine residues on a protein molecule.
2. *Serine threonine kinases* phosphorylate serine and threonine residues on a protein molecule.

Examples of Receptor Signaling by Activation of Tyrosine Kinases

Typically, cell surface receptor molecules for hormones and growth factors would consist of an extracellular hormone binding domain and a cytoplasmic catalytic (enzyme) domain with protein kinase activity or some other enzyme activity. In either case, the signaling pathway begins with hormone binding to the receptor site that is located at the extracellular domain. After ligand binding, the resulting change in the conformation of the receptor molecule activates the enzyme (tyrosine kinase) in the cytosolic domain.

EGF Receptor Activation

EGF receptor is a good example of a receptor that has a tyrosine kinase in the cytoplasmic domain. When the receptor is not active, it exists as a *monomer.* Upon binding of EGF to the receptor at the extracellular domain, the conformation of the receptor changes. The change in the conformation converts EGF receptor from its inactive *monomeric* form to an active *dimeric* form (Figure 11.12) and at the same time activates the tyrosine kinase in the cytoplasmic domain. The tyrosine kinase from one receptor molecule phosphorylates its dimeric partner and stabilizes the activity (tyrosine kinase). This kind of phosphorylation is called *cross-phosphorylation*. Activated tyrosine kinase then stimulates the cells, through a sequence of intracellular events, to divide by inducing DNA, RNA, and protein synthesis. The receptor activity will persist until the receptor protein remains phosphorylated and terminate as soon as dephosphorylated. (The consequence of uncontrolled EGF receptor activation is unregulated cell multiplication and cancer development.)

Insulin Receptor

Insulin receptor is another good example of a tyrosine kinase activity–coupled receptor molecule. When insulin binds to the α-subunit of the receptor molecule, the conformation of receptor molecule changes, which in turn activates the tyrosine kinase in the cytoplasmic domain of the β-subunit. Activated tyrosine kinase then phosphorylates four specific tyrosine residues in the β-subunit of the receptor molecule, which stabilizes the receptor activity. This kind of phosphorylation (phosphorylation of its own protein molecule) is called *autophosphorylation*. The tyrosine kinase activity of the autophosphorylated insulin receptor persists even after insulin is removed from the binding site. Activated insulin receptor tyrosine kinase:

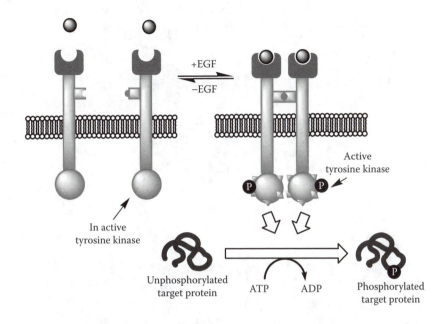

Figure 11.12   Activation of the EGF receptor involves stimulation of receptor kinases, which serve as good examples of receptor-linked tyrosine kinases. The receptor has an extracellular EGF binding domain and a cytoplasmic tyrosine kinase domain. Once activated by EGF binding, the receptor converts from its monomeric state to an active dimeric state in which the receptor molecules associate noncovalently and cross-phosphorylate each other. Once phosphory-lated, the receptor-linked tyrosine kinases become active and in turn phosphory-late their substrates to further conduct the signal.

1. Induces glucose uptake by activating the glucose transporter (Figure 11.13)
2. Triggers glycogen synthesis by phosphorylating a *protein phosphatase*

The activated protein phosphatase removes three phosphates from an inactive *glycogen synthetase* and thereby activates this enzyme to initiate glycogen synthesis.

Phosphorylation-Induced Receptor Down Regulation and Receptor Desensitization

Down Regulation

Down regulation is a very common mechanism by which the receptors from the cell surface are taken inside the cell by *endocytosis*. The purpose of down regulation is to minimize the receptor response after reaching

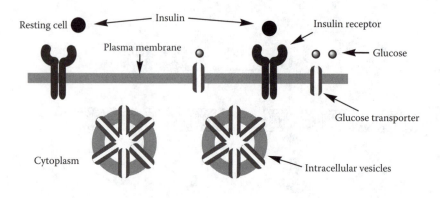

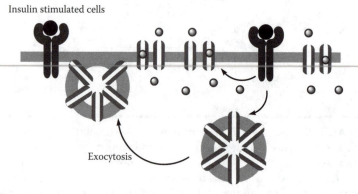

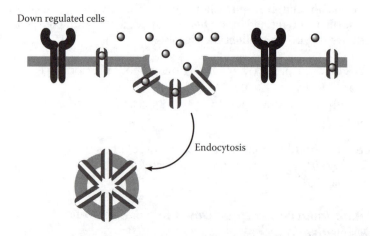

Figure 11.13 Up regulation and down regulation of glucose transporters follow-ing insulin regulation. When there is insulin stimulation, increasing quantities of glucose transporters are transported to the plasma membrane, causing up regu-lation. On removal of insulin, glucose transporters are internalized, resulting in down regulation (decreased number) of transporters.

an initial high level and eventually stop the hormone action or agonist action. Down regulation can stop the receptor-mediated response even in the continued presence of endogenous factors or agonists. In the down regulation process, there is an actual decrease in the number of cell surface receptors, which will come back to normal once the excess agonist is removed from the system. Down regulation of the insulin receptor shown in Figure 11.13 is a good example for understanding this phenomenon.

Desensitization

Desensitization can be caused either by down regulation of receptors or by uncoupling of receptor–effector molecules. Desensitization is normally a reversible process. Phosphorylation of the receptor molecules is one of the important steps that initiate down regulation or desensitization mechanisms. This may be because when receptors such as insulin and EGF receptors are activated by phosphorylation, the cell can recognize phosphorylated receptors as *active receptors* and down regulates only those that are phosphorylated (Figure 11.14).

A second type of desensitization occurs by simply inhibiting the receptor function without inducing endocytosis. For example in the case of β-*adrenoceptor* activation, binding of agonists causes the receptors to activate G_s (GTP binding protein-stimulatory) proteins and stimulate the synthesis of cAMP. The activated β-adrenoceptor also initiates the phosphorylation of a serine residue on its carboxy terminus by a specific β-adrenoceptor kinase (termed βARK). The presence of phosphorylated serine in the receptor molecule increases the affinity of β-adrenoceptor for a protein called β-*arrestin,* which is present in the cells. Binding of β-arrestin results in the termination of β-adrenoceptor interaction with G-proteins, which is also called desensitization. The desensitized receptors will be sensitized when cellular *phosphatases* remove phosphate from the serine residue of the β-adrenoceptor molecule, as shown in Figure 11.15.

RECEPTOR-COUPLED (MEMBRANE-BOUND) GUANYLATE CYCLASE (GC)

Guanylate cyclase is an enzyme that converts GTP (guanosine triphosphate) to cGMP, another important second messenger in mediating vasodilatory actions of hypotensive drugs and hormones. There are two types of guanylate cyclases in the body. One is called soluble guanylate cyclase; the other is called membrane-bound guanylate cyclase. The membrane-bound guanylate cyclase is part of a receptor protein called *atrial natriuretic peptide* (ANP) receptor, which is bound to the plasma membrane of cells such as vascular smooth muscle cells. This receptor is activated

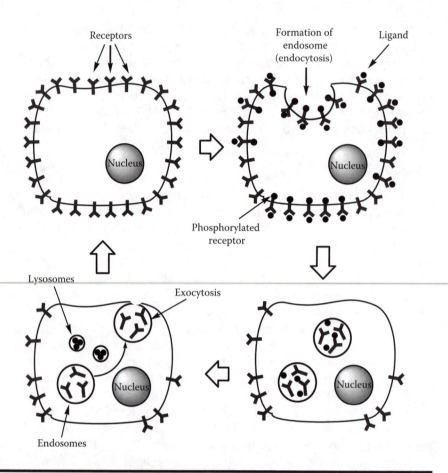

Figure 11.14 Down regulation of receptors by internalization (endocytosis) is triggered by receptor phsophorylation. After internalization, the receptor and the ligand dissociate and are segregated for degradation and recycling. Degradation of ligands occurs in the lysosomes.

by atrial natriuretic peptide, a hormone that is secreted from the right atrium of the heart. When ANP binds to its receptors, the guanylate cyclase enzyme in the cytosolic portion of the protein is activated, which converts GTP to cGMP (Figure 11.16). The cGMP that is produced by the guanylate cyclase mediates several responses in the body, including vasodilation.

SOLUBLE GUANYLATE CYCLASE

This enzyme is called soluble guanylate cyclase because it is present in the cytoplasm and not bound to the plasma membrane of the cells. Soluble guanylate cyclase is a *heme-containing* enzyme. The enzyme is not directly

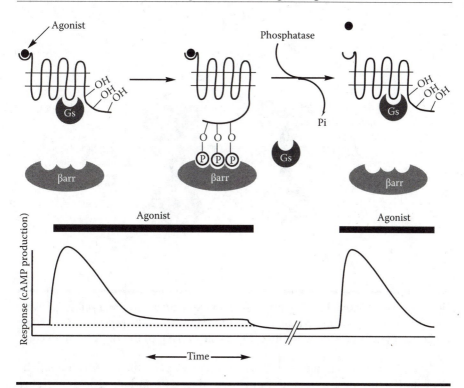

Figure 11.15   Desensitization of β-adrenergic receptors by β-arrestin. Phosphorylation of the serine residues in the carboxy terminus of the β-adrenergic receptors attracts the binding of β-arrestin, which terminates the interaction with G-proteins and also the receptor response. The ligand can produce an effect only after the phosphates are removed from the carboxy terminus by phosphatase.

coupled to any receptors but is activated as a result of NO (nitric oxide) binding to the heme moiety of the enzyme molecule. Compounds such as *sodium nitroprusside, sodium nitrite,* and *nitroglycerine* activate this enzyme by releasing NO. The effect of NO producing NTG (nitroglycerine) on norepinephrine and K$^+$ induced smooth muscle contraction is depicted in Figure 11.17. Endothelium-dependent relaxing factor (EDRF) also activates soluble guanylate cyclase. The cGMP produced by this enzyme also mediates vasodilatory responses by inhibiting the increase in free intracellular calcium concentration and also by blocking smooth muscle contraction through cGMP-dependent protein kinases.

RECEPTORS LINKED TO G-PROTEINS AND SECOND MESSENGER PRODUCTION

Many extracellular ligands activate the cells and tissues by increasing the intracellular concentration of second messengers such as cAMP, IP$_3$, DAG,

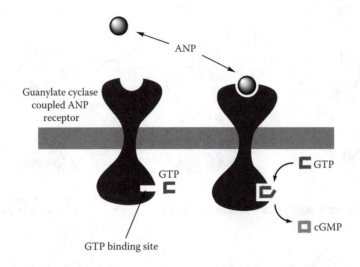

Figure 11.16 Ligand binding initiates activation of guanylate cyclase activity, which is coupled to the Atrial Natriuretic Peptide (ANP) receptor. Guanylate cyclase activity is present with the cytoplasmic domain of the receptor molecule.

and Ca^{2+} ion via activation of a class of proteins called G-proteins. The G-protein–mediated transmembrane signaling is conducted in three separate stages:

1. Extracellular ligand is bound by cell surface receptors.
2. The ligand-bound receptor activates the G-proteins that are located in the cytoplasmic side of the plasma membrane.
3. The activated G-proteins then regulate enzymes such as *adenylate cyclase*.

A wide variety of receptors utilize the G-proteins as transducers of their signals. G-protein–regulated effects include activation of adenylate cyclase, activation of phospholipase C, and activation of plasma membrane ion channels. The G-proteins are composed of a GTP-binding α subunit, an intermediate β subunit, and a plasma memberane–anchoring γ subunit. Typically, G-protein–coupled receptors span the plasma membrane as a bundle of seven alpha helices, and they interact with G-proteins through their cytoplasmic domain. Subsequent to activation of an associated receptor, GTP binds to the α subunit of the G-proteins and activates them to produce one of the above-mentioned signaling effects. The G-proteins remain active until the GTP on α is hydrolyzed to GDP. A cell may express as many as twenty different kinds of G-proteins, some of which are listed in Table 11.2.

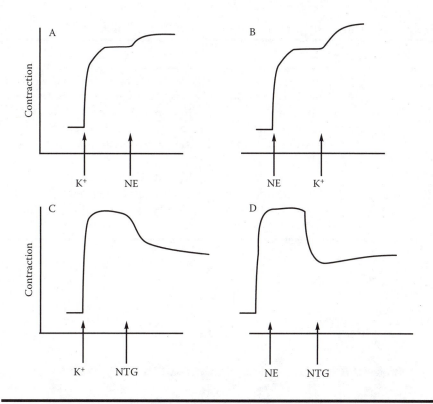

Figure 11.17 Effects of vasodilators on contraction of smooth muscle from human vein segments studied *in vitro*. Panel A shows the contraction initiated by K+, which is augmented by norepinephrine. Panel B shows the contraction initiated by norepinephrine, which is augmented by K+. Panel C and Panel D show the effects of a vasodilator (NTG: nitroglycerine) on K+- and norepinephrine-induced contraction. (Reproduced with some modification with permission from Mikkelsen E., Anderson, K.E., and Bengtsson, B., Effects of verapamil and nitroglycerin on contractile responses to potassium and noradrenaline in isolated human peripheral veins. *Acta Pharmacol. Toxicol.,* 1978; 42:14.)

ACTIVATION OF ADENYLATE CYCLASE AND G-PROTEIN FUNCTION

Adenylate cyclase is a large transmembrane protein that synthesizes cAMP. Adenylate cyclase has two homologous catalytic domains in the cytoplasm that retain enzyme activity function. The transmembrane domains of adenylate cyclase anchor the enzyme to the plasma membrane. Vertabrates produce at least 10 different adenylate cyclases with similar activities, but they are diverse and often have multiple regulatory mechanisms that act synergistically. GTP binding to G-proteins such as G_s and G_i regulates the

Table 11.2 Different Types of G-Proteins and Their Cellular Effects

G-Protein Type	Activators	Cellular Effects
G_s	β-Adrenergic, histamine, serotonin	Stimulates adenylate cyclase (AC) and activates Ca^{2+} channels
G_i	α2-Adrenergic, muscarinic, opioids	Inhibits adenylate cyclase (AC) and activates K^+ channels
G_q	Muscarinic, serotonin ($5-HT_{1C}$)	Activates phospholipase C (PLC)
G_o	Not yet fully defined	Inhibits Ca^{2+} current
G_t	Photons (rhodopsins and color opsins in the retinal rod)	Stimulates adenylate cyclase (AC) in the eye

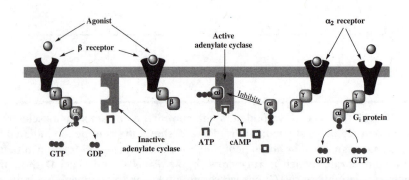

Figure 11.18 Schematic representation of receptor interaction with G-proteins. G-proteins are comprised of α, β, and γ subunits, among which γ and β serve to anchor the G-protein to the membrane. When an agonist binds to the G_s protein–linked receptor, change in the conformation releases the αs subunit, which activates adenylate cyclase after exchanging GTP for GDP. Instead, activation of the G_i; protein–coupled receptor would result in inhibiting the adenylate cyclase through the αi subunit.

adenylate cyclase in response to appropriate receptor activation, as shown in Figure 11.18. The $α_s$ subunit of G_s proteins is released from the trimeric complex in response to activation of appropriate receptors such as β-*adrenergic* receptors and binds to the adenylate cyclase. Binding of the GTP-attached $α_s$ subunit to a site somewhat closer to the catalytic activity region of adenylate cyclase induces a conformational change that stimulates the enzyme activity. On the other hand, when G_i protein that is coupled to α_2 receptors is activated, the binding of the α_i subunit to the cytosolic domain of the adenylate cyclase leads to inhibition of the enzyme activity. These kinds of diverse regulatory mechanisms allow adenylate cyclase to integrate with a variety of input signals.

DOWNSTREAM CAMP SECOND MESSENGER PATHWAY

The second messenger cAMP produces a cellular response by activating an intracellular signaling cascade via activation of cAMP-dependent protein kinases (PKA) or via opening the cAMP-dependent ion channels, which consequently produce specific cellular functions. The cAMP concentration normally found in resting cells is so low, in the range of 10^{-8} M, which is insufficient to activate the signaling cascade. However, subsequent to the stimulation of appropriate receptors (such as the β-adrenergic receptors) the cytoplasmic cAMP concentrations could increase more than 100-fold, which is sufficient to saturate the regulatory subunit of PKA and initiate the intracellular signaling cascade (Figure 11.19).

CA²⁺/PHOSPHOINOSITIDE/PKC SIGNALING PATHWAY

Phosphoinositides are major players in the intracellular signaling pathways. The parent compound that is required to initiate an important cascade of signals is *phosphatidylinositol* (PI), which is a phosphoglyceride with a cyclohexanol head group called *inositol*. Both phosphatidylinositol-4-phosphate (PIP) and phosphatidylinositol-4,5-biphosphate (PIP$_2$) are produced by phophorylation of 4- and 5-hydroxyl groups of phosphatidylinositol by specific kinases. PIP$_2$ is the substrate for *phospholipase C* (PLC), which is controlled by a series of receptors either directly or through G-proteins. When PLC is activated, it cleaves PIP$_2$ into IP$_3$ and DAG, which are the two other most important second messengers participating in intracellular signaling. The water-soluble IP$_3$ diffuses rapidly through cytoplasm and binds to the receptors on the *endoplasmic reticulum* (ER), thereby releasing Ca²⁺, which is stored in the ER, to increase the cytoplasmic concentration. Lipid-soluble DAG binds to protein kinase C (PKC) in the regulatory domain and activates PKC, while DAG binding also helps in translocating the activated PKC from the cytoplasm to the plasma membrane. By increasing the cytoplasmic Ca²⁺ concentration and also by activating PKC, the cells will accomplish a series of synergetic signaling cascades that will end up producing pathway-specific final effects. After conducting the signal, both IP$_3$ and DAG are degraded, into inositol and IP$_3$ phosphatidic acid, respectively, which are utilized by the cells for restoring PIP levels (Figure 11.20).

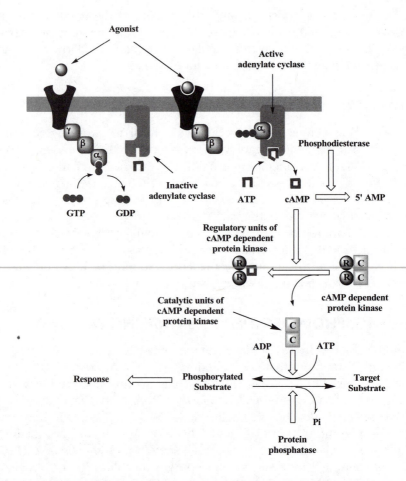

Figure 11.19   The cAMP second messenger pathway, which includes receptor, G-proteins, adenylate cyclase, phosphodiesterase, and cAMP-dependent protein kinase (PKA). PKA is activated subsequent to cAMP binding to the regulatory subunits of the adenylate cycalse. Phosphorylation of the substrate protein by PKA leads to initiation of response, while phosphatases can terminate cellular response.

As mentioned earlier, the PKC enzymes that are activated by DAG are serine/threonine kinases, which are essential for mediating many of the common intracellular signaling cascades. In fact, PKCs exist in more than 10 isoforms (Table 11.3), among which many are DAG-dependent (Figure 11.21). Some of the PKC isozymes also require Ca^{2+} for activation, and a binding site for Ca^{2+} also exists in the regulatory domain of PKC. The existence of PKC in several isoforms offers the capability of providing

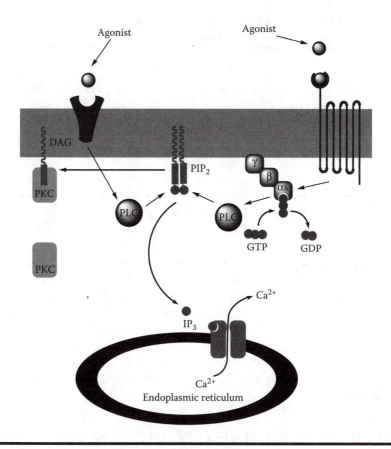

Figure 11.20 Pathways showing activation of phospholipase C (PLC) through and independent of G-proteins and production of diacylglycerol (DAG) and inositol triphosphate (IP$_3$) from phosphoinositol-biphsophate (PIP$_2$). IP$_3$ acts on the endoplasmic reticulum and releases Ca^{2+} to increase the cytoplasmic Ca^{2+} concentration. Increase in the cytoplasmic concentration can contribute to opening of some of the voltage-sensitive calcium channels and finally produce a strong cellular response.

selective responses for various stimuli, depending on the type of second messengers generated in the cells.

The PKCs have the serine/threonine kinase activity domain that is commonly referred as the catalytic domain in the C-terminal portion of the enzyme protein. The N-terminal portion of the enzyme contains the regulatory domain that includes both the DAG binding site and the Ca^{2+} binding site. A pseudosubstrate sequence that exists in the N-terminal portion of the PKC enzyme keeps the enzyme inhibited by binding intramolecularly to the active site. Pseudosubstrates typically contain alanine

Table 11.3 Different Isoforms of Protein Kinase C (PKC), Tissue Distribution, and Activity Regulators

PKC Type	Tissue Distribution	Enzyme Activity Regulators
α	Ubiquitous	Ca^{2+}, DAG, PS, FFA, Lyso-PC[a]
β	Many tissues	Ca^{2+}, DAG, PS, FFA, Lyso-PC
γ	Brain only	Ca^{2+}, DAG, PS, FFA, Lyso-PC
δ	Ubiquitous	DAG, PS
ε	Brain and other tissues	DAG, PS
η	Lung, skin, and heart	—
ζ	Ubiquitous	PIP_3

[a] Free fatty acid (FFA), Lyso-phosphatidylcholine (Lyso-PC).

in the phosphorylation site instead of serine or threonine. When DAG binds to the regulatory domain (C1 region), the pseudosubstrate is released from the binding site that allows the normal substrates to bind and becomes phosphorylated. The Ca^{2+}-dependent PKC isozymes have a binding site in the C2 regions of the regulatory domain that enhances the binding of phospholipids such as phosphatidyl serine (PS) to this region and activates PKC. Activated PKCs have many potential targets in cells that have been implicated in the regulation of cellular activities, ranging from gene expression to cell motility to the generation of other second messengers.

WHAT IS THE PURPOSE OF G-PROTEINS OR ANY OTHER SECOND MESSENGER SYSTEM?

The purpose of G-proteins and second messengers is to amplify and strengthen the signal initiated by ligands. For example, a neurotransmitter such as norepinephrine may encounter its membrane receptor for a very short time, only a few milliseconds. When the encounter generates GTP-bound G_s molecules, that will activate adenylate cyclase. At that moment, the activation of adenylate cyclase depends upon the longevity of G_s protein rather than receptor binding. Characteristically the G_s proteins remain active for about 10 seconds, which further amplifies the original signal.

LIGAND-GATED ION CHANNELS

Opening the ion channels is one other way of transducing signals from extracellular sources to intracellular locations. Many drugs in clinical

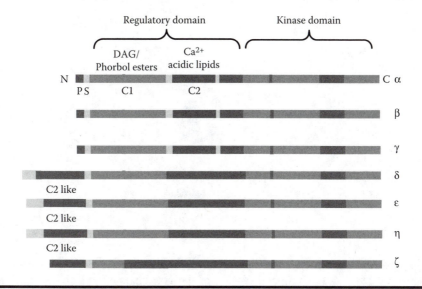

Figure 11.21 **The members of the protein kinase C (PKC) family. In the diagram, the regulatory domain and kinsase domain are indicated, along with binding sites within those domains for diacylglycerol (DAG), phosphatidylserine (PS), and Ca^{2+}.**

Table 11.4 Various Ion Channels and Activating Ligands

Activating Ligand	Type of Ion Channel
Acetylcholine	Na^+ channel
GABA	Cl^- channel
Glutamate	Ca^{2+} channels
NMDA[a]	Ca^{2+} channels

[a] N-methyl-D-asparate (NMDA).

medicine act by mimicking or blocking the actions of endogenous ligands that regulate the flow of ions through plasma membrane channels. The natural ligands include acetylcholine, gamma-aminobutyric acid, and the excitatory amino acids (glycine, aspartate, and glutamate). Receptors of these ligands transmit their signal across the plasma membrane by increasing the transmembrane conductance of the relevant ion and thereby altering the electrical potential across the membrane. The agonists and the corresponding ion channels are as shown in Table 11.4.

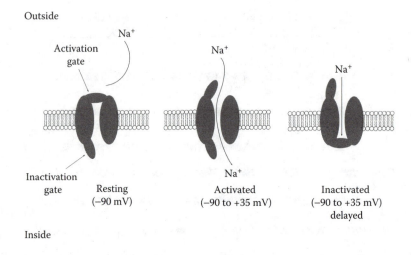

Figure 11.22 The opening and closing of the Na⁺ channel, and the changes in the membrane potential during those events.

SIGNALING THROUGH VOLTAGE-DEPENDENT ION CHANNELS

Voltage-Dependent Sodium (Na⁺) Channel

This type of sodium channel is present on the membranes of excitable nerve, cardiac, and skeletal muscle cells and is subjected to voltage-controlled channel opening, also termed *gating*. In their resting state, the above-mentioned cells maintain an intracellular Na⁺ concentration much lower (more negative voltage) than that of the extracellular environment. When the membrane is depolarized, the voltage-dependent Na⁺ channel will be opened, allowing a transient influx of Na⁺ ions to take place before closing. The local anesthetic agents bind to the sodium channels and block the transient Na⁺ ion permeability, thereby also blocking the nerve conduction. (The net result is the brain does not sense the pain.)

The structure of a voltage-gated sodium channel is schematically shown in Figure 11.22. Depolarization of the membrane causes voltage-driven conformational changes in the sodium channel, which is called the *activated state*, and opens an activation gate. During this state, sodium ions can literally pour inward through the channel and increase the Na⁺ concentration inside the cell. The same increase in voltage that opens the activation gate also closes the inactivation gate. However, closure of the inactivation gate occurs in a few ten thousandths of a second after the activation gate opens allowing the Na⁺ to go through for a few ten thousandths of a second. Once the inactivation gate is closed, the membrane

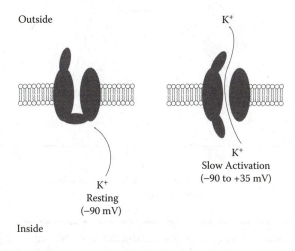

Figure 11.23   **The opening and closing of the K⁺ channel, and the changes in the membrane potential during those events.**

potential begins to recover back towards the resting state. A very important characteristic of a Na⁺ channel inactivation process is that the inactivation gate will not reopen until the membrane potential returns either to or near resting membrane potential.

Voltage-Gated Potassium (K⁺) Channel

The figure illustrates the K⁺ channel in two separate states: during resting and toward the end of the action potential. During the resting state, the K⁺ channel is closed, as shown in Figure 11.23; therefore, K⁺ ions are prevented from passing through this channel to the exterior of the cell. When the membrane potential rises from –90 mV toward zero, the change in the membrane potential causes a slow conformational opening of the gate that allows K⁺ diffusion outward. However, because of the slowness of the channel, these open just at the same time when the sodium channels are beginning to close. The timing of these events is illustrated in Figure 11.24. Thus, the decrease in sodium entry and a simultaneous potassium exit from the cell speeds up the repolarizarion process.

LIGAND-GATED SODIUM CHANNEL

Many endogenous ligands transmit signals across the plasma membrane by increasing the conductance of specific ions across the membrane. For example, acetylcholine causes the opening of an ion channel by binding to the nicotinic receptor, which allows Na⁺ to flow down its concentration

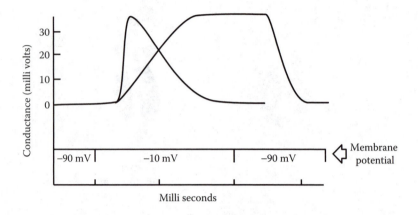

Figure 11.24 Typical changes in the conductance of Na⁺ and K⁺ ion channels when these channels are opened and closed during depolarization and repolarization of the membrane. The Na⁺ channels are opened and closed in milliseconds when the resting potential (–90 mV) increases.

gradient into the cells (Figure 11.25). The Na⁺ influx produces a *localized depolarization,* causing the membrane potential to rise and create a local potential called *end-plate potential.* This end-plate potential can initiate an action potential that will cause many voltage-dependent sodium channels to open. Thus, the membrane potential will be further raised, opening more sodium channels (as illustrated in Figure 11.26), creating a *positive-feedback vicious cycle.* Once this cycle is initiated, it will continue until all the sodium channels have become completely activated (opened).

CALCIUM CHANNELS

It is well recognized that calcium (Ca²⁺) is an important regulatory element for many cellular processes. The extracellular Ca²⁺ level is estimated to be in the 1 to 2 mM range, and the intracellular Ca²⁺ level is estimated to be between 0.1 and 10 μM, depending on the state of the cell.

Different types of Ca²⁺ channels are known to exist and are characterized by fundamental differences in the mechanisms governing their opening and closing (Figure 11.27). Some Ca²⁺ channels are voltage dependent and open in response to an appropriate membrane depolarization. Within this category are three subclasses of Ca²⁺ channels that differ in their voltage sensitivities, kinetic properties, and pharmacological activities. Specific details of these Ca²⁺ channels are given in Table 11.5 and Table 11.6.

The three different types of Ca²⁺ channels are referred to as:

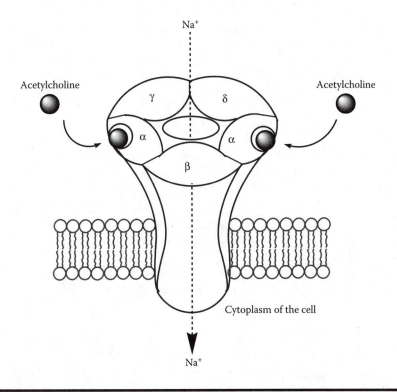

Figure 11.25 An illustration of the nicotinic (acetylcholine) receptor that regulates the Na⁺ channel. The receptor complex is composed of five subunits (two α, one β, one γ, and one δ). The receptor opens the channel and allows Na⁺ influx when acethylcholine or nicotine binds to the ligand binding domain on the α subunit.

1. The *L-type channels* — high voltage–activated, slow channels that conduct a long-lasting current (flow)
2. The *T-type channels* — low voltage–activated channels characterized by transient currents with relatively small conductance
3. The *N-type channels*, which are neither T nor L, but are activated at higher voltage than required for the N type and which conduct relatively transient current of intermediate size

LOCATION(S) OF THE VOLTAGE-SENSITIVE CA²⁺ CHANNELS (VSCC)

1. Both L and N but not T channels are present in the sympathetic neurons of superior cervical ganglia.

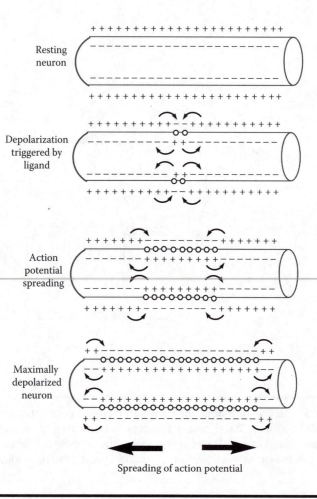

Resting neuron

Depolarization triggered by ligand

Action potential spreading

Maximally depolarized neuron

Spreading of action potential

Figure 11.26   An illustration showing the propagation of action potential in both directions from the point of origin.

2. Both L and T type but not N channels are present in cardiac and skeletal muscles.
3. Both L and T type but not N channels are present in smooth muscles.

The second major category of Ca^{2+} channels is operated through receptor-dependent mechanisms (Figure 11.27). These channels are opened in response to activation of an associated receptor. A typical channel of this type includes an ion channel associated with a nicotinic acetylcholine receptor. Some of the Ca^{2+} channel blockers are shown in Figure 11.28.

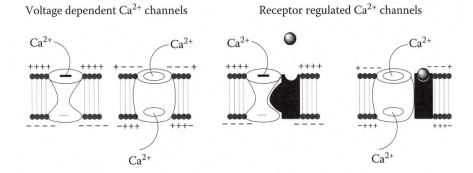

Voltage dependent Ca²⁺ channels   Receptor regulated Ca²⁺ channels

Figure 11.27   A diagram showing the hypothetical models of both the voltage-dependent and receptor-operated Ca²⁺ channels. The diagram also indicates the voltage ranges that would open the three kinds of voltage-dependent Ca²⁺ channels.

Table 11.5   Ranges of Membrane Potential Required for Activation, Conductance, and Blockers for Voltage-Dependent Ca2+ Channels

Function	T Type	N Type	L Type
Activation range (mV)	>–70	>–30	>–10
Conductance	Tiny	Moderate	Large
Duration	Transient	Transient	Long-lasting
Sensitivity to DHPs[a] (dihydropyridine)	No	No	Yes
Sensitivity to conotoxin	No	Yes	Yes

[a] Dihydropyridines (DHPs).

Table 11.6   Examples of Ligand-Activated Ca²⁺ Channels

Receptor Type	Cell/Tissue Type
ATP	Smooth muscle
Vasopressin	Smooth muscle
Mitogens	Lymphocytes
Parathyroid hormone	Osteoclasts
NMDA	Neurons
Glutamate	Neurons

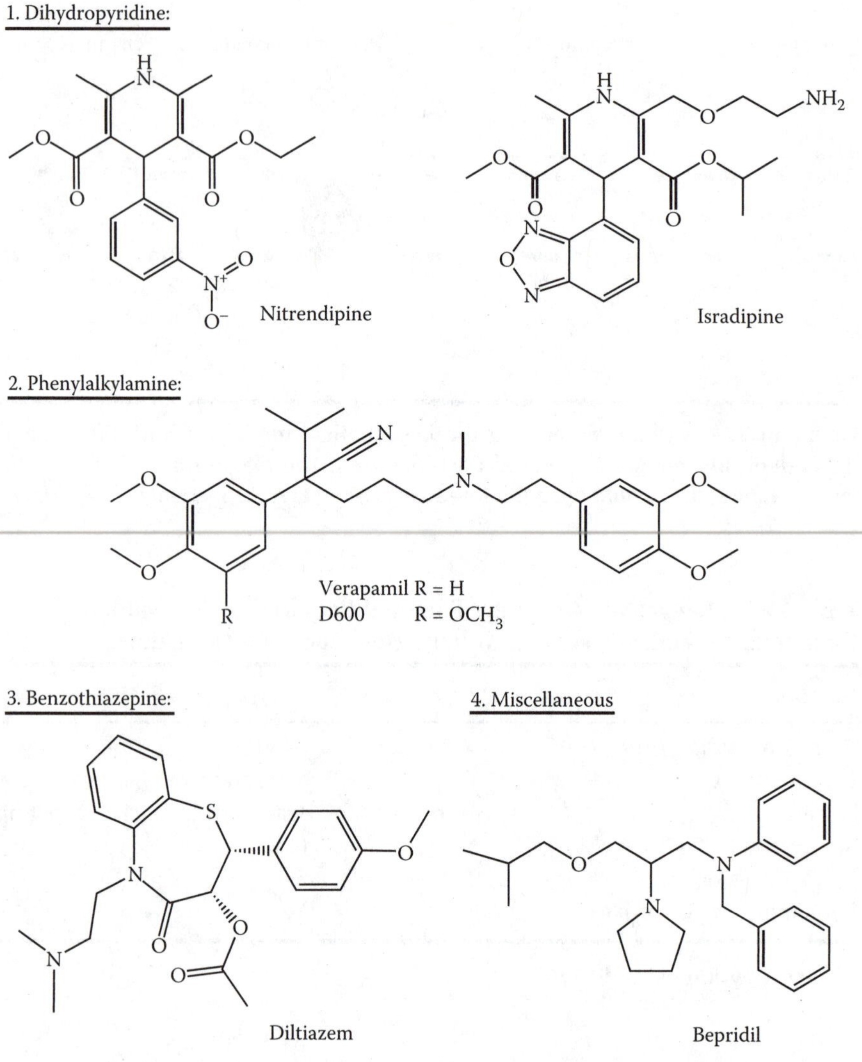

1. Dihydropyridine:

Nitrendipine

Isradipine

2. Phenylalkylamine:

Verapamil R = H
D600   R = OCH$_3$

3. Benzothiazepine: 4. Miscellaneous

Diltiazem   Bepridil

Figure 11.28   Structure of different classes of calcium channel blockers.

HOW DOES CALCIUM CONTRACT THE SKELETAL MUSCLES AND THE VASCULAR SMOOTH MUSCLES?

Increase in the cytoplasmic Ca^{2+} triggers various intracellular events that ultimately produce specific physiological effects. For example, in smooth muscle cells as well as in striated muscles, Ca^{2+} plays a major role in causing muscle contraction. A pathway leading to smooth muscle contraction is illustrated in Figure 11.29, which also indicates the site of action for Ca^{2+} channel blockers, use of which would lead to muscle relaxation.

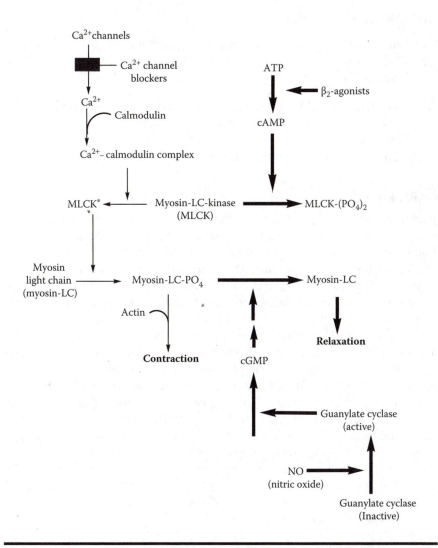

Figure 11.29 A pathway showing various intracellular events that lead to smooth muscle contraction. The contraction is triggered by an influx of Ca^{2+} through opening of the transmembrane Ca^{2+} channels. The Ca^{2+} combines with calmodulin to form a complex that converts myosin light chain kinase (MLCK) from an inactive form to an active form (MLCK*). Activated MLCK* phosphorylates the myosin light chain (MLC), thereby initiating the interaction of myosin with actin. Relaxation of smooth muscle can occur when phosphorylation of myosin light chain (MLC) is reversed by removal of phosphates by cGMP-activated enzymes.

CHLORIDE CHANNEL

The function of Cl– channel protein is to regulate the transport of chloride ion (Cl–) across the plasma membrane. There are two major kinds of Cl– channels:

1. Those activated by binding of a transmitter such as γ-aminobutyric acid (GABA), glycine, or glutamate, which are receptor-activated ion channels
2. Those activated by membrane depolarization or by Ca^{2+}

GABA Receptors

γ-Aminobutyric acid (GABA) is an inhibitory neurotransmitter. These GABA receptors are molecular targets for many drugs prescribed in the United States, such as sedative barbiturates and anxiety-relieving (anxiolytic) benzodiazepines (e.g., Valium). There are three basic subtypes of GABA receptors: $GABA_A$, $GABA_B$, and $GABA_C$; among these $GABA_A$ is the most prevalent in the mammalian brain. The $GABA_A$ receptor is similar to the acetylcholine receptor in that it is linked to an ion channel, particularly the Cl^- channel. The inhibitory effect of GABA on the neuronal cells is the result of its interaction with membrane-associated $GABA_A$ receptors that are located at the postsynaptic sites of the neuronal junction. The action of GABA on neurons is described as an *ionotropic effect* because it results in a brief (~1 msec) opening of a Cl^- channel. The rapid influx of Cl^- from the extracellular fluid hyperpolarizes the postsynaptic membrane and thus inhibits the ability of the neuron to fire. The other subtype of receptor is $GABA_B$, which are located in the presynaptic autonomic and central nerve terminals. The similarity in the effects seen with certain drugs and the operation of Cl^- channels suggests that there is a degree of homology between the subunits of $GABA_A$ and glycine receptors and voltage-dependent Cl^- channels.

Structure of GABA$_A$ Receptors

The $GABA_A$ receptor is widely distributed in the central nervous system (CNS). It is a macromolecular complex that has different binding sites for diverse drugs and also a channel for Cl^- ions. This receptor is a heterooligomer consisting of five subunits, each of which in turn consists of four membrane-spanning domains (Figure 11.30). One or more of these membrane-spanning domains (cylinders shown in Figure 11.30) contribute to the wall of the chloride channel. The subunits are classified as the benzodiazepine-binding α subunit and GABA-binding β subunit. Binding of a drug to one site induces a change in the three-dimensional structure (conformation) of the receptor that changes the affinity of the other sites.

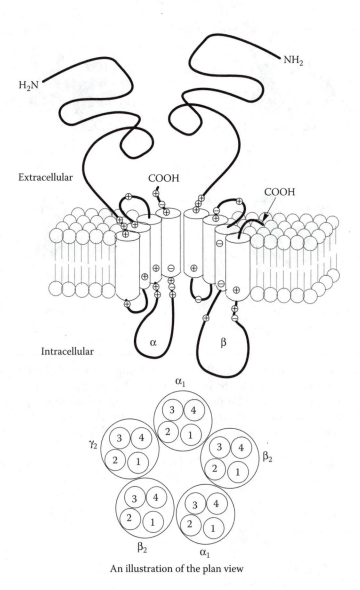

Figure 11.30 An illustration showing a portion of the GABA (γ-aminobutyric acid) receptor complex in the cell membrane. The illustration also depicts the extracellular, transmembrane, and cytoplasmic domains of α and β subunits of the GABA receptor complex. The plan view shows all the subunits of the GABA receptor complex forming the channel in the middle. According to this model, each subunit has four membrane-spanning domains. (From Olsen R.W. and Tobin, A.J., Molecular biology of GABA receptors, FASEB J., 1990; 4:1469–1480).

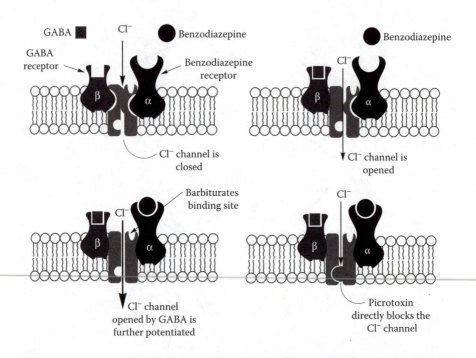

Figure 11.31 A model of the GABA receptor complex showing binding sites for GABA (γ-aminobutyric acid), benzodiazepines, barbiturates, and convulsants. GABA binding opens the chloride channel, the opening further potentiated by benzodiazepine binding. Similary, barbiturates can also potentiate the GABA effect. Convulsants such as picrotoxin block the chloride channel directly.

For example, GABA and benzodiazepines allosterically modulate the binding of each other. Therefore, $GABA_A$ receptors can be functionally altered by a variety of compounds that bind to the receptor–ionophore complex at different sites such as the GABA site, the benzodiazepine site, the picrotoxin site, and the barbiturate site.

GABA Binding Site

Electrophysiological studies have shown that benzodiazepines potentiate GABA-ergic neurotransmission by allosteric regulation. Activation of $GABA_A$ receptors by GABA agonists results in the opening of the chloride channel. The ensuing influx of chloride anions inhibits the firing of the neurons by causing hyperpolarization. The activation and modulation of chloride flux by GABA is achieved by dynamic alterations in the protein configuration of the receptor–ionophore complex. Directly acting GABA agonists usually bear some structural resemblance to GABA. Some of the agonists, that directly bind to the GABA binding site are shown in Table 11.7.

Table 11.7   Different Kinds of GABA_A Receptor Agonists and Antagonists

Types of Agonists/Antagonists	Properties/Effects
Direct-acting GABA mimetics	
3-Aminopropane sulfonic acid	Direct-acting GABA agonists but do
β-Guanidinopropionic acid	not pass the blood–brain barrier
4-Aminotetrolic acid	
Muscimol	Direct-acting GABA agonists,
THIP (gabaxadol)	readily pass the blood–brain
Isoguvacine	barrier
Progabide	
Indirectly acting GABA mimetics	
Gabaculine	Cause the release of GABA from
Baclofen	intracellular stores
Nipecotic acid	
GABA antagonists	
Bicuculline	Competitive antagonist
Picrotoxin	Does not inhibit GABA binding;
	instead, blocks Cl^- channel
Benzodiazepines	
Diazepam	Allosterically potentiate the effect
Oxazepam	of GABA
Flurazepam	
Nitrazepam	
Triazolam	
Chlordiazepoxide	
Benzodiazepine antagonists	
Flumazenil	Blocks actions of benzodiazepines
	but does not affect the action of
	barbiturates
Inverse agonist	
Ethyl β-carboline-3-carboxylate (β-CCE)	Blocks the effect of
	benzodiazepine
Barbiturates	
Phenobarbital	Can potentiate GABA effect and
Secobarbital	also allosterically relieve
Pentobarbital	picrotoxin-inhibited Cl^- channel
Glutethimide	

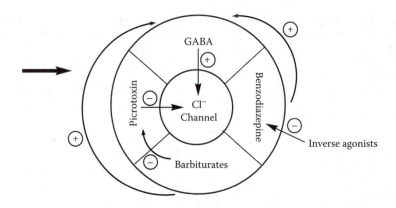

Figure 11.32 A diagrammatic representation of GABA (γ-aminobutyric acid) receptor complex with different sites of drug action. The diagram also shows the positive (+) and negative (−) influence of the drugs on GABA-initiated Cl⁻ channel opening.

Benzodiazepine Binding Site

The binding sites for GABA, benzodiazepines, barbiturates and picrotoxin, their possible interaction are depicted in the diagram (Figure 11.32). Benzodiazepines binding to the receptor complex increase the frequency of Cl⁻ channel opening without altering the channel conductance or duration of opening. Benzodiazepines binding to the receptor site at the α-subunit of the receptor complex allosterically enhance the binding affinity of the GABA receptors at the β-subunit and facilitate the frequency of Cl⁻ channel opening. On the other hand, binding of GABA to its own sites can also allosterically enhance the binding of benzodiazepines to their receptors by increasing the receptor affinity. Therefore, drugs that bind to the benzodiazepine site and enhance the electrophysiological effects of GABA are called *benzodiazepine agonists*; compounds that bind to the benzodiazepine site and decrease the effects of GABA are called *inverse agonists*. Figure 11.33 shows the chemical structures of benzodiazepines.

Barbiturates Binding Site

Barbiturates also enhance the actions of GABA by allosterically enhancing GABA binding to receptors. In contrast to benzodiazepines, barbiturates prolong the Cl⁻ channel opening rather than intensifying the frequency of GABA-activated Cl⁻ channel opening. Barbiturates interact allosterically with picrotoxin binding sites and inhibit the binding of *convulsants* such as picrotoxin. Figure 11.34 shows the chemical structures of barbiturates.

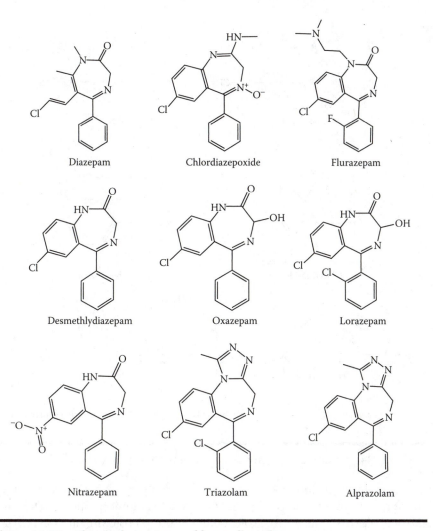

Figure 11.33 **Chemical structures of benzodiazepines.**

Picrotoxin Binding Site

Picrotoxin is another type of inhibitor for the GABA-regulated Cl- channel. This compound does not inhibit GABA binding; instead, it blocks Cl⁻ ion transport by binding to a distinct site in the ionophore (Figure 11.31). Drugs that can displace the binding of picrotoxin to the receptor–ionophore complex are called *ionophore agonists*.

GABA Antagonists

The action of GABA at the receptor–ionophore complex may be antagonized by GABA antagonists by directly competing with GABA for its

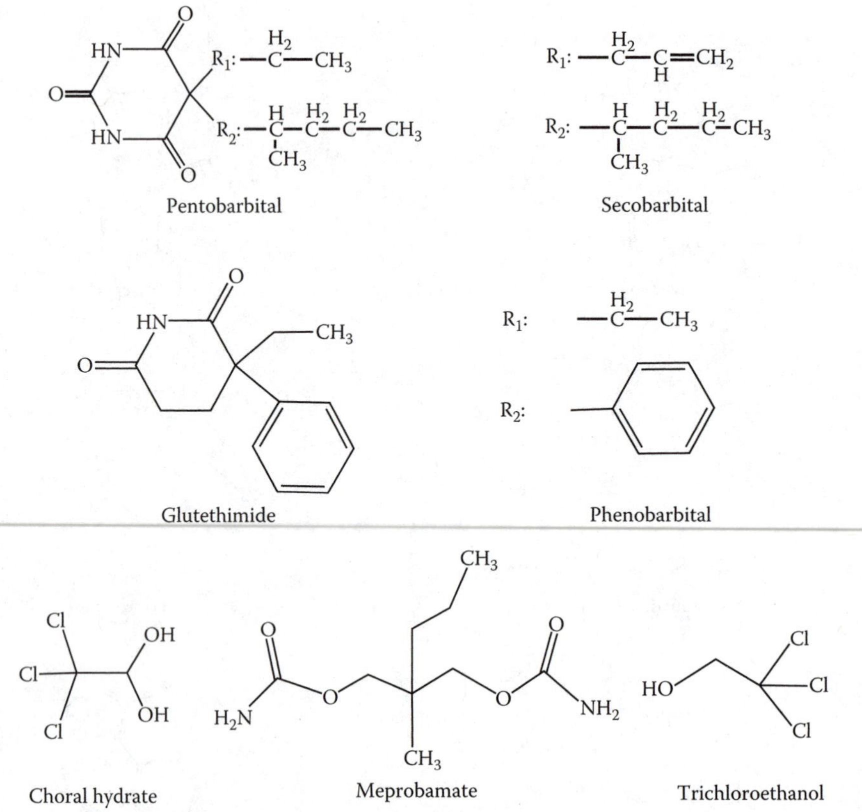

Figure 11.34 Chemical structures of barbiturates.

receptor. Indirect inhibition occurs by modifying the GABA receptor allosterically or by inhibiting the GABA-activated ionophore. The two classical GABA antagonists, bicuculline and picrotoxin, appear to act through different mechanisms. Bicuculline acts as a direct competitive antagonist of GABA at the receptor level, while picrotoxin acts as a noncompetitive antagonist by blocking the GABA-activated ionophores. Various GABA agonists (mimetics) and antagonists are listed in Table 11.7.

REFERENCES

1. Basic & Clinical Pharmacology by Bertram G. Katzung, 8th edition, Chapter 2 (Drug Receptor and Pharmacodynamics), Chapter 22 (Sedative-Hypnotic Drugs) (2001, Lang Medical Books/McGraw-Hill, New York, St. Louis, San Francisco, Lisbon, London, Madrid, Montreal, New Delhi, Singapore, Tokyo, and Toronto.
2. Textbook of Pharmacology by W.C. Bowman and M. J. Rand; Chapter-39 (Principles of Drug Action), 1980, Blackwell Scientific Publications, Edinburgh, London, Melbourne, and Oxford.

3. Molecular Biology of The Cell by Bruce Alberts, Dennis Bray, Julian Lewis, Martin Raff, Keith Roberts, James D. Watson, Chapter 13 (Chemical Signaling Between cells), Garland Publishing Inc, New York & London.
4. Textbook of Pharmacology by Smith and Reynard, Chapter 20 (Antianxiety drugs).
5. The Pharmacological Basis of Therapeutics by Joel G. Hardman and Lee E. Limbard, 10th Edition, Chapter 2 (Pharmacodynamics: Mechanisms of Drug Action and the Relationship Between Drug Concentration and Effect), 2001, McGraw-Hill Medical Publishing Division, New York, Chicago, San Francisco, Lisbon, Madrid, Mexico City, Milan, New Delhi, San Juan, Seoul, Singapore, Sydney and Toronto.
6. Cell Biology by Thomas D. Pollard and William C. Earnshaw, Chapters 25-29, (Reception and Transduction of Environmental Information), 2004, Saunders An Imprint of Elsevier, Philadelphia.

INDEX

A

Absorption, *see also* Administration, drugs
  active transport, 104
  basics, 93, 101–103, *102*
  bioavailability, 108–109
  blood flow, 107
  body compartment pH, *100,* 105–107,
    106–107
  contact time, 108
  endocytosis, 105
  exocytosis, 105
  facilitated transport, 104–105
  first-pass metabolism, 108–109, *109*
  ion pair transport, 105
  membranes, crossing, 103–105
  passive diffusion, 103–104
  pH, body compartments, *100,* 105–107,
    106–107
  phagocytosis, 105
  physiochemical factors, 103–108
  physiological factors, 103–108
  pinocytosis, 105
  surface area available, 108
Acetaminophen
  dose-dependent toxicity, 178–180, *185*
  ether glucuronide, *173*
  sulfate conjugation, 178, *183*
  weak acids, 45–46, *46*
Acetone, *62, 160*
Acetophenetidine, *159*
Acetylation, 172, 174, *175*
N-acetylbenzoquinoneimine, 179
Acetylcholine
  binding sites, 232, *232*

  cholinergic neurotransmission, 210–214,
    212–215
  hydrolysis, 233, *233*
  structure, *217*
Acetylcholine chloride, 218
Acetylcholinesterase, *224,* 230–242
Acid-base properties
  basics, 37–38
  conjugate acids and bases, *9,* 41–43,
    42–43
  Henderson-Hasselbach equation, 53–59,
    55, 57, 59–60
  inductive effects, 47–49, *48*
  resonance effects, 47, 49–51, *50–52*
  salt hydrolysis, 38–41
  strengths, acids and bases, 43–46, *45–46*
Acidic form, drugs, 53
Acquired tolerance, 312
Action onset and duration, 100, *101,* 297
Activated state, 336
Active receptors, 325
Active transport, 104
Acyclovir, 127, *127*
Acyl intermdiate, 246
Adenine, *72*
Adenylate cyclase, 320, 328–331, *330*
Administration, drugs, *see also* Absorption
  action onset, 100, *101*
  basics, 93–94
  local site restriction, 101
  long-term administration, 100–101
  onset of action, *101*
  particle size, 98, *99*
  pK_a, 98–100, *100*

polymorphism, 97–98, *98*
properties, drugs, 94–100
solubility, 94–95, *95–97*
therapeutic objective, 100–101
Adrenelin, 203
Adrenergic agonists and antagonists,
 205–206, 205–208, *208–210*
β-Adrenergic receptors, 330
β-Adrenoceptor, 325
Adrenocorticotropic hormone, 192
Adriamycin, 87, *89*
Affinity activity, 200
Agonists, 201–209, *205–206, 208–210*, 215,
 216
Alcohol and aldehyde oxidation, 163, *165*
Alcohols, 234, *235*
Aldehyde reduction, 166, *166–168*
Aldo-keto reductases, 166
Aliphatic oxidation, 153, 155, *155–157*
Alkaloids, 215, 219–221
Alkylating agents, 81, *81–84*, 83
Allopurinol, 255, *257–258*
Allosteric regulation, 228, *229*
Alloxanthine, 255, *257*
Alprazolam, *349*
Aluminum hydroxide, *63*
Aluminum magnesium hydroxide sulfate, *63*
Amantadine, 161, *181*
Amide hydrolysis, 167, *170*
Amikacin, 127, *127*
Amino acids, 104
P-Aminobenzoic acid, 174
γ-Aminobutyric acid, *see* GABA (γ-
 aminobutyric acid)
7-Amino metabolite, *169*
Aminopterin, 71, *72*
Ammonia, 25
Amoxicillin, *22*, 247
Amphetamine
 aromatic hydroxylation, *152*
 oxidative deamination, *160*
 weak acids, *46*
 weak bases, 45–46
Ampicillin, 105, 247
Anesthetics, volatile, 61–63, *64–65*
Aniline, *62*
Anion, 18
Anionic site, 232
ANP (atrial natriuretic peptide) receptors,
 325–326

ANP-C (atrial natriuretic peptide clearance)
 receptors, 196–197
Antagonists
 cholinergic neurotransmission, 215, *216*
 differential effects, agonists, *205–206,*
 205–208, *208–210*
 drug-receptors, dynamics and theories,
 270–274
 folate acid, 86
 GABA, *347, 349–350*
 pharmacodynamics, drug-receptors, 201,
 215, *216*
Antibacterials, *71*
Anticancer drugs
 alkylating agents, 81, *81–84*, 83
 antimetabolites, 83–84, *85–88*, 86
 basics, 80
 chemotherapy, 78–80, *79–80*
 crosslinking agents, DNA, 89, *90*
 intercalators, DNA, 87, 89, *89*
 mustards, 79–80, *79–80*
Anticholinesterase drugs, *see also*
 Irreversible anticholinesterases;
 Reversible anticholinesterases
 basics, 234
 effects, 236–238
 glaucoma, 238–239, *239*
 myasthenia gravis, 239–240, *240*
 uses, 238
Antimalarial drugs, *see* Pyrimethamine
Antimetabolites
 anticancer drugs, 83–84, *85–88*, 86
 isosteric replacements, 71, *72*
Antimuscarinic blocking agents, *220*, 221
Antipsychotic drugs, *71*
Area under the curve (AUC), 129, *129*
Argon, 18
Aricept, 4, 22, *23*
Ariëns theory, 264, 270, 282
Arithmetic mean dose, 291
Aromatic oxidation, *148*, 149–153, *151–154*
Aromatic rings, 70, *71*
β-Arrestin, 325
Aspirin
 hydrolysis reactions, *170*
 salt hydrolysis, 39
 weak acids, 45–46, *46*
Association, drugs, 264–265
Atomic radius, 14, 16
Atomic structure, *see* Periodic table

Atrial natriuretic peptide (ANP) receptors, 325–326
Atrial natriuretic peptide clearance (ANP-C) receptors, 196–197
Atropine, *220*, 221
Atypical receptors, 208–209, *211*
AUC (area under the curve), 129, *129*
Autocoids, 192, *193*
Autocrine function, 190, 192, *193*
Autophosphorylation, 322
Autoreceptors, 208
Azathioprine, 176
Aziridinium ion, 81, *82–83*
Azo group reduction, 167, *169*

B

Bacilli bacteria, 251
Bacterial cell wall synthesis, 243–244, *244*
Barbiturates
    chemical structures, *350*
    chloride channels, 348, *350*
    GABA, *348*
    intracellular binding, 117
Baroreceptors, 208
Bases, *see* Acid-base properties
Basic form, 53
Benozoic acid, *174*
Benzene, *71*
Benzethonium chloride, *26*
Benzodiazepine
    binding site, 348, *348–349*
    chemical structures, *349*
    GABA, *348*
Benzothiazepine, *342*
Bepredil, *342*
Beta-lactam antibiotics, 247, *247*, 250
Beta-lactamase inhibitors, 251–254, *254*
Bethanechol, *217*, 218–219
Binding sites
    chloride channels, 346, *346–350*, 348–349
    pharmacodynamics, drug-receptors, 198
Bioavailability
    absorption, 108–109, *109*
    distribution, 127–129, *128–129*
Bioisosteres, 70
Biopharmaceutics
    absorption and administration, 93–109
    distribution and excretion, 111–132
    metabolic changes, 135–185

Blood-brain barrier
    basics, 102–103
    capillary permeability, 112
    muscarine, 219
Blood capillaries, 103
Blood flow, absorption, 107
Blood perfusion, 114, *114*
Blood pressure, *205–206*, 205–208, *208–210*, 237
Body compartment pH
    absorption, *100*, 105–107, *106–107*
    distribution, 116
    partitioning process, 58, *59*
Bonds
    chemical properties, 16–18, *17*
    polarity, 33–34, *34*, 47
Bowman's capsule, 131
Brain capilliaries, 112, *113*, 114
Brodie studies, 99
Bromocriptine mesylate, *21*
Brønsted-Lowry theory, 37, 41, 43
Butryaldehyde, *62*
Butyrylcholinesterase, 231–232
B vitamins, 104

C

Calcium
    active transport, 104
    channels, receptor regulation, 338–340, *341*, 341–342, 342, *343*
    cytoplasm, 316
    metals, 14
    muscles effect, 342, *343*
Calcium carbonate, *63*
Calcium channel blockers, 340, 342, *342*
Calcium/phosphoinositide/PKC signaling pathway, 331–334, *333–335*
cAMP, *317*, 331, *332*
Cancer, chemical treatments
    alkylating agents, 81, *81–84*, 83
    anticancer drugs, 80–89
    antimetabolites, 83–84, *85–88*, 86
    basics, 77
    cell cycles, 78–79, *79*
    chemotherapy, 78–80, *79–80*
    DNA crosslinking agents, 89, *90*
    DNA intercalators, 87, 89, *89*
    malignant cells, 77–78
    mustards, 79–80, *79–80*
    normal cells, 77–78
Capillary permeability, 112, *113*, 114

Carbachol, *217,* 238
Carbamates, *233,* 234, *235–236*
Carbamazepine, 167
Carbinolamine, *160*
Cardiac glycosides, 104
Carryover, 297
Cation, 18
Ceiling effect and dose, 289
Celebrex, 4, *5,* 30–31, *31*
Celecoxib, 4
Cell-cell communication, 191, *193*
Cells
    bacterial cell wall synthesis, 243–244, *244*
    cycles, 78–79, *79*
    drug-receptors, 196
    malignant, 77–78
    normal, 77–78
    surface, 192
Cephalosporin, 250
Cetelpyridinium chloride, *26*
cGMP, *317,* 325–327
Channels
    CA²⁺, 339–340, *341–342*
    calcium, 338–339, *341,* 342, *343*
    chloride, 344–350
    ion, 334–337, *335–338*
    ligand-gated, 334–335, *335,* 337–338,
        339–340
    L-type, 339–340
    N-type, 339–340
    potassium, 337, *337–338*
    sodium, *336,* 336–338, *339–340*
    T-type, 339–340
    voltage-dependent ions, 336–337,
        336–338
    voltage-sensitive CA²⁺, 339–340, *341–342*
Chemical properties
    basics, 3
    bonds, 16–18, *17*
    chemical reactivity, *10–13,* 10–16, *15*
    coordinate covalent bonds, 25, *26*
    covalent bonds, 20–24, *21–26*
    electronegativity, 33
    ionic charge magnitude, 18–19
    molecular polarity, *34,* 34–35
    molecule shapes, 28–31, *29–32*
    periodic table, 3–16
    polarity, 33–34, *34*
    polyatomic ions, 19, *19*
    properties, 3–4, *5–9,* 6–7, 10
    resonance structures, 27–28, *27–29*

Chemical reactivity, *10–13,* 10–16, *15*
Chemical scalpels, 280
Chemical signaling, 189–191, *191*
Chemoreceptors, 208
Chemotherapy, 78–80, *79–80*
Chirality, 67
Chlorambucil, 81, *81,* 83
Chloride channels
    antagonists, GABA, *347,* 349–350
    barbiturates binding site, 348, *350*
    basics, 344
    benzodiazepine binding site, 348,
        348–349
    binding sites, 346, *346–350,* 348–349
    GABA receptors, 344–350
    picrotoxin binding site, *346,* 349
    receptor regulation, signaling
        mechanisms, 344–350
Chlorine, 18
Chlorodiazepoxide, *349*
Chloropheniramine, *168*
Chlorophentermine, 161
Chloropromazine, *162*
Chloropromazine sulfone, *162*
Chloropromazine sulfoxide, *162*
Chloroquine
    distribution patterns, 117, 120
    distribution volume, *121*
    half-life and steady state, 126, *127*
    intracellular binding, 117
Chlorpromazine, *153*
Chlorpropamide, 116
Chlortetracycline, *74*
Chlorthizide, 55
Cholamphenicol, *76*
Choline acetyl transferase, 210
Choline esters, 215
Cholinergic neurotransmission
    acetylcholine, 210–214, *212–215*
    antagonists, 215, *216*
    antimuscarinic blocking agents, *220,*
        221
    cholinomimetics, 214–215, *216–219,*
        217–221
    direct-acting cholinomimetics, 215,
        216–219, 217–221
    function, *215*
    location, 213–214, *215*
    mucarinic actions, 212
    nicotinic actions, 212
    pharmacodynamics, 209–221

Cholinesterase
   enzyme inhibition, 232–233, *232–233*
   regenerating compounds, 241–242,
      242–243
Cholinomimetics, 212, 214–215, *216–219,*
   217–221
Choral hydrate, *350*
Chymotrypsin, *224*
Cimetidine, 161
Cipro, 6–7, *7*
Ciprofloxacin, *121,* 144
Cisplatin, *90*
Claritin, *21,* 22, *24*
Clark's theory, 259–263, *260, 262–263*
Classical isosteres, 69–70
Clathrin, 310
Clavulanic acid, 253
Clearance, distribution, 122–125
Clonazepam, *169*
Cloxacillin, 251
Clozapine, 107, *107,* 142
Coated pits, 310
Cocaine, *170*
Codeine, 143, *159*
Colchicine, 130
Competitive antagonism, 271–272, *273–275,*
   274
Competitive inhibition, 225–226, *225–226*
Concentration-effect curves, *269,* 269–270,
   271–273
Concentration relation, 269
Confidence limits, 292
Conjugate acids and bases, *9,* 41–43, *42–43*
Conjugated estrogens, 101
Contact time, 108
Contraction, muscles, 342, *343*
Convulsants, 348
Cooperativity, 229, *230*
Coordinate covalent bonds, 25, *26*
Corticosteriods, 318
Coumarin anticoagulants, 117
Covalent bonds, 16, 20–24, *20–26*
Crosslinking agents, DNA, 89, *90*
Cross-phosphorylation, 322
Cumulative percentage responding, 291
Cycles, CYP450 families, 147–149, *148*
Cyclophosphamide, 81, *84*
Cyclosporin, 144
CYP450
   basics, 136–137, *137*
   clozapine, 142

codeine, 143
   cycle, 147–149, *148*
   CYP3A family, 143–144
   CYP2C19, 143
   CYP2D6, 142–143
   diazepam-omeprazole interaction, 143
   environmental factors, metabolism, 139,
      142
   enzyme complex, 144–145
   enzymes, 149–163
   genetic factors, metabolism, 139,
      142
   grapefruit juice, 144
   induction, 138–139, *140–141*
   inhibition, 138
   omeprazole-diazepam interaction,
      143
   polymorphism, genetic, 142–143
   redox reactions, 144–145
   substrates, *137*
CYP3A, 143–144
CYP3A4, 144
CYP2C19, 143
CYP2D6, 142–143
Cysteine, 223, *224*

D

D600, *342*
DAM (diacteylmonoxime), 241, *242*
DAO (diamine oxidase), 165
Dapsone, 174
Dehalogenation, 162–163, *164*
Delocalization, 28
Demecarium, 238
Deprotonated form, drugs, 53
Desensitization, 325, *326–327*
Desflurane, *64*
Desmethyldiazepam, *349*
Desulfuration, 162, *163*
Diacteylmonoxime (DAM), 241, *242*
Diamine oxidase (DAO), 165
Diazepam
   aromatic hydroxylation, *153*
   chemical structures, *349*
   omeprazole interaction, 143
   onset of action, 100
   weak acids, *46*
   weak bases, 45–46
Dibenzodiazepine derivatives, *71*
Dicloxacillin, 251
Diethyl ether, 102–103

Differential effects, agonists
   adrenergic agonists and antagonists,
      205–206, 205–208, *208–210*
   atypical receptors, 208–209, *211*
   epinephrine, 202–205, *203–204*
Digitoxin, 130
Digoxin, 100
Dihydrofolic acid, 86, *88*
Dihydrophyridine, *342*
Diisopropyl-phosphofluoridate (DIPF), 223,
   224
Diltiazem, 144, *342*
Dimeric form, 322
Dimethylphenylpiperazinium, *217*
DIPF (diisopropyl-phosphofluoridate), 223,
   224
Direct-acting cholinomimetics, 215,
   216–219, 217–221
Dissociation, drugs, 264–265
Distribution, *see also* Excretion
   basics, 111–112
   bioavailability, 127–129, *128–129*
   blood perfusion, 114, *114*
   body compartment pH, 116
   capillary permeability, 112, *113,* 114
   clearance, 122–125
   elimination rate, 122
   half-life, *125,* 125–127, *127*
   intracellular binding, 117
   maintenance dose rate, 122–125,
      123–124
   patterns, 117–120, *118–119*
   permeability, 112, *113,* 114–116,
      115–116
   pH, body compartments, 116
   plasma protein binding, 116
   steady state, *125,* 125–127, *127*
   volume determination, *120–121,*
      120–122
DNA crosslinking agents, 89, *90*
DNA intercalators, 87, 89, *89*
Dobutamine, *181*
Donepezil, 4, *5*
Dopamine, 178
Dosage schedule, optimum, 296
Dose-dependent toxicity, acetaminophen,
   178–180, *185*
Dose rate, maintenance, 122–125, *123–124*
Dose ratio, 276
Dose-response curves, 288–292

Down regulation, 309–310, *311,* 312, 323,
   324, 325
Doxorubicin, 87, *89,* 105
Drug action mechanism, 189, *190*
Drug effects, 223, *224,* 225
Drug-receptor and drug-enzyme interactions
   dynamics and theories, 259–305
   enzyme inhibition, drug-induced,
      223–258
   pharmacodynamics, 189–221
   regulation and signaling mechanisms,
      307–350
Drug-receptors, dynamics and theories
   action onset and duration, 297
   antagonism, 270–274
   Ariëns theory, 264
   basics, 259
   Clark's theory, 259–263, *260, 262–263*
   competitive antagonism, 271–272,
      273–275, 274
   concentration-effect curves, *269,*
      269–270, *271–273*
   concentration relation, 269
   dose-response curves, 288–292
   duration of action, 297
   effect regulation factors, 284–292
   efficacy, 286–287, *289–290*
   exercises and samples, 297–305
   graded dose-response curves, 288–290,
      291
   irreversible antagonism, 280–281,
      281–282
   mathematical relationship importance,
      278–279
   modified occupation theory, 264
   noncompetitive antagonism, 281–282,
      283
   occupation theory, 259–263, *260,*
      262–263
   onset of action, 297
   partial agonists, 282–284, *284–287*
   Paton's theory, 264–268, *266–267*
   peak effect, 297
   potency, 286–287, *288*
   quantal dose-response curves, 290–292,
      292–293
   rate theory, 264–268, *266–267*
   residual effects, 297
   response relation, 269
   samples and exercises, 297–305
   Schild's equation, 275–278, *279*

therapeutic index, *293–295*, 293–296
time-action curves, *296*, 296–297
Drug-receptors, pharmacodynamics, *see also*
    Receptors
    acetylcholine, 210–214, *212–215*
    adrenergic agonists and antagonists,
        205–206, 205–208, *208–210*
    affinity activity, 200
    agonists, 201–209, 215, *216*
    antagonists, 201, 215, *216*
    antimuscarinic blocking agents, *220*, 221
    atypical receptors, 208–209, *211*
    autocrine function, 192, *193*
    binding sites, 198
    chemical signaling, 189–191, *191*
    cholinergic neurotransmission, 209–221
    cholinomimetics, 214–215, *216–219*,
        217–221
    differential agonists, 202–209
    direct-acting cholinomimetics, 215,
        216–219, 217–221
    drug action mechanism, 189, *190*
    endocrine function, 192, *193*
    ephinephrine, differential effects,
        202–205, *203–204*
    extracellular receptors, 196
    function, acetylcholine receptors, *215*
    induced fit, 199–200, *200*
    interactions, 198
    intracellular receptors, 196
    intrinsic activity, 200–201
    ligand structure and activity relationship,
        201
    location, acetylcholine receptors,
        213–214, *215*
    lock-and-key fit, 198–199, *199*
    models, 198–200
    mucarinic actions, acetylcholine, 212
    nicotinic actions, acetylcholine, 212
    paracrine function, 192, *193*
    partial agonist, 201, *202*
    plasma membrane-bound receptors,
        196–197, *197*
    receptor concept importance, 202
    receptor types, 194, *195*, 196–197
    signaling molecules, 192–193, *194–195*
Drug taste, 75
Dualists, 264
Duration of action, 297

E

Echothiophate, 238, *240*, 241
Edrophonium, 234, 240, *240*
Effective dose, 293
Effector molecule, 228
Effect regulation factors, 284–292
Efficacy, 286–287, *289–290*
Electron configuration, periodic table, *12, 15*
Electronegativity, 16, 33
Electrostatic interactions, 117
Elimination, *see* Excretion
Elimination rate, 122
Enalapril, *121*
Endocrine function, 190, 192, *193*
Endocytosis, 105, 310, *311, 323*
Endoplasmic reticulum, 331
Endosomes, 310
End-plate potential, 338
Enflurane, *64*
Enteral administration, 93
Enterohepatic cycle, 130, *130*
Environmental factors, metabolism, 139, 142
Enzyme complex, 144–145
Enzyme inhibition, drug-induced, *see also*
    Inhibition
    acetylcholinesterase interaction, 230–242
    allosteric regulation, 228, *229*
    anticholinesterase drugs, 234, 236–240,
        239–240
    bacterial cell wall synthesis, 243–244, *244*
    beta-lactamase inhibitors, 251–254, *254*
    butyrylcholinesterase, 231–232
    cholinesterase, 232–233, *232–233*
    cholinesterase-regenerating compounds,
        241–242, *242–243*
    competitive inhibition, 225–226,
        225–226
    cooperativity, 229, *230*
    drug effects, 223, *224*, 225
    feedback inhibition, 229–230, *231*
    glaucoma, 238–239, *239*
    inhibitors, 234, 248, *249–250*, 250
    interaction examples, 230–242
    irreversible anticholinesterases, 235, 241
    myasthenia gravis, 239–240, *240*
    noncompetitive inhibition, 228, *228*
    penicillinases, 251, *253*
    penicillins, 250–251, *252*
    peptidoglycans, 245–246, *245–246*
    reversible anticholinesterases, 234–235
    suicide inhibition, 254–255

thymidylate synthetase, 254–255, *255–256*

transpeptidase-penicillinase inhibition, 243–255

uncompetitive inhibition, 226–227, *227*

xanthine oxidase, 255, *257–258*

Ephedrine, 67, *67*

Epidermal growth factor, 192

Epinephrine
  biosynthesis, *180, 204*
  competitive antagonism, 279
  differential effects, agonists, 202–205, *203–204*
  three-point model, 69

Epoxide hydration, *154,* 171

Epoxide hydrolase, 151

Equilibrium, 37

Erythromycin
  beta-lactamase inhibitor, 252
  CYP3A family, 144
  enterohepatic cycle, 130
  half-life and steady state, 126–127, *127*

Eseroline, 28, *29*

Esteractic site, 232

Ester hydrolysis, 167, *170*

Estradiol, 66, *66,* 104

Ethanol, *62,* 165

Ethinyl estradiol, 130, *152*

Ethylmorphine, *159*

Ethylphenidate, *68*

Excretion, *see also* Distribution
  basics, 111, 130
  enterohepatic cycle, 130, *130*
  renal excretion, 131–132, *131–132*

Exocytosis, 105

Extensive metabolizers, 142

Extent of distribution, 112

Extracellular receptors, 196

F

Facilitated transport, 104–105

FAD/FADH system, 147, *147*

Family defined, 137

Feedback inhibition, 229–230, *231*

Fick's first law of diffusion, 103–104, 106

First messengers, 190, 315, *see also* Second messenger systems

First-pass metabolism, 108–109, *109*

Fluconazole, 97–98, *98*

Fluorine, 10, 16, 84

Fluorodeoxyuridine, 254

Fluorodeoxyuridylate (F-dUMP), 254–255, *255–256*

5-Fluorourcil (5-FU), 84, 86, *87,* 104

Fluoxetine, 120, *121*

Flurazepam, *349*

Folate acid antagonists, 86

Folic acid, *72*

Function, acetylcholine receptors, *215*

Functional groups
  amine, 28
  basics, 4
  benazepril, 6, *6*
  Cipro, 6–7, *7*
  common, *8–9*
  cyano group, 23
  donepezil, *5*
  electron-withdrawing and electron-donating, 47, 49
  hydroxyl, 28
  imide, 42
  inductive effect, *48*
  ionizable molecules, 55
  nitrile, 23
  resonance effects, 49, *50*

Functionalization, *see* Phase I reactions (functionalization)

Furan, *71*

Furosemide, *121*

G

GABA (γ-aminobutyric acid), 62

GABA (γ-aminobutyric acid) receptors
  antagonists, *347,* 349–350
  basics, 344
  binding site, 346, *347*
  chloride channels, 344–350
  structure, 344, *345,* 346

Gaddum equation, 272, 274, 279

Gastric antiacids, 61, *63*

Gastro-Intestinal Therapeutic System (GITS) tablet, 101

Gating, 336

Genetic factors, metabolism, 139, 142

Geomtric isomers, 64, 66, *66*

GITS (Gastro-Intestinal Therapeutic System) tablet, 101

Glaucoma, 238–239, *239*

Glomerular filtration, 132

Glucocorticoid receptors, 318

Glucose, 104

Glucurondiation, 171–172, *172–174*

Glutathione conjugation, 174, 176, *176–177*, 178
Glutethimide, *350*
Glyceraldehyde, 199–200
Glyceryl trinitrate, 128
Glycogen synthetase, 323
G phases, 78
G-proteins, 320, 327–331, *330, 334*
Graded dose-response curves, 288–290, *291*
Gram, Christian, 243
Grapefruit juice, 144
Guanine, 81, *82–83*
Guanylate cyclase, 320, 325–327, *328–329*

H

Half-life, *125,* 125–127, *127*
Halogens, 22
Halothane, *64,* 102–103
HAM (hydroxylamine), 241, *242*
Heart rate, *205–206,* 205–208, *208–210*
Heidelberger studies, 87
Heme-containing enzyme, 326
Henderson-Hasselbach equation
    acid-base properties, 53–59, *55, 57, 59–60*
    compartment pH, 116
    pK_a, 99
Heteroreceptors, 208–209
Heterotrophic cooperatvity, 229
Hexetal, *74*
Hexobarbital, 167
HGPRTase (Hypoxanthine-Guanine PhosphoRibosyl Transferase), 84
Histamine
    acetylation, 174
    autocoids, 192
    methylation, 178
Homotrophic cooperatvity, 229
Hormones, 318–325
Hydralazine, 174
Hydrogen, 22, 25
Hydrogen bonding, 117
Hydrolysis reactions, 40, 167–171
Hydrophilic nature, signaling molecules, 192
Hydrophobic (lipophilic) signaling molecules, 192
4-Hydroxycyclophosphamide, *84*
Hydroxylamine (HAM), 241, *242*
Hypnotic glutethimide, 130
Hypoxanthine, *72,* 255, *257*

Hypoxanthine-Guanine PhosphoRibosyl Transferase (HGPRTase), 84

I

Ibuprofen, *155*
Idiosyncratic drug response, 313
Individual tolerance, 312
Indomethacin, 167
Induced fit, 199–200, *200*
Induction, 138–139, *140–141*
Inductive effects, 47–49, *48*
Inhalation, *see* Volatile anesthetics
Inhibition, *see also* Enzyme inhibition, drug-induced
    competitive, 225–226, *225–226*
    CYP450 families, 138
    feedback, 229–230, *231*
    noncompetitive, 228, *228*
    suicide inhibition, 254–255
    thymidylate synthetase, 254–255, *255–256*
    transpeptidase-penicillinase, 243–255
    uncompetitive, 226–227, *227*
    xanthine oxidase, 255, *257–258*
Inhibitors
    beta-lactamase, 251–254, *254*
    cholinesterase, 234
    transpetidase, 248, *249–250,* 250
Inner transition, 14
Inositol, 331
Insulin, 4, 192
Integral receptors, 196, *197*
Interaction examples, 230–242
Intercalators, DNA, 87, 89, *89*
Intestines, 108
Intracellular binding, 117
Intracellular receptors, 196
Intranasal administration, 94
Intrathecal administration, 94
Intrinsic activity, 200–201, 264
Inverse agonists, 348, *348*
Iodine, 104, 117
Ion channels, 334–337, *335–338*
Ionic bonds
    basics, 16, 18
    covalent bond comparison, *20*
    polarity, 34
Ionic charge magnitude, 18–19
Ionizing, drug dissolution, 37
Ionophore agonists, 349
Ionotropic effect, 344

Ion pair transport, 105
Ipratropium bromide, 115, *116*
Iron, 104
Irreversible antagonism, 280–281, *281–282*
Irreversible anticholinesterases, 235, *237,*
    241, *see also* Anticholinesterase drugs;
    Reversible anticholinesterases
Isoflurophate, 238
Isoleucine, 229–230, *231*
Isomerism, 66
Isoniazid, 174
Isoproterenol, *181*
Isosteric replacements, 71, *72*
Isosterism and isosteres, 69–71, *71–72*
Isradipine, *342*
Izumenolide, 251–252

K

Ketamine, 159
Ketoconazole, 144
Ketones, 166, *166–168*
Kidneys, 103, 131–132, *131–132*

L

Langmuir studies, 69–70
Lethal dose, 293
Levodopa, 114
Lidocaine, 167
Ligand-gated channels, 334–335, *335,*
    337–338, *339–340*
Ligands, 320–325
Ligand structure and activity relationship,
    201
Linear electron arrangement, 29, *29*
Lipid-soluble ligands, 313
Lipid theory, 62
Lipophilicity, *74*
Lithium, 11, 126–127
Localized depolarization, 338
Local site restriction, 101
Location, acetylcholine receptors, 213–214,
    215
Lock-and-key fit, 198–199, *199*
Long-term administration, 100–101
Lorazepam, *349*
L-type channels, 339–350
Lymphokines, 192

M

Magnesium, 11, 14
Maintenance dose rate, 122–125, *123–124*
Malignant cells, 77–78
MAO (monoamine oxidase), 165
Mathematical relationship importance,
    278–279
Maximal efficacy, 286
Mechlorethamine, 80–81, *80–83*
Median dose, 290, 292
Median effective dose, 294
Median lethal dose, 294
Membrane-bound guanylate cyclase,
    325–326, *328*
Membranes, crossing, 103–105
Meprobamate, *155, 350*
6-Mercaptopurine, 84, *85, 181*
Mesalamine, *76*
Mesculine, 174
Metabolic changes, drugs
    acetaminophen, 178–180, *185*
    basics, 135–136
    clozapine, 142
    codeine, 143
    conjugation, 171–178
    CYP3A4, 144
    CYP3A family, 143–144
    CYP2C19, 143
    CYP450 cycle, 147–149, *148*
    CYP2D6, 142–143
    CYP450 enzyme complex, 144–145
    CYP450 family, 136–144, *137*
    diazepam-omeprazole interaction, 143
    dose-dependent toxicity,
        acetaminophen, 178–180, *185*
    environmental factors, 139, 142
    FAD/FADH system, 147, *147*
    genetic factors, 139, 142
    grapefruit juice, 144
    hydrolysis reactions, 167–171
    induction, 138–139, *140–141*
    inhibition, 138
    NAD+/NADH system, 145, *145–146*
    omeprazole-diazepam interaction, 143
    Phase II reactions, 149, 171–178
    Phase I reactions, 149–171, *150*
    polymorphism, genetic, 142–143
    redox reactions, 144–145
    reduction, 166–167
Metabolism, drug, *76*
Metalloenzymes, 251

Metals, 14
Methacholine, *217,* 238
Methamphetamine, 159
Methicillin, 251
Methotrexate, 71, *72,* 86
Methoxyflurane, *64*
Methyldopa, *181, 184*
6-Methylthipurine, *159*
Meyer and Overton studies, 62
Midazolam, *155*
Milrinone, 24, *24*
Mineralocorticoids, 318
Miochol, 218
Mode, 290
Models, 198–200
Modified occupation theory (Ariën), 264
Molecular formula, 4
Molecular polarity, *34,* 34–35
Molecule changes, 72–73, *74–76*
Molecule shapes, 28–31, *29–32*
Monoamine oxidase (MAO), 165
Monomer, 322
Monomeric form, 322
Monosaccharides, 104
Morphine, *121*
M phase, 78–79
Mucarinic actions, acetylcholine, 212
Multiple bonds, 22
Muscarine, *217,* 219
Muscles, 342, *343*
Mustards, 79–80, *79–80*
Mustargen, 81, *82–83*
Myasthenia gravis, 238–240, *240*

N

NAD$^+$/NADH system, 145, *145–146*
Naficillin, 251
N-dealkylation, 156–157, *158–159*
Neon (gas), 18
Neostigmine, 240, *240*
Neurotransmission, 191, *193*
Neurotransmitters, 210
Nicotinamide adenine dinucleotide (NAD), 145, *145–146*
Nicotine
  alkaloids, 219–221
  methylation, *181*
  structure, *217*
Nicotinic actions, acetylcholine, 212
Nifedipine, 101
Nitrazepam, *169, 349*

Nitrendipine, *342*
Nitrogen, 22–23, *24,* 25
Nitrogen mustards, 79, *79*
Nitroglycerine, 327
Nitro group reduction, 167, *169*
Nitrous oxide, *64*
N-methylation, 178, *179–181*
Noble gases, 14, 17
Nonclassical isosteres, 70
Noncompetitive antagonism, 281–282, *283*
Noncompetitive inhibition, 228, *228*
Nonlinear (angular) triatomic H_2O molecule, 35
Nonmetals, 14
Nonpolar convalent bonds, 33–34
Nonspecific drugs, structurally, 61, *62–63*
Norepinephrine, *180, 204,* 279
Normal cells, 77–78
N-oxidation, 161, *161–162*
N-type channels, 339–340

O

Occupation theory (Clark), 259–263, *260, 262–263*
n-Octanol, *105*
Octet rule, 17
O-dealkylation, 156–157, *158–159*
Olsalazine, *76*
Omeprazole-diazepam interaction, 143
O-methylation, 178, *179–181*
Onium cation formation, 80, *80*
Onium charge, 234
Onset of action, *101,* 297
Optimum dosage schedule, 296
Oral administration, 94
Orbitals, 10–11, *11*
Organophosphates, 235, *237*
Overshoot, 308–309
Overton, Meyer and, studies, 62
Oxacillin, 251
Oxazepam, *349*
Oxidative deamination, 157, 159, *160,* 165, *165*
Oxisuran, 161
Oxygen, 14, 22

P

PAM (pralidoxime), 241, *242*
PAPS (3'-phosphoadenosyl-5'-phosphate), 178, *182*

Paracrine function, 190, 192, *193*
Parenteral administration, 94
Partial agonists, 201, *202, 282–284, 284–287*
Particle size, 98, *99*
Partition coefficient, *64,* 105, *105*
Passive diffusion, 103–104
Paton's theory, 264–268, *266–267,* 270
Patterns, distribution, 117–120, *118–119*
Pauling, L., 33
Peak effect, 297
Penicillinases, 251, *253*
Penicillin benzathine, 95
Penicillin calcium, 13, *13*
Penicillin G, 95, *95*
Penicillins
    basics, 250–251, *252*
    body compartment pH, 107, *107*
    permeability, 115, *115*
    renal processes, 132
Penicillin salts, 95, *95–97*
Penicillin sodium, 13, *13*
Penicilloic acid, 251
Pentaglycines, 246
Pentavalent phosphorus compounds, 241
Pentobarbital
    aliphatic hydroxylation, *155*
    aliphatic oxidation option, *156*
    chemical structures, *350*
    desulfuration, 162, *163*
Peptide bond hydrolysis, 171
Peptidoglycans, 245–246, *245–246*
Periodic table
    chemical reactivity, 10–11, *10–13,* 13–14,
        15, 16
    drug properties, 3–4, *5–9,* 6–7, 10
Peripheral receptors, 196, *197*
Permeability, 112, *113,* 114–116, *115–116*
pH, body compartments
    absorption, *100,* 105–107, *106–107*
    distribution, 116
    partitioning process, 58, *59*
Phagocytosis, 105
Pharmacodynamics, drug-receptors
    acetylcholine, 210–214, *212–215*
    adrenergic agonists and antagonists,
        205–206, 205–208, *208–210*
    affinity activity, 200
    agonists, 201–209, 215, *216*
    antagonists, 201, 215, *216*
    antimuscarinic blocking agents, *220,* 221
    atypical receptors, 208–209, *211*

autocrine function, 192, *193*
binding sites, 198
chemical signaling, 189–191, *191*
cholinergic neurotransmission, 209–221
cholinomimetics, 214–215, *216–219,*
    217–221
differential agonists, 202–209
direct-acting cholinomimetics, 215,
    216–219, 217–221
drug action mechanism, 189, *190*
drug-receptor interactions, 198
endocrine function, 192, *193*
ephinephrine, differential effects,
    202–205, *203–204*
extracellular receptors, 196
function, acetylcholine receptors, *215*
induced fit, 199–200, *200*
intracellular receptors, 196
intrinsic activity, 200–201
ligand structure and activity relationship,
    201
location, acetylcholine receptors,
    213–214, *215*
lock-and-key fit, 198–199, *199*
models, 198–200
mucarinic actions, acetylcholine, 212
nicotinic actions, acetylcholine, 212
paracrine function, 192, *193*
partial agonist, 201, *202*
plasma membrane-bound receptors,
    196–197, *197*
receptor concept importance, 202
receptor types, 194, *195,* 196–197
signaling molecules, 192–193, *194–195*
Pharmacologic potency, 286
Phase I reactions (functionalization)
    alcohol and aldehyde oxidation, 163, *165*
    aldehyde reduction, 166, *166–168*
    aliphatic oxidation, 153, 155, *155–157*
    amide hydrolysis, 167, *170*
    aromatic oxidation, *148,* 149–153,
        151–154
    azo group reduction, 167, *169*
    basics, 135–136, 149, *150*
    CYP450 enzymes, 149–163
    dehalogenation, 162–163, *164*
    desulfuration, 162, *163*
    epoxide hydration, *154,* 171
    ester hydrolysis, 167, *170*
    hydrolysis reactions, 167–171
    ketone reduction, 166, *166–168*

N-dealkylation, 156–157, *158–159*
nitro group reduction, 167, *169*
N-oxidation, 161, *161–162*
O-dealkylation, 156–157, *158–159*
oxidative deamination, 157, 159, *160, 165, 165*
peptide bond hydrolysis, 171
reduction, 166–167
S-dealkylation, 156–157, *158–159*
sulfoxide/sulfone formation, 161, *162*
Phase II reactions (conjugation)
acetylation, 172, 174, *175*
basics, 135–136, 149, *150,* 171
glucurondiation, 171–172, *172–174*
glutathione conjugation, 174, 176, *176–177,* 178
N-methylation, 178, *179–181*
O-methylation, 178, *179–181*
S-methylation, 178, *179–181*
sulfate conjugation, 178, *182–184*
Phenelzine, 174
Phenformin, *152*
Phenobarbital
aromatic hydroxylation, *152*
chemical structures, *350*
lipophilicity, *74*
therapeutic index example, 295
Phenol, *62*
Phenothiazine derivatives, *71*
Phenotypes, 142
Phenoxybenzamine, 280–281
Phensuximide, 167
Phentermine, *162*
Phenylacetone, *160*
Phenylalkyamine, *342*
Phenylbutazone, *152*
5-Phenylhydantoin, 167
Phenytoin, *152, 181*
Phosphatases, 325
Phosphatidylinositol, 331
3'-Phosphoadenosyl-5'-phosphate (PAPS), 178, *182*
Phosphoinositides, 331–334, *333–335*
Phospholipase, 331
Phosphoramide mustard, *84*
Phosphorylated active site, 235
Phosphorylation, 320, *321*
pH partition theory, 99–100, *100*
Physicochemical properties
acid-base properties, 37–60
cancer treatments, 77–89

chemical properties, 3–35
structural determinants, 61–73
Physiochemical factors, 103–108
Physiological factors, 103–108
Physostigmine, 238, *240*
Picrotoxin
barbiturates binding site, 348
binding site, *346,* 349
chloride channels, *346*
GABA, *348*
Pilocarbine, *217,* 219, 238
Pinocytosis, 105
pK$_a$, 98–100, *100*
PKC signaling pathway, 331–334, *334–335*
Plasma membrane-bound receptors, 196–197, *197*
Plasma protein binding, 116
Polar convalent bonds, 33–34
Polarity, 33–34, *34*
Polyatomic ions, 19, *19*
Polymorphism, 97–98, *98,* 142–143
Poor metabolizers, 142
Positional isomer, 64, *65*
Positive feedback vicious cycle, 338
Postganglionic sympathetic nerve terminals, 203
Potassium
active transport, 104
channels, receptor regulation, 337, *337–338*
metals, 14
subshell, 11
Potassium acetylsalicylate, 39
Potassium salt, 39
Potency, 286–287, *288*
Pralidoxime (PAM), 241, *242*
Premarin vaginal cream, 101
Procainamide, 174
Procainamide hydrolysis, *170*
Procaine hydrolysis, *170*
Procardia XL, 101
Propanolol, *160*
Properties, drugs, *5–9, 6–7, 10,* 94–100, *see also* Chemical properties; Physicochemical properties
Propranolol, 116, *116, 152*
Propylthiouracil, *181*
Prostaglandin E$_2$, 192
Protein kinases, 320–321
Protein phosphatase, 320, 323
Protonated form, drugs, 53

Protonsil, *169*
Pseudocholinesterase, 230–231
Pyridine, *71*
Pyridostigmine, 240
Pyrimethamine, 55–58, *57*
Pyrimidine bases, 104
Pyrrole, *71*

Q

Quantal dose-response curves, 288,
    290–292, *292–293*
Quaternary ammonium compounds, 25, 105
Quinine HCl, 105

R

Ranitidine, 132
Rate of distribution, 112
Rate theory (Paton), 264–268, *266–267*
Receptor-coupled guanylate cyclase,
    325–326, *328*
Receptor regulation, signaling mechanisms
    adenylate cyclase, 328–331, *330*
    antagonists, GABA, *347,* 349–350
    barbiturates binding site, 348, *350*
    benzodiazepine binding site, 348,
        348–349
    binding sites, 346, *346–350,* 348–349
    CA^{2+} channels, 339–340, *341–342*
    calcium channels, 338–339, *341,* 342,
        343
    cAMP, 331, *332*
    CA^{++}/phosphoinositide/PKC signaling
        pathway, 331–334, *333–335*
    chloride channels, 344–350
    contraction, muscles, 342, *343*
    desensitization, 325, *326–327*
    down regulation, 309–310, *311,* 312, *324,*
        325
    GABA receptors, 344–350
    G-proteins, 327–331, *330,* 334
    guanylate cyclase, 325–327, *328–329*
    hormones, 318–325
    idiosyncratic drug response, 313
    ion channels, 334–337, *335–338*
    ligand-gated channels, 334–335, *335,*
        337–338, *339–340*
    ligands, 320–325
    membrane-bound guanylate cyclase,
        325–326, *328*
    overshoot, 308–309

phosphoinositides, 331–334, *333–335*
phosphorylation, 320, *321*
picrotoxin binding site, *346,* 349
potassium channels, 337, *337–338*
protein kinases, 320–321
receptor-coupled guanylate cyclase,
    325–326, *328*
receptor signaling, 313–317, *314*
second messenger systems, 313–316,
    327–328, 331, 334
sodium channels, *336,* 336–338,
    339–340
soluable guanylate cyclase, 326–327, *329*
spare receptors, 307–308, *309–310*
tachyphylaxis, 312
tolerance, 312
tyrosine kinases, 322–323, *323–324*
voltage-dependent ion channels,
    336–337, *336–338*
voltage-sensitive CA^{2+} channels, 339–340,
    341–342
Receptors, *see also* Drug-receptors,
    pharmacodynamics
    acetylcholine, 211–214, *214–215*
    atypical, 208–209, *211*
    chemical signaling and function, 189–197
    concept importance, 202
    GABA receptors, 344–350
    second messenger systems, 327–328, *330*
    signaling mechanisms, 313–314, *314*
    types, 194, *195,* 196–197
Redox reactions, 144–145
Reduction, 166–167
Renal excretion, 131–132, *131–132*
Renal glomerular membranes, 103
Renal tubules, 103
Representative elements, 14
Residual effects, 297
Resonance effects, 47, 49–51, *50–52*
Resonance structures, 27–28, *27–29*
Response relation, 269
Reversible anticholinesterases, 234–235, *see
    also* Anticholinesterase drugs;
    Irreversible anticholinesterases
Ritalin, *68*

S

Safety margin, 295
Salbutamol, *184*
Salt hydrolysis, 38–41
Salycilic acid, *170*

Schild's equation, 275–278, *279*
S-dealkylation, 156–157, *158–159*
Secobarbital, *350*
Second messenger systems, *see also* First
    messengers
  basics, 313
  cAMP, 331, *332*
  purpose, 334
  receptors, 327–328, *330*
  types, 315–316, *315–318*
Sensory receptors, 208
Serine threonine kinases, 321
Serotonin, *165*, 178
Sertaline, 98, *99*
Sevoflurane, *64*
Sex steroids, 318
Signaling mechanisms, receptor regulation
  adenylate cyclase, 328–331, *330*
  antagonists, GABA, *347*, 349–350
  barbiturates binding site, 348, *350*
  benzodiazepine binding site, 348,
    348–349
  binding sites, 346, *346–350*, 348–349
  CA^{2+} channels, 339–340, *341–342*
  calcium channels, 338–339, *341, 342,*
    343
  cAMP, 331, *332*
  CA^{++}/phosphoinositide/PKC signaling
    pathway, 331–334, *333–335*
  chloride channels, 344–350
  contraction, muscles, 342, *343*
  desensitization, 325, *326–327*
  down regulation, 309–310, *311,* 312, *324,*
    325
  GABA receptors, 344–350
  G-proteins, 327–331, *330,* 334
  guanylate cyclase, 325–327, *328–329*
  hormones, 318–325
  idiosyncratic drug response, 313
  ion channels, 334–337, *335–338*
  ligand-gated channels, 334–335, *335,*
    337–338, *339–340*
  ligands, 320–325
  membrane-bound guanylate cyclase,
    325–326, *328*
  overshoot, 308–309
  phosphoinositides, 331–334, *333–335*
  phosphorylation, 320, *321*
  picrotoxin binding site, *346,* 349
  potassium channels, 337, *337–338*
  protein kinases, 320–321

receptor-coupled guanylate cyclase,
    325–326, *328*
  receptor signaling, 313–317, *314*
  second messenger systems, 313–316,
    327–328, 331, 334
  sodium channels, *336,* 336–338,
    339–340
  soluable guanylate cyclase, 326–327, *329*
  spare receptors, 307–308, *309–310*
  tachyphylaxis, 312
  tolerance, 312
  tyrosine kinases, 322–323, *323–324*
  voltage-dependent ion channels,
    336–337, *336–338*
  voltage-sensitive CA^{2+} channels, 339–340,
    341–342
Signaling molecules, 192–193, *194–195*
Skeletal muscles, 342, *343*
S-methylation, 178, *179–181*
Sodium
  active transport, 104
  channels, receptor regulation, *336,*
    336–338, *339–340*
  metals, 14
  noble gas comparison, 18
  subshell, 11, 13
Sodium bicarbonate, *63*
Sodium nitrite, 327
Sodium nitroprusside, 327
Sodium tolbutamide, 100
Soluable guanylate cyclase, 326–327, *329*
Solubility, 94–95, *95–97*
Solvated anions and cations, 39
Somatropin, 192
Sorting endosomes, 310
Spare receptors, 307–308, *309–310*
Specific drugs, structurally, 63–64, *65–70,*
    66–68
S phase, 78
Spironolactone, 106–107, *107*
Standard safety margin, 295
Staphylococci bacteria, 251
Staphylococcus aureus, 247
Steady state, *125,* 125–127, *127*
Steroidal allene acetate, *26*
Steroid hormones, 319–320
Steroid pyrrolate, 107, *107*
Strengths, acids and bases, 43–46, *45–46*
Strong acids, 44–45, *45,* 47
Structural determinants
  isosterism and isosteres, 69–71, *71–72*

molecule changes, 72–73, *74–76*
structurally nonspecific drugs, 61, *62–63*
structurally specific drugs, 63–64, *65–70*, 66–68
volatile anesthetics, 61–63, *64–65*
Structural formula, 4
Structurally nonspecific drugs, 61, *62–63*
Structurally specific drugs, 63–64, *65–70*, 66–68
Subfamily defined, 137
Subshell, 11, 13
Substrates, *137*
Succinate dehydrogenase, 226, *226, 231*
Succinylcholine, 240
Suflonic acids, 105
Suicide inactivators, 253
Suicide inhibition, 254–255
Sulfamethazine, 174
Sulfamethoxazole, 174
Sulfanilamide, *169*
Sulfapyridine, 174
Sulfate conjugation, 178, *182–184*
Sulfisoxazole, 174
Sulfoxide/sulfone formation, 161, *162*
Sulfur, 14, 25
Sulfur dioxide, 27
Sulfur mustards, 79, *79*
Surface area available, 108
Synapse, 209
Synaptic cleft, 209

T

Tachyphylaxis, 312
Taxol, *75, 79*
TBG (thyroxine binding globulins), 196
Terbutaline, *184*
Testosterone, 104
Tetracycline, *74,* 117
Tetrahedral electron arrangement, 29, *30*
Thalidomide, 67–68, *68*
Theophylline, 121
Therapeutic dose, 293
Therapeutic index, *293–295, 293–296*
Therapeutic objective, 100–101
Thiopental, 115, *115,* 162, *163*
Thiophene, *71*
Thioridazine, 161
Threonine, 229–230
Threshold dose, 289
Thymidylate synthetase, 254–255, *255–256*
Thyroid hormone, 318

Thyroid stimulating hormone (TSH), 192–193
Thyroxine binding globulins (TBG), 196
Time-action curves, *296, 296–297*
Timolol, 238
Tolbutamide, *121, 155*
Tolerance, 312
Topical administration, 94
Toxic dose, 293
Toxicity, aromatic oxidation, 151
Transition elements, 14
Transmembrane ion-channels, 313
Transmembrane receptors, 196, *197,* 314
Transmission, 210
Transpeptidase-penicillinase inhibition, 243–255
1,2,3-Triaminobenzene, *169*
Triazolam, *349*
Tricarcillin, 251
Trichloroethanol, *350*
Trigonal planar electron arrangement, 29, *30*
TSH (thyroid stimulating hormone), 192–193
T-type channels, 339–340
Tubocurarine, 240
Tubular reabsorption, 132
Tubular secretion, 132
Tyrosine kinases, 321–323, *323–324*

U

UDPGA (uridine diphosphate glucuronic acid), 171–172, *172*
Uncompetitive inhibition, 226–227, *227*
Urecholine, 219
Uridine diphosphate glucuronic acid (UDPGA), 171–172, *172*

V

Valence electrons, 16–17, 20
van der Waals interactions, 89, 117
Vascular smooth muscles
   anticholinesterases, 237
   calcium, 342, *343*
   receptor-coupled guanylate cyclase, 325–326
Vasodilators, 327, *329*
Verapamil, *342*
Vinylene system, 70, *71*
Vitamin B, 104
Volatile anesthetics, 61–63, *64–65,* 162–163

Voltage-dependent ion channels, 336–337, *336–338*
Voltage-sensitive CA²⁺ channels, 339–340, *341–342*
Volume determination, *120–121,* 120–122
VSEPR (valence-shell-electron-pair-repulsions), 29–32, *29–32*

W

Warfarin, 116–117, *152*
Water-soluable ligands, 313
Water solubility, *76*

Weak acids
  pK$_a$, 99–100
  pyrimethamine, 58–59
  strengths, 44–45, *45,* 47
Weak bases
  pK$_a$, 99–100
  pyrimethamine, 58–59
  strengths, 45–46
Wild type (CYP2D6 gene), 142

X

Xanthine oxidase, 255, *257–258*